D1406075

Alternative Medicine Guide to

Women's Health 2

BURTON GOLDBERG

and the Editors of

ALTERNATIVE MEDICINE

FUTURE MEDICINE PUBLISHING

TIBURON, CALIFORNIA

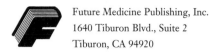

Future Medicine Publishing, Inc.
1640 Tiburon Blvd., Suite 2
Tiburon, CA 94920

Editor: Richard Leviton
Senior Editor: Stephanie Marohn
Writers: Richard Leviton & Stephanie Marohn
Research Editor: Keri Brenner
Associate Editor: John Anderson

Art Direction/Cover Design: Janine White
Production Manager: Gail Gongoll
Interior design: Amparo Del Rio Design
Cover Photo: © 1997, Telegraph Colour Library/FPG International LLC
Illustrations (pp. 16, 17, 29, 49, 58, 59, 85, 115, 116):
LifeART Images Copyright © 1989-1998 by TechPool Studios, Inc. USA

Manufactured in the United States of America.

10 9 8 7 6 5 4 3 2 1

Library of Congress Cataloging-in-Publication Data

Goldberg, Burton, 1926-
    Alternative Medicine Guide to Women's Health 2 / Burton Goldberg and the Editors of Alternative Medicine.
            p.   cm.
    Includes bibliographical references and index.
    ISBN 1-887299-30-0 (paperback)
    1. Women—Health and hygiene 2. Alternative Medicine 3. Self-care, Health.   I. Alternative Medicine. II. Title. III. Title: Women's health.
RA778.G683   1998
616.5'082--dc21   98-18382
                                                              CIP

Portions of this book were previously published, in a different form, in
Alternative Medicine: The Definitive Guide and *Alternative Medicine* magazine.

Contents

Success Stories

Throughout this book, we illustrate the effectiveness of alternative medicine therapies for women's health problems with actual patient cases. Use this handy guide to quickly locate these "success stories."

Important Information

BURTON GOLDBERG and the editors of *Alternative Medicine* are proud of the public and professional praise accorded Future Medicine Publishing's series of books. This latest book continues the groundbreaking tradition of its predecessors.

The health of you and your loved ones is important. Treat this book as an educational tool that will enable you to better understand, assess, and choose the best course of treatment when women's health problems strike, and how to prevent these problems from striking in the first place. It could save your life.

Remember that this book on women's health is different. It is not another catalog of mainstream medicine's conventional treatments and drugs used to treat these problems. This book is about *alternative* approaches to women's health–approaches generally not understood and, at this time, not endorsed by the medical establishment. We urge you to discuss the treatments described in this book with your doctor. If your doctor is open-minded, you may actually educate him or her. We have been gratified to learn that many of our readers have found their physicians to be open to new ideas.

Use this book wisely. Because many of the treatments described in this book are, by definition, alternative, they have not been investigated, approved or endorsed by any government or regulatory agency. National, state, and local laws may vary regarding the use and application of many of the treatments that are discussed. Accordingly, this book should not be substituted for the advice and care of a physician or other licensed healthcare professional. Pregnant women, in particular, are especially urged to consult with a physician before commencing any therapy. Ultimately, you, the reader, must take responsibility for your health and how you use the information in this book.

Future Medicine Publishing and the authors have no financial interest in any of the products or services discussed in this book, other than the citations to Future Medicine's other publications. All of the factual information in this book has been drawn from the scientific literature.

User's Guide

One of the features of this book is that it is interactive, thanks to the following 8 icons:

This means you can turn to the listed pages elsewhere in this book for more information on the topic.

This tells you where to contact a physician, group, or publication, or how to obtain substances mentioned in the text. This is an editorial service to our readers. Most importantly, the use of this icon empowers you right now, by giving you a source to acquire something vital to your health, quickly and easily. Whenever possible, we give you complete contact information for all substances mentioned in the text. All items are based on recommendations from the clinical practice of physicians in this book. The publisher has no financial interest in any clinic, physician, or product discussed in this book.

Many times the text mentions a medical term that requires explanation. We don't want to interrupt the text, so instead we put the explanation in the margins under this icon. This gives you the option of proceeding with the text or taking a moment to learn more about an important term. You will find some of the key definitions repeated at different places in the book so you don't have to search for the definition.

This sign tells you there may be some risks, uncertainties, side effects, or special contraindications regarding a procedure or substance.

This icon will alert you to an article published in our bimonthly magazine, *Alternative Medicine*, that is relevant to the topic under discussion.

This icon asks you to give a particular point special attention in your thinking. It is important to the overall discussion at hand.

Here we refer you to our book, *Alternative Medicine Definitive Guide to Cancer,* for more information on a particular topic.

Here we refer you to our book, *Alternative Medicine Guide to Women's Health 1,* for more information on a particular topic. The first book in the Women's Health Series covers infertility, endometriosis, vaginitis, menstrual problems, ovarian cysts, PMS, fibroids, yeast infections, and urinary tract infections.

You Don't Have to "Put Up" With Your Health Problems

MANY PEOPLE HAVE COME to understand that illness and disease are not something you have to live with, that alternative medicine has practical solutions for identifying and treating the underlying causes and thus can reverse the illness itself. Many have learned this the hard way, living with discomfort and pain for years before discovering that there is another option.

The operative word here is *causes*—not one cause, but multiple factors which alone might not be too much for your body to handle, but together overload your body systems, resulting in a health condition such as breast cancer or osteoporosis. Looking at health in this way makes for more effective and long-lasting treatment than the single-cause focus of conventional medicine. Health problems such as those included in this book are rarely caused by one factor alone and treatment must address all of the contributing causes if it is going to be successful.

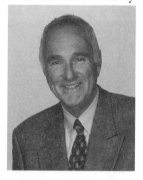

In this book, you will learn that once you identify the hidden factors which are combining to produce a health problem, you can systematically treat each one and permanently eliminate conditions as complex and resistant to conventional treatment as chronic fatigue syndrome. Patient success stories throughout the book provide practical details on how dozens of women were able to restore their health.

Although the conditions in this book are different from each other, they share many of the same underlying causes. Two of the most prominent are hormonal imbalances and an underactive thyroid gland. These two causal factors are also notoriously overlooked by conventional medicine. While doctors frequently prescribe estrogen for various women's ailments, not enough estrogen is rarely the problem. Instead, too much estrogen *in relation* to the level of progesterone is most often behind the hormonal havoc occurring in the body. Unfortunately, conventional medicine does not usually consider the ratio of the hormones. The role of the thyroid in hormonal imbalance and a host of health disorders is similarly ignored.

The conventional medical establishment (the American Medical Association, medical schools, the drug industry, and government "oversight" bodies, all of which have financial ties to their type of medicine) has a literal investment in relying on prescriptive palliatives rather than in addressing the underlying causes for long-lasting solutions to health conditions. In 1997 alone, American women bought 33.6 million prescriptions of Premarin (a synthetic estrogen derived from the urine of female horses), making it the nation's best-selling drug. Women now account for 59% of prescription drug purchases overall. Pharmaceutical companies, recognizing the potential of the women's market, are currently developing 372 medicines to treat a range of women's health conditions—up from only 263 experimental drugs in 1991. Drugmakers are also expanding the clinical testing of their products to include more women participants.

While reaping huge cash benefits for the drug industry, these drugs are not going to solve your health concerns. At best, they may temporarily relieve your symptoms, but between side effects and a tendency to worsen the original problem by masking it and driving it deeper into the body, it's hardly worth it—especially when you have a choice.

Alternative medicine physicians focus on finding the root causes, rather than merely trying to alleviate symptoms so you can live with the problem. In this book, you will learn how hormonal imbalances, an underactive thyroid gland, and a range of other causal factors can be reversed with natural therapies that don't give you even more uncomfortable symptoms in the form of side effects.

This book is here to tell you that you don't have to live with your health problems and that you owe it to yourself not to. By treating what is really causing the condition, be it depression or fibrocystic breast disease, not only can the original disorder be eliminated, but further health problems which might otherwise emerge from the same source can be deterred. With your overall health improved in the process, taking care of the condition you're suffering from today is good preventive medicine for your future. God bless.

—Burton Goldberg

Fibrocystic breast disease
could be called a disease of congestion and
toxicity. Lumps form in the breast when toxins and
excess estrogen build up in the body
because blood and lymph circulation is poor and
the body's normal detoxification systems
are overloaded.

1

Fibrocystic Breast Disease

IBROCYSTIC BREAST DISEASE (FBD) is the most common disorder of the breasts, occurring, by conservative estimates, in nearly 50% of premenopausal women.[1] Other estimates, including that of the American Academy of Pathology, range as high as 80% of North American women.[2] The symptoms of FBD—a misnomer because it is a characteristic not a disease—include breast pain and tenderness and lumps or cysts in the breast detectable to the touch. Some women only experience discomfort before menstruation, while others suffer considerable pain throughout the menstrual cycle. An estimated 30% of women with fibrocystic breast disease are incapacitated by severe pain interfering with their sleep and daily life.[3]

Fibrocystic breast disease, sometimes called cystic mastitis, is a benign (noncancerous) condition and is not considered a risk factor for breast cancer. (However, the fibrous lumpiness makes it more difficult to detect a cancerous tumor in the breast, so you need to have a physician monitor the condition.)

Many physicians regard breast pain and tenderness as a normal premenstrual symptom. But the late William Ghent, M.D., former Professor Emeritus of Surgery at Queen's University in Kingston, Ontario, Canada, and one of the foremost researchers of FBD, dis-

---

Causes of Fibrocystic Breast Disease

- Estrogen dominance
- Poor blood and lymphatic circulation
- Toxic accumulation
- Underactive thyroid gland
- Nutritional deficiencies
- Poor digestion and elimination
- Dietary factors
- Emotions and stress

---

agreed with this view. "Premenstrual breast pain and tenderness is not normal. If it's painful, premenstrually, it's sick," he stated. "I am sure that males would not accept sore testicles for seven to ten days of each month as normal."

There are three categories of benign breast lumps. The first type, cysts, are the ones most associated with fibrocystic breast disease, but the other two types may be present as well. The three categories are:[4]

■ Cysts—Round or oval in shape, cysts are fluid-filled and range from soft and squeezable to firm. They can be painful, but tend to come and go rapidly, often appearing during premenstrual periods (the last two weeks of the menstrual cycle) and then disappearing. They move freely under the touch.

■ Fibroadenoma—Also round or oval in shape, fibroadenomas are, however, relatively solid, rubbery to the touch. Like cysts, they move freely, but, unlike cysts, are not painful. These lumps are the kind usually found in younger women.

> ## Alternative Medicine Therapies for FBD
>
> ■ Castor oil packs
> ■ Chelation therapy
> ■ Detoxification therapy
> ■ Dietary recommendations
> ■ Glandular extracts
> ■ Herbal medicine
> ■ Homeopathy
> ■ Intestinal cleansing
> ■ Iodine therapy
> ■ Natural progesterone therapy
> ■ Nutritional supplements
> ■ Thyroid treatment
> ■ Traditional Chinese medicine

■ Lipoma, or fatty tumor—These lumps are irregularly shaped, range from soft to firm in consistency, and are usually painless. They are fixed and do not move freely. Occurring in women of all ages, lipomas are often caused by a trauma or injury to the breast.

The classification of fibrocystic breast disease actually gives us little information about an individual's condition because FBD encompasses such a broad range of conditions. The symptom common to all women is sore, lumpy breasts, but the nature of the lumps and the soreness varies hugely: some women have FBD cyclically while others experience it all month long; some are in extreme pain, some only mild; some women have cysts and scar tissue while others have only fibroadenomas. Carolyn DeMarco, M.D., of Toronto, Ontario, Canada, concurs that the classification tells us little, adding further that "the severity of the pain does not necessarily correlate with the amount of lumpiness."[5]

Along with the pain and discomfort of FBD, worry over whether a lump is cancerous or not can make fibrocystic breast disease a dev-

Fibrocystic breast disease (FBD) is the most common disorder of the breasts, occurring, by conservative estimates, in nearly 50% of premenopausal women. Other estimates range as high as 80% of North American women.

astating experience. A general rule to apply to ease the anxiety is that a breast lump that is painful is likely to be a cyst rather than a cancerous tumor, which usually is not tender. However, as noted above, the other categories of fibrocystic lumps—lipomas and fibroadenomas— are not painful and yet are benign. This makes it difficult to distinguish whether a lump is benign or cancerous so, again, consultation with a physician is advisable.

According to women's health expert Christiane Northrup, M.D., of Yarmouth, Maine, the first thing to determine about any lump is whether it is a cyst (here, the term is used loosely to describe all types of fibrocystic lumps). The physician can insert a needle in the lump and withdraw the fluid contents, a process called needle aspiration. If it is a cyst, the fluid will come out readily and the lump will disappear once the fluid is removed. If it is a solid lump, and not a cyst, the physi-

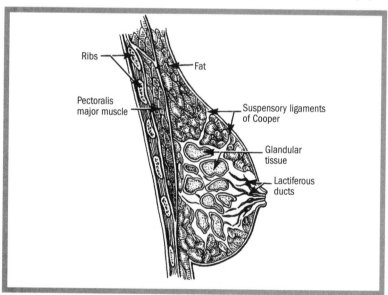

Ribs
Fat
Pectoralis major muscle
Suspensory ligaments of Cooper
Glandular tissue
Lactiferous ducts

THE INSIDE OF A HEALTHY BREAST. Inside the female breast there are layers of fat, glandular tissue, and milk ducts.

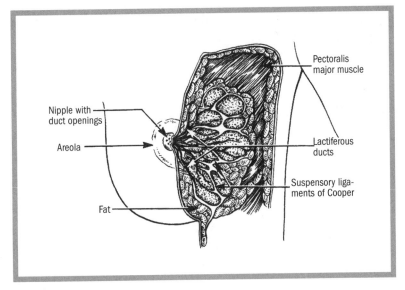

ANOTHER VIEW OF THE BREAST.

cian will not be able to withdraw fluid. (To avoid needling a lump that is not a cyst, the physician may choose to do an ultrasound first—a screening method using pictures of sound waves coming from the tissue—to see if the lump is solid.) If it is a cyst, the fluid tends to be yellow or greenish-brown, Dr. Northrup says. Even though cysts are normally benign, as a precaution, Dr. Northrup always sends the fluid to a laboratory to be checked for cancer cells.[6]

For more about **mammograms, thermography**, and **AMAS**, see Chapter 2: Breast Cancer, pp. 84-94.

If the lump is solid and not a cyst, Dr. Northrup usually suggests the woman get a second opinion from a surgeon or other specialist. A conventional surgeon will generally recommend a mammogram (breast X ray).[7] However, alternative medicine offers safer, more accurate screening tests, such as thermography (heat-sensitive photographs of breast tissue) and a blood test called AMAS, which do not involve irradiating the breast.

Once it is established that you don't have cancer and instead have benign breast lumps or fibrocystic breast disease, then you can proceed with some type of treatment. The common conventional medical approach relies on diuretic drugs, painkillers, and synthetic hormone therapy, particularly the steroid danazol. The diuretics, which increase urine and, therefore, fluid elimination, can actually produce more pain and lumpiness.[8] Danazol can be effective, but may entail disturbing side effects, including masculinization (facial and body hair growth

For a discussion of **estrogen dominance**, see this chapter, pp. 25-27. For more about **environmental estrogens** or **xenoestrogens**, see this chapter, pp. 29-31.

Estrogen is a female "sex" hormone, produced mainly in the ovaries (some in the fat cells), which regulates the menstrual cycle. Estrogen is important for adolescent sexual development, prepares the uterus for receiving the fertilized egg by stimulating the uterine lining to grow, and affects all the body's cells; its levels decline after menopause. Estrogen slows down bone loss which leads to osteoporosis, and it can help reverse the incidence of heart attacks; estrogen also improves skin tone, reduces vaginal dryness, and can act as an antiaging factor. For the first ten to 14 days in a woman's cycle, the uterus is mainly under the influence of estrogen. Estrogen levels begin to climb right before menstruation, from about days seven to 14, and peak at ovulation. There are three natural types of estrogen: estradiol (produced directly from the ovary); estrone (produced from estradiol); and estriol (formed in smaller amounts in the ovary). Estradiol is the most potent of the three. It prepares the uterus for the implantation of a fertilized egg, and also helps mature and maintain the sex characteristics of the female organs.

and deepening of the voice), weight gain, acne, decreased sex drive, fluid retention, vaginal dryness, reduction in breast size, liver dysfunction, menstrual disturbances, moodiness, and nervousness.[9] Further, the pain-relieving benefit is often temporary.[10]

Alternative medicine, on the other hand, offers a wide range of treatment options—from acupuncture and homeopathy to natural progesterone and detoxification—for eliminating the often hidden causes of fibrocystic breast disease. As with any disorder, especially chronic ones, more than a single cause is usually involved, as the following medical history graphically shows.

Toxic buildup, dietary factors, and poor circulation leading to a relative estrogen excess were all part of Barbara's severe, long-term FBD. However, through a comprehensive treatment program consisting of natural hormone therapy, nutritional supplements, dietary changes, detoxification, castor oil compresses, and a special exercise to support lymphatic drainage, Barbara was able to completely eliminate her breast lumps and pain.

Success Story: Ten-Year Fibrocystic Breast Disease Reversed

Barbara, 45, had endured lumpy, painful breasts for about ten years. In recent years, the pain had become so severe that, in the yoga classes she taught, she was unable to do the poses requiring her to lie on her stomach because the pressure on her breasts was unbearable. Barbara also had chronic, intermittent irritable bowel syndrome. Irritable bowel syndrome refers to an irregular and painful bowel elimination pattern; in Barbara's case, she alternated between constipation, with dry stools, and regular bowel movements, but with a lot of bloating and abdominal cramping at all times. Finally, Barbara had chronic sinus congestion to the degree that the sinus cavities around her eyes and nose were consistently blocked up, leaving her feeling stuffy and congested in her face and head.

Barbara had consulted a conventional physician to have the lumps, some of which were quite hard, checked for cancer. The physician ordered a mammogram. The mammogram was quite painful because Barbara had to squeeze her breasts to flatten them for the X-ray machine. After that trauma, the physician performed a manual breast palpation to check the lumps, followed by a needle biopsy, and a second mammogram. By the time Barbara left the doctor's office, she was crying in pain. Fortunately, none of the lumps were found to be malignant.

At that point, Barbara sought help from chiropractor and nutritional consultant Katrina Kulhay, D.C., director of the Kulhay Wellness Center in Toronto, Ontario, Canada. Barbara filled out Dr. Kulhay's Nutrition/Organ Survey, a comprehensive 55-section questionnaire on the patient's symptoms and habits, grouped according to their relevance to disturbances in major organs, such as stomach, liver, or kidneys.

The results of Barbara's questionnaire confirmed what Dr. Kulhay suspected: Barbara's symptoms of breast lumpiness and soreness, her irritable bowel syndrome, and her sinus congestion were the result of a hormonal imbalance, specifically, an excess of estrogen (SEE QUICK DEFINITION) relative to her progesterone (SEE QUICK DEFINITION) level. Dr. Kulhay could have performed a blood test to check Barbara's hormone levels, but Barbara's symptoms, combined with her answers to the survey, made it clear that this was a contributing factor.

The Nutrition/Organ Survey also revealed poor blood and lymph circulation (see this chapter, pp. 27-29), which can lead to estrogen buildup in the body. As a yoga instructor, Barbara was getting plenty of exercise, but it was not aerobic and therefore did not contribute as much to keeping her circulation operating optimally. Exposure to environmental estrogens (SEE QUICK DEFINITION) may also have added to the estrogen accumulation. Dr. Kulhay notes that breasts, with their fatty tissue and extensive lymph channels, easily become a repository for toxins in the form of lumps.

Toxic accumulation was revealed by two tests: darkfield microscopy (SEE QUICK DEFINITION) showed mercury toxicity, probably from Barbara's mercury amalgam dental fillings; and hair analysis indicated higher than normal levels of aluminum. In addition, the

QUICK DEFINITION

Environmental estrogens are foreign compounds and/or chemical toxins that mimic the effects of estrogen. Environmental estrogens, also called xenoestrogens, are present primarily in man-made chemicals ("greenhouse gases," herbicides, and pesticides such as DDT) and industrial by-products (from manufacture of plastics and paper, as well as from the incineration of hazardous wastes). Environmental estrogens often cause an imbalance of estrogen relative to progesterone, another key hormone. When a woman's body has too much estrogen (a condition called estrogen dominance), a variety of health problems can result, including breast cancer, fibroids, and endometriosis, among others. According to some researchers, environmental estrogens also affect men, and may contribute to testicular cancer, urinary tract disorders, and low sperm count. Dioxins are one kind of xenoestrogen. The World Health Organization puts the "tolerable" intake of dioxins for a human being at 10 picograms a day; at that rate, one gram of dioxins would provide every person in the United States with their "safe" daily intake for 100 years.

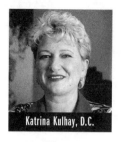

Katrina Kulhay, D.C.

"The breasts are full of lymphatic drainage," Dr. Kulhay says. "To cleanse the lymph, you have to get the main organs involved in elimination—the liver, kidneys, and bowels—detoxified and working efficiently."

darkfield microscopy also showed evidence of parasitic infection. However, Dr. Kulhay concluded that it was not extensive enough to warrant a full-scale parasite elimination program. Her conclusion was borne out when Barbara's FBD was cleared up without addressing this issue. The same was true of the elevated mercury and aluminum. If Barbara had failed to respond to the other therapies, these components would have been the next focus of treatment.

Barbara's questionnaire also indicated that the toxic buildup and congestion were blocking her body from absorbing the nutrients (particularly trace minerals such as iodine) it needed to digest and eliminate food properly—a condition called malabsorption syndrome. Dr. Kulhay cites malabsorption syndrome as a quite common problem in women with fibrocystic breast disease and other estrogen-excess conditions.

Detoxification therapies are essential in most cases of FBD, reports Dr. Kulhay. "The breasts are full of lymphatic drainage," she says. "But in order to cleanse the lymph, you have to get the main organs involved in elimination—the liver, kidneys, and bowels—detoxified and working efficiently."

However, before starting Barbara on a detoxification program, Dr. Kulhay took immediate steps to begin balancing her hormones. Twice daily, Barbara was to rub ¼ teaspoon of natural progesterone cream on her breasts, belly, or other soft-tissue skin. The progesterone cream would help restore the proper progesterone-estrogen ratio. After only one month of using the natural progesterone, Barbara reported a 50% improvement in her symptoms.

Dr. Kulhay also prescribed the following supplements:

■ Aqueous iodine: to supplement trace minerals and reduce breast inflammation and swelling; 1-10 drops daily

■ Evening primrose oil: to reduce breast inflammation and swelling and stimulate prostaglandin (SEE QUICK DEFINITION) production; two capsules, three times daily

■ Vitamin E: to help hormone balance; 1,000 IU daily

■ GreenAlive: a powdered supplement (contains *acidophilus*, ginseng, apple pectin, and the liver-cleansing herb milk thistle) to aid in digestion; 1 tbsp daily, mixed in water

At the same time, Dr. Kulhay worked with Barbara to improve her diet. The first step was to eliminate caffeine products, which research has linked to FBD. Caffeine is one of several methylxanthines (a group of drugs derived from xanthine and including caffeine, theophylline, and theobromine), stimulants which irritate the digestive tract, Dr. Kulhay says. If the intestines are irritated, they cannot eliminate properly, nor can they absorb nutrients, perpetuating the malabsorption syndrome, irritable bowel syndrome, and toxic buildup.

Barbara also reduced her intake of estrogenic foods such as beef, chicken, dairy, and soy. These foods in themselves tend to increase the body's own estrogen production, but beef, chicken, and dairy products are doubly estrogenic because they often contain residues from hormones fed to the animals to speed their growth or increase their egg or milk production.

After three months of the natural progesterone cream, the supplements, and the dietary changes, Barbara's bowel function and sinus congestion were improved.

At this point, Dr. Kulhay decided Barbara was ready for an internal cleansing program to help the organs involved in detoxification—liver, kidneys, and bowels—function more efficiently. She started Barbara on the liver-cleansing herbs dandelion and licorice, along with more milk thistle. In addition, Dr. Kulhay prescribed castor oil packs (SEE QUICK DEFINITION) applied to the breasts and the liver area (upper right abdomen) in the first half of the menstrual cycle (the estrogen-dominant phase). The castor oil helps pull out toxins, reduce inflammation, and improve circulation.

Barbara did a three-day rotation, positioning the castor oil packs on

A **prostaglandin** is a hormone-like, complex fatty acid which affects smooth muscle function, inflammatory processes, and constriction and dilation of blood vessels, particularly in the lungs and intestines. In women, prostaglandins have a stimulating effect on the uterus. Essential fatty acids in the diet (omega-3 and omega-6, found in fish oils) provide the raw material for prostaglandin production; once ingested, these essential fatty acids can be converted to prostaglandins by nearly any cell in the body. Omega-6-derived prostaglandins (the most common type) can have either pro-inflammatory or anti-inflammatory properties, while most prostaglandins converted from omega-3 sources help reduce pain and inflammation. For proper body function, an appropriate balance of both types of prostaglandins must be maintained. Eating too many trans-fatty acids (found in processed foods such as margarine), for example, can interfere with fatty acid metabolism and thus reduce production of prostaglandins.

For more about **detoxification**, see this chapter, pp. 35-39. For more about **natural progesterone cream**, see this chapter, pp. 39-42.

Barbara's symptoms of breast lumpiness and soreness, her irritable bowel syndrome, and her sinus congestion were the result of a hormonal imbalance, specifically, an excess of estrogen relative to her progesterone level, says Dr. Kulhay.

her breasts the first day and on her liver area the second day, and on the third day, she rubbed *Phytolacca* (pokeweed) oil on her breasts to ease the pain and break up the cystic formations. *Phytolacca* (*Phytolacca americana*) is a plant that is often used as a laxative because of its cathartic properties. (Dr. Kulhay says *Phytolacca* ointment is also acceptable, if oil is not available.)

To improve blood and lymphatic circulation and thereby aid the detoxification process, Dr. Kulhay advised Barbara to start using a Rebounder mini-trampoline. She bounced gently on it, beginning with two minutes a day and working up to 40 minutes daily.

Barbara continued on this program for six months, gradually weaning off all supplements and decreasing progesterone cream use to only the last two weeks of her menstrual cycle. Within a year of beginning treatment with Dr. Kulhay, all Barbara's breast lumps and pain had disappeared. Four years later, they have not returned. Whenever Barbara feels cysts may be forming, she takes evening primrose oil and that takes care of it.

Dr. Kulhay's Master List for FBD Treatment

What follows is an outline of all the therapies and nutritional supplements that Dr. Kulhay can use in treating women with fibrocystic breast disease. She emphasizes that most women do not need all of these and that she chooses which would be most effective with each woman based on the woman's responses to Dr. Kulhay's 55-section Nutrition/Organ Survey.

Dietary Recommendations:
- Decrease estrogenic foods such as beef, poultry, and dairy.
- Decrease caffeine, cola, chocolate, and black tea (methylxanthines).
- Decrease alcohol, trans-fatty acids (SEE QUICK DEFINITION), and saturated fats, such as those found in margarine and processed food.
- Increase fiber (grains, nuts, seeds) to clean the colon.
- Take GreenAlive powder (mixed in water and taken daily) to

support liver detoxification and improve digestion.

■ Drink only "good" water (water with all chemicals and other toxins removed). Dr. Kulhay recommends reverse osmosis ozonated water because it has the greatest number of toxins filtered out. Two separate units are required: the reverse osmosis unit (portable ones that attach to the tap are available) which filters out 98% of toxins including viruses, bacteria, and parasites (the average carbon filter device does not filter microorganisms, according to Dr. Kulhay); and a unit to ozonate the water (available through your local water company) which uses ultraviolet light to kill contaminants.

Supplements:

■ Aqueous liquid iodine: supplies essential trace mineral often deficient in women with FBD (available only by prescription); 1-10 drops daily

■ Coenzyme Q10: antioxidant, aids circulation; 100 mg daily

■ Kelp: rich in iodine, supports thyroid function; six tablets daily

■ Vitamin E: antioxidant, helps hormonal balance; 1,000 mg daily for one month

■ Beta carotene: vitamin A precursor, antioxidant; 150,000 IU (short-term dose for special cases)

■ Germanium: trace element, improves stability of cell walls so they are less likely to absorb toxins, increases oxygen to tissues; 100 mg per day in tablets

■ Vitamin C: antioxidant, increases tissue repair, for hormonal (adrenal) balance; 2,000-7,000 mg, powdered and buffered, daily

■ Vitamin B6: for fluid retention and hormonal regulation; 50 mg, three times daily

■ Evening primrose oil: reduces inflammation, stimulates prostaglandin production; two capsules, three times daily

Homeopathy:

Dr. Kulhay states that the choice of remedy often depends on if the pain is present before, during, or after menstruation and if cysts are hard or soft. Some of the common remedies for fibrocystic breast disease (all of which have extensive lists of symptoms that a homeopath considers in determining a remedy for a given individual) are: *Calcarea carbonica, Conium maculatum, Mercurius solubilis Hahnemanni,*

QUICK DEFINITION

A **trans-fatty acid** is a chemically and structurally altered hydrogenated vegetable oil (such as margarine), which is combined with hydrogen to lengthen shelf-life. The double bonds linking hydrogen atoms are changed from a "cis" (atoms bonded on the same side of a chain) to a "trans" form (atoms bonded on opposite sides of a chain), a chemical structure which is considered more stable. Commercially prepared hydrogenated fats are from 8% to 70% trans-fatty acids (TFAs) which and comprise about 60% of the fat found in processed foods. It is estimated that Americans consume over 600 million pounds annually of TFAs in the form of frying fats. TFAs can increase the risk of heart disease by 27% when consumed as at least 12% of the total fat intake. TFAs also reduce production of prostaglandins (hormones that act locally to control all cell-to-cell interactions) and interfere with fatty acid metabolism.

Phosphorus, Phytolacca, Apis, Arsenicum album, Baryta carbonica, Silicea, and *Sulphur.*

Herbal Medicine:

■ Liver cleansing herbs such as dandelion (liquid extract), milk thistle (powdered and mixed in liquid), and licorice. Dr. Kulhay recommends liquid forms rather than encapsulated herbs because many women do not have enough hydrochloric acid in their stomachs to dissolve the capsule shell.

■ *Phytolacca* (herbal pokeroot) oil or ointment, applied topically for five nights per week for 1-2 months. This helps break up the lumps, draws the toxins out, and is anti-inflammatory.

Hormone Therapy:

■ Natural progesterone cream: ¼ tsp rubbed into soft tissues (breasts, face, inside upper arms, abdomen), twice daily. Some physicians advise using the cream only during the last two weeks of the menstrual cycle, but Dr. Kulhay and others recommend using it the full month.

■ Progesterone tablets (wild yam extract): only if a woman prefers not to use cream, 50 to 250 mg daily.

Other Therapies:

■ TENS (transcutaneous electric nerve stimulation) unit applied to breasts to improve energy circulation

■ Balancing movement and bodywork such as yoga, *tai chi, qigong,* acupuncture, chiropractic, massage

■ Mini-trampoline (Rebounder) for lymphatic drainage and to improve circulation

■ Colonics (using ozonated water) to help remove toxins and excess estrogen from the intestines

■ Castor oil packs used in the pre-ovulatory phase (first two weeks) of the cycle to draw out toxins and excess estrogen, improve circulation in the breasts and chest (to further aid in the elimination of estrogen), and reduce inflammation

■ Darkfield microscopy to check blood for parasites or toxins, such as mercury and other heavy metals

To contact **Katrina Kulhay, D.C.**: The Kulhay Wellness Centre, 2 St. Clair Avenue West, Suite 607, Toronto, Ontario, M4V1L5 Canada; tel: 416-961-1900; fax: 416-961-9578. To receive Dr. Kulhay's Nutrition/Organ Survey and have it analyzed, send $50 and a note with the request to the above address. For **GreenAlive**, contact: Bioquest Imports, P.O. Box 27014-1395, Marine Drive, Vancouver, B.C., V7T2X8 Canada; tel: 604-922-0285; fax: 604-922-4649. For **Phytolacca** ointment and **liquid herbal extracts**, contact: Seroyal, 44 East Beaver Creek Hill Road, Unit 17, Richmond, Ontario, L4B1G8 Canada; tel: 800-263-5861 or 905-764-6355; fax: 905-764-6357. **Natural progesterone cream** is available at health food stores. One brand, ProGest, is available from: Transitions for Health, 621 S.W. Alder St., Suite 900, Portland, OR 97205-3627; tel: 800-888-6814 or 503-226-1010; fax: 800-944-2495. For a **portable reverse osmosis unit**, contact: Nimbus, 2 Manor Road East, Unit 4, Toronto, Ontario, M4S1P8 Canada; tel: 416-488-7072.

Eight Causes of Fibrocystic Breast Disease

The case of Barbara highlights the role of relative estrogen excess and the accumulation of toxins in fibrocystic breast disease. There are a number of factors that can contribute to both and, as you will learn in the eight causes of FBD covered here, they are often interconnected.

1) Estrogen Dominance

A key causal factor in breast lumps is an excess of estrogen in relation to progesterone, a condition known as estrogen dominance.[11] Estrogen causes breast stimulation, fluid retention, and cell proliferation which, if occurring excessively, lead to lumpy deposits.[12]

According to enzyme therapist and biochemist Lita Lee, Ph.D., of Lowell, Oregon, estrogen dominance is a primary cause in almost all female conditions, including fibrocystic breast disease, PMS, mood swings, excessive bleeding, endometriosis, fibroids, infertility, and ovarian cysts. "The healthy ratio of progesterone to estrogen is ten to one," states Dr. Lee. "The lower the ratio, the more health problems." Women's health specialist Jesse Lynn Hanley, M.D., of Malibu, California, concurs. "A relative estrogen excess is a significant cause of female reproductive problems in the Western world," she states.

Other consequences of estrogen dominance can include increased fat storage, tissue damage, bruising and pigment discoloration on the face, and aging of the skin. It can also damage the pituitary gland and put stress on liver function, reports Dr. Lee. The liver is required to detoxify estrogen and to convert thyroid hormone to its active form. If the liver is not working properly, it will perpetuate the estrogen excess cycle by allowing estrogen to build up.

Estrogen dominance can be created by numerous factors. An accumulation of estrogen frequently results, as it did in the case of Barbara, from poor blood and lymph circulation and sluggish elimination, which in turn means the liver, kidneys, and bowels are unable to process and get rid of excess estrogen. The excess estrogen is then reabsorbed by the body instead of being eliminated, further adding to the imbalance of the hormonal ratio.

Another source of inflated estrogen levels is eating foods that increase the body's natural estrogen production (meat, poultry, dairy, and soy). As Barbara learned, a diet high in estrogenic foods is often double exposure because many of the foods that naturally contain estrogen are from animals which have also been pumped full of synthetic hormones.

Are Your Hormones the Problem?— A Saliva Test Can Tell You

If you want to know if a relative estrogen excess or other hormonal imbalance is a possible factor in your fibrocystic breast disease, you can find out through a simple saliva test. Called the Aeron LifeCycles saliva assay report, the test can be ordered by both laypeople and physicians and measures up to eight different hormones. The results are plotted on graphs for easy interpretation, and changing levels can be plotted over time on the same graph, if supplementation or subsequent testing is done.

Although hormones are present in saliva only in fractional amounts compared to that in the blood, "clinically relevant and highly accurate levels of hormones can be determined in saliva," says John Kells, president of Aeron LifeCycles in San Leandro, California. "Saliva testing provides a means to establish whether or not your hormone levels are within the expected normal range for your age."

Kells says most of the key hormones at play in a man's or woman's body decline as we age, leaving us more susceptible to reduced physiological functioning and possibly disease. The goal of hormone replacement is to prevent illness and enhance the quality of

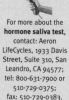

For more about the **hormone saliva test,** contact: Aeron LifeCycles, 1933 Davis Street, Suite 310, San Leandro, CA 94577; tel: 800-631-7900 or 510-729-0375; fax: 510-729-0383.

life, says Kells, but he notes that "there is a fair bit about this that is not yet known."

The saliva assay has several advantages over traditional blood testing for hormones. It is painless and noninvasive, and tests can be performed simply at any time or place. As DHEA, cortisol, estrogen, progesterone, and testosterone levels are highest in the morning, it is far more convenient to be able to test them at home (and then immediately ship the saliva sample to Aeron's laboratory) than to drive to a physician's office possibly later in the day when hormone levels have naturally fallen off a little.

As the test is less expensive than blood testing, you can do frequent testing to monitor changes (brought on by interventions such as diet, exercise, herbs, stress reduction, or acupuncture) and to adjust dosages of over-the-counter hormones such as natural progesterone or melatonin, Kells says. In general, Kells explains that it is best to establish a baseline level of saliva hormones first, then after intervention (which can include hormone supplementation) test a second time to measure the changes.

Estrogen dominance can also be the result of exposure to any of a class of estrogen-mimicking chemicals, known as xenoestrogens or environmental estrogens, which are increasingly prevalent in our food and in our environment. Once in the body, these chemicals—commonly found in pesticides, herbicides, and certain fuels, as well as in the by-products of incineration of plastics and hazardous wastes—act in the same way as estrogen and, in so doing, throw the estrogen-progesterone ratio off balance.

Finally, estrogen dominance can be the result of a low level of progesterone. Chronic stress depletes this essential hormone and production can decline during perimenopause (the ten to 15 years before the cessation of menses) or as a corollary of an underactive thyroid gland (hypothyroidism).

Rather than artificially manipulating your estrogen levels with synthetic hormones and ignoring the reasons behind the imbalance, it is more valuable to determine why you have the estrogen buildup or progesterone deficiency in the first place. Depending on the source of the relative estrogen excess, restoring hormonal balance can be more effectively achieved with dietary changes, nutritional supplements, natural progesterone cream, bowel detoxification, and eliminating exposure to environmental toxins as much as is possible.

People living today carry within their bodies a "chemical cocktail" made up of industrial chemicals, pesticides, food additives, heavy metals, and other toxins which tend to accumulate in the fatty tissue and lymph drainage channels in the female breast.

2) Poor Blood and Lymph Circulation

Next to hormonal levels, circulation is possibly the central issue in FBD, a disease of congestion. Given that there is a network of lymphatic channels in the breasts, when circulation is sluggish, toxins and excess estrogen will accumulate there. In addition, as Dr. Kulhay explained, fatty tissue, such as that found in the breasts, is where the body deposits toxins it cannot eliminate. Stimulated by excess estrogen, these toxins form lumps in the breast tissue. Thus, fibrocystic lumps can be regarded as toxic storehouses.

For more about **dietary estrogens**, see this chapter, p. 33. For more about **underactive thyroid**, see this chapter, p. 31, Chapter 4: Chronic Fatigue Syndrome, pp. 180-183, and Chapter 5: Depression, pp. 218-223.

Poor blood circulation functions in a similar manner. Toxins travel in the bloodstream and are either destroyed there by immune system cells and enzymes or transported to the lymph system for elimination from the body. With decreased blood flow, toxins may accumulate beyond the point that the body can handle them. Toxic overload is the result and the body attempts to relieve the circulating burden by storing toxins in tissue. Again, the end product may be fibrocystic breast lumps.

The Lymph System At a Glance

The human body has three circulatory systems—blood, nerve impulses, and lymph. The lymphatic system, which is largely ignored by mainstream medicine, includes a vast network of capillaries that transport the lymph; a series of nodes throughout the body (primarily in the neck, groin, and armpits) that collect the lymph; and three organs, namely, the tonsils, spleen, and thymus gland, which produce white blood cells (called lymphocytes) vital to the immune system.

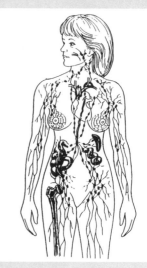

The space between cells occupies about 18% of the body. Fluid in this space, containing plasma proteins, foreign particles, and bacteria which accumulate between cells, is called lymph. Thus the purpose of the lymphatic system is to collect the lymph and to return its contents to the bloodstream. More specifically, the lymph system collects waste products and cellular debris from the tissues.

The lymph flows *slowly* upward through the body to the chest (at the rate of three quarts per 24 hours) where it drains into the bloodstream through two large ducts. Lymph also flows down from the head and neck into this drainage site. Unlike the heart, the lymphatic system does not have a pump to move it along; rather, its movement depends on such factors as muscle contraction or manual manipulation. The lymph circulation is also a *one-way* circulation: it only *returns* fluid to the bloodstream. The lymph system becomes particularly active during times of illness (such as the flu), when the nodes (particularly at the throat) visibly swell with collected waste products.

Poor circulation in the blood and lymph system can result from lack of exercise or chronic stress which tightens muscles and blood vessels and hinders organs from operating freely. Exposure to too many environmental chemicals or other toxins can also interfere with smooth flow of lymph fluid and blood which then creates a circular effect: poor circulation leading to decreased ability to eliminate the toxins which further slows circulation. A buildup of mucus in the digestive system, which can result from eating a diet high in mucus-producing foods such as dairy products, creates congestion, impeding circulation.

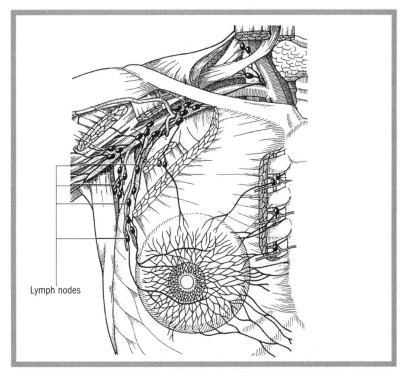

Lymph nodes

LYMPHATIC DRAINAGE AROUND THE BREAST. There are many lymph nodes located around the breast; their purpose is to collect waste products and cellular debris from the tissues and return these to the bloodstream for elimination from the body. A healthy lymphatic system is one guarantee that breasts will remain healthy and free of lumps or cysts, but when circulation of lymph and blood in this area is sluggish, toxins and excess estrogen will accumulate there and start contributing to poor breast health.

3) Toxic Accumulation

People living today carry within their bodies a "chemical cocktail" made up of industrial chemicals, pesticides, food additives, heavy metals, general anesthetics, and the residues of conventional pharmaceuticals, as well as of legal (alcohol, tobacco, caffeine) and illegal (heroin, cocaine, marijuana) drugs. In women, as mentioned above, these toxins tend to accumulate in the fatty tissue and lymph drainage channels in the breast. Whether the toxins evolve into the cysts and lumps of fibrocystic breast disease is a function of other influences, some of which were mentioned in the profile of Barbara. These include estrogen excess, poor circulation, nutrient

For more about **toxic overload** and **mucus production**, see Chapter 2: Breast Cancer, pp. 68-70, 78-79. For more about **detoxification**, see this chapter, pp. 35-39.

A Primer on the Thyroid

The thyroid gland, one of the body's seven endocrine glands, is located just below the larynx in the throat, with interconnecting lobes on either side of the trachea. The thyroid is the body's metabolic thermostat, controlling body temperature, energy use, and, in children, the body's growth rate. The thyroid controls the rate at which organs function and the speed with which the body uses food; it affects the operation of all body processes and organs. Of the hormones synthesized in and released by the thyroid, T3 (tri-iodothyronine) represents 7% and T4 (thyroxine) accounts for almost 93% of

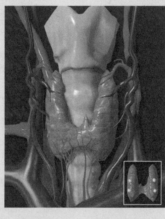

the thyroid's hormones active in all of the body's processes. Iodine is essential to forming normal amounts of thyroxine. The secretion of both these hormones is regulated by thyroid-stimulating hormone, or TSH, secreted by the pituitary gland in the brain. The thyroid also secretes calcitonin, a hormone required for calcium metabolism.

Hypothyroidism is a condition of low or underactive thyroid gland function that can produce numerous symptoms. Among the 47 clinically recognized symptoms: fatigue, depression, lethargy, weakness, weight gain, low body temperature, chills, cold extremities, general inappropriate sensation of cold, infertility, rheumatic pain, menstrual disorders (excessive flow, cramps), repeated infections, colds, upper respiratory infections, skin problems (itching, eczema, psoriasis, acne, dry, coarse, or scaly skin, skin pallor), memory disturbances, concentration difficulties, paranoia, migraines, oversleep, "laziness," muscle aches and weakness, hearing disturbances, burning/prickling sensations, anemia, slow reaction time and mental sluggishness, swelling of the eyelids, constipation, labored or difficult breathing, hoarseness, brittle nails, and poor vision. A resting body temperature (measured in the armpit) *below* 97.8° F may indicate hypothyroidism; menstruating women should take the underarm temperature only on the second and third days of menstruation.

deficiencies, poor diet, underactive thyroid gland, stress, and emotional elements.

Toxins now accumulate in the human system faster than they can be naturally eliminated, which means the body now needs assistance in detoxifying. Everyone has an individual level of tolerance for toxins that cannot be exceeded if good health is to be maintained. When the system gets overwhelmed with toxins beyond this level, immune system mechanisms malfunction and health problems, such as fibrocystic breast disease, manifest. As Dr. Kulhay emphasized, toxic overload is usually a factor in FBD and detoxification is therefore an essential part of FBD treatment.

4) Underactive Thyroid Gland

When the thyroid is underfunctioning (hypothyroidism, see "A Primer on the Thyroid," p. 30), metabolic processes in the body do not work well and fatigue, weight gain, sluggishness, constipation, mood swings, and depression are some of the consequences. Hormone levels are also affected; without sufficient thyroid hormones, the production of progesterone is disrupted and the estrogen-progesterone ratio is thrown askew. In addition, the constipation caused by an underactive thyroid gland allows a buildup of estrogens, toxins, viruses, bacteria, and parasites in the intestines and the reabsorption of estrogens into the bloodstream, further elevating estrogen levels.

The thyroid is particularly susceptible to chemical exposure. Pesticides and other environmental toxins can cause hypothyroidism, according to Dr. Lita Lee. Thus, with toxins accumulating in the breasts and the thyroid damaged by similar toxic invasion, the FBD cycle is potentially deepened, with each contributing factor worsening the others.

Nearly all conventional doctors ignore this endocrine gland's complex role in human health and still far too few alternative medicine physicians pay the thyroid the attention it warrants. Yet it's been known since the early 1960s that an underactive thyroid gland can be responsible for at least 47 medical conditions. In that decade, researchers estimated that perhaps 40% of the U.S. population had hypothyroidism. Today, some physicians put that figure at closer to 90%.

Unfortunately, many patients fall through the cracks of medicine's obliviousness to thyroid function or, if they're fortunate enough to have a thyroid test, they may get "normal" results because most standard tests are not sensitive enough to identify hypothyroidism. More sensitive tests that can accurately measure thyroid function are discussed in the chapter on chronic fatigue syndrome.

5) Nutritional Deficiencies

In addition to nutritional deficiencies in general, which weaken body systems and open the way for the development of a wide range of disorders, a lack in two specific nutrients is associated with fibrocystic

For more about the **thyroid gland**, see Chapter 4: Chronic Fatigue Syndrome, pp. 180-183, and Chapter 5: Depression, pp. 218-223. For **thyroid testing**, see Chapter 4: Chronic Fatigue Syndrome, pp. 181-183. For more about **essential fatty acids**, see Chapter 5: Depression, pp. 224-231. For information on **testing your nutritional status**, see Chapter 4: Chronic Fatigue Syndrome, pp. 190-192.

Essential fatty acids (EFAs) are unsaturated fats required in the diet. Omega-3 and omega-6 oils are the two principal types. The primary omega-3 oil is alpha-linolenic acid (ALA) and is found in flaxseed (58%), canola, pumpkin, walnut, and soybeans. Fish oils, such as salmon, cod, and mackerel, contain the other important omega-3 oils, DHA (docosahexaenoic acid) and EPA (eicosapentaenoic acid). Linoleic acid or cis-linoleic acid is the main omega-6 oil and is found in most plants and vegetable oils, including safflower (73%), corn, peanut, and sesame. The most therapeutic form of omega-6 oil is gamma-linolenic acid (GLA), found in evening primrose, black currant, and borage oils. Once in the body, omega-3 and omega-6 are converted to prostaglandins, hormone-like substances that regulate many metabolic functions, particularly inflammatory processes.

breast disease. These nutrients are iodine and gamma-linolenic acid (GLA).

Gamma-linolenic acid, an essential fatty acid (SEE QUICK DEFINITION) found in evening primrose, flaxseed, and borage oils, is a building block of prostaglandins. A particular type of prostaglandin called PGE1 has proven helpful in preventing and reversing fibrocystic breast disease.[13] Prostaglandins are necessary for a wide variety of biological processes, including strengthening the immune system, controlling inflammation, and preventing tumor growth. Thus, a GLA deficiency has implications for the swelling and soreness of fibrocystic breast disease, inflammation due to congestion, and toxic accumulation in breast tissue.

Iodine is an essential trace element found in table salt (potassium iodide is added), seafood, and seaweed. People need at least 160 mcg daily, but in 1993, for example, the average North American consumed only about 150 mcg daily, most of it from table salt, according to Dr. Carolyn DeMarco. "Recent evidence suggests that at least 25% of women in North America are iodine deficient at some point in their lives," says Dr. DeMarco.[14]

The main function of iodine is as a component of thyroid hormone and, as such, it plays a role in cellular oxidation and metabolism. Inadequate iodine intake, continuing over several months, can result in hypothyroidism[15] which, as mentioned in the previous section, can result in breast lumps because of sluggish body functions, congestion, and toxic accumulation.

According to noted women's health specialist Tori Hudson, N.D., of A Woman's Time: Menopause Options and Natural Health Clinic in Portland, Oregon, researchers have long been aware that the thyroid gland requires iodine to make thyroxine (a thyroid secretion), essential for thyroid activity. However, it is only in recent years, Dr. Hudson reports, that researchers have discovered that the reproductive system, especially breast and ovarian tissue, requires iodine as well.[16]

The exact mechanism of the action of iodine on breast tissue is not understood, she says. The one established fact is that iodine is only found in certain areas of the breast, the terminal and interlobular duct cells.

These areas, while small compared to the whole breast, are the same areas responsible for cystic and malignant changes.[17] The theory, says Dr. Hudson, is that iodine protects the breast tissue from oversensitivity to estrogen stimulation.

However, simply eating more iodized salt may not provide this protective effect, as breast tissue does not contain enough of an enzyme necessary to extract iodine from circulating iodides. This enzyme, called peroxidase, is rife in thyroid tissue but not in the breasts. For this reason, supplemental iodine, prepared in a way that the breast tissues can absorb, is the form of iodine therapy needed in fibrocystic breast treatment, explains Dr. Hudson.

6) Poor Digestion and Elimination

With the buildup in the intestines due to problems digesting food, a diet high in mucus-producing foods, chronic constipation, or toxic overload, absorption of nutrients is compromised and the body is even less able to process and eliminate toxins and intestinal buildup. The result is further toxicity and nutritional deficiencies, including of key nutrients which could reduce the pain and inflammation of fibrocystic breast disease.

As Dr. Kulhay mentioned, reduced absorption of nutrients is called malabsorption syndrome and deprives the body of the fuel it needs to prevent and reverse developing health problems. The result is, again, a vicious cycle, with each element worsening the others involved: less nutrients, even poorer digestion, more toxic accumulation, further sluggishness or congestion in all body systems.

In addition, as discussed previously, poor intestinal elimination contributes to estrogen dominance, which is a primary cause of fibrocystic breast disease.

7) Dietary Factors

Diet is a causal factor in most chronic health conditions and fibrocystic breast disease is no exception. Estrogenic foods (meats, poultry, dairy, and soy) and meat and dairy products containing hormone residues have already been pinpointed in this chapter as contributors to excess estrogen in the body.

These foods, along with mucus-producing foods (dairy, refined white flour products, fried foods, high-fat baked goods, and processed foods), combine to create general body congestion, excess estrogen, and stress on liver, kidneys, and intestines, interfering with the body's natural detoxification mechanisms. Reducing estrogenic and mucus-

Is There an FBD Personality?

In a recent study comparing the personality characteristics of women with FBD, women with breast cancer, and healthy women, both the women with FBD and those with breast cancer demonstrated a greater need for neatness and order and were less curious and analytical than women in the healthy group. As for self-perception, women with FBD described themselves as "tense, restless, outgoing, expressing anger." Those with breast cancer self-described as "timid, nonassertive, noncompetitive, calm, easygoing, keeping anger inside" while women in the healthy group characterized themselves as "calm, relaxed, outgoing, able to express anger."[19]

forming foods will help address the problems of poor circulation and toxic buildup. A high-fiber diet will also help reduce estrogen and toxin levels by promoting proper elimination.

Based on these known dietary factors, Jonathan Wright, M.D., director of the Tahoma Clinic in Kent, Washington, recommends a primarily vegetarian, high-fiber, low-fat, dairy-free diet for fibrocystic breast disease patients. Similarly, Dr. Christiane Northrup advises a diet low in fat and high in whole grains and fiber. She suggests giving up dairy for three months and then slowly reintroducing low-fat dairy products while monitoring for tolerance. Carolyn Dean, M.D., of New York City, concurs with a low-fat diet, high in whole grains, vegetables, and beans because this regimen helps excrete estrogen from the body. She also cites this diet as helpful for weight loss which can, in turn, benefit FBD. "Overweight women have too much estrogen which can stimulate the breasts," she states.[18]

As Dr. Kulhay advised Barbara, another dietary link to FBD is caffeine products. For some women, simply giving up caffeine is enough to make the lumpiness in their breasts disappear. In addition, since FBD is a disease of toxic buildup, avoiding pesticides by eating organically grown produce is highly advisable. Similarly, as healthy thyroid function is important to reducing breast lumps, adding seaweed or other sources of iodine to your diet is recommended. Finally, sprinkling ground flaxseeds on salads and other foods is an easy dietary change that can provide essential fatty acids often deficient in women with FBD.

8) Emotions and Stress

Finally, chronic stress, unresolved emotions, or emotional trauma can contribute as much to congestion in the body as can sluggish digestion and toxic overload. Muscles and blood vessels tend to constrict when you are tense, sad, angry, or depressed. This slows the circulation of your energy, blood, and lymph, promoting the further buildup of toxins and the development of FBD.

Alternative Medicine Therapies for Fibrocystic Breast Disease

To treat all of the causes involved in an individual case of fibrocystic breast disease, multiple therapies will likely be required. The following is a selection of useful alternative medicine solutions for FBD, some of which were mentioned in Barbara's case. Additional case histories are also included to illustrate how other practitioners incorporate these therapies in their treatment plans.

Detoxification Therapy

"A body with a healthy immune system, efficient organs of elimination and detoxification [SEE QUICK DEFINITION], and a sound circulatory and nervous system can handle a great deal of toxicity," states Leon Chaitow, N.D., D.O., of London, England. "But if a person's immune system has been damaged from chronic exposure to environmental pollutants, restoring these functions, organs, and systems can be accomplished only through detoxification therapies, including fasting, chelation [SEE QUICK DEFINITION], and nutritional, herbal, and homeopathic methods, which accelerate the body's own natural cleansing processes." Intestinal detoxification is also an important method for removing toxins from the body.

Ridding the body of toxins, which tend to accumulate in breast tissue, is one powerful step a woman can take in preventing and treating breast disorders such as FBD. In Barbara's case, herbs and supplements, castor oil packs, and exercise on a mini-trampoline flushed toxins and cleansed and strengthened her natural detoxifying mechanisms (intestines, liver, kidneys, and lymph system). In addition to these therapies, the seven-step detoxification program and parasite elimination protocol covered here can help in FBD treatment.

Seven Steps to Promote Detoxification

William Lee Cowden, M.D., co-author of *Alternative*

Detoxification involves a variety of techniques to rid the body of poisons accumulated as a result of a polluted environment (air, water, and food), exposure to toxic chemicals and pesticides, chronic stress, faulty dietary practices, and chronic constipation or poor elimination, among other factors. Detoxification methods include fasting, intestinal cleansing, enemas and colonics, lymph drainage procedures, chelation, biological dentistry, water and heat therapies, therapeutic massage, and bodywork techniques.

Chelation therapy refers to a method of binding up ("chelating") toxins (e.g., heavy metals) and metabolic wastes and removing them from the body while at the same time increasing blood flow and removing arterial plaque. One type of chelation therapy involves the chelating agent disodium EDTA given as an intravenous infusion over a 3½ hour period. Usually 20 to 30 treatments are administered at the rate of one to three sessions per week. Chelation therapy is especially beneficial for all forms of atherosclerotic cardiovascular disease including angina pectoris and coronary artery disease.

35

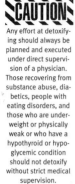

Medicine Definitive Guide to Cancer, suggests seven steps anyone can adopt starting today to assist their body in eliminating toxins and to promote immune and digestive health.

First, make some dietary changes. Start eating a diet that is high in fiber and fresh raw vegetables and fruits, and very low in mucus-producing foods. It would be preferable to completely stop eating all milk products from cows and all refined white flour products, such as pastas, breads, and baked goods. At least for the duration of this program, it is also advisable to reduce your intake of sugar, eggs, meats, fowl, most fish, nuts, seeds, and unsprouted beans and grains.

Second, reduce your stress load. Practice stress-reduction techniques before each meal. These might include muscle relaxation, deep breathing, or the visualization of a favorite and pleasant natural setting. Listening to a stress-reduction audiotape before the meal can be helpful. It is also advisable to eat in a calm, pleasant environment, either by yourself or with a companion whose presence does not produce stress or discomfort in you.

Third, practice lymphatic drainage. It is important to take steps to clean out your lymphatic system, especially the lymph vessels that attach to the intestines. You can do this by gently bouncing on a mini-trampoline (Rebounder) for five to 15 minutes once daily. This will stimulate the numerous lymph nodes in your neck, chest, and groin to start draining toxins into the bloodstream for removal from the body.

Fourth, brush your skin. In the early morning, soon after you get up, take a wooden brush with stiff natural bristles and lightly brush your skin. Move the brush across the skin toward the center end of each collarbone, as important lymph drainage sites are located here. Spend eight to ten minutes dry brushing your entire body. This procedure will mechanically aid your lymph system in its detoxification efforts. Do the dry brushing before taking the bath below, but be aware that skin brushing just before bedtime can make it difficult to fall asleep.

Fifth, try ozonated bathing. Many of the toxins that build up in the body (and especially the breasts) are fat soluble and gather in the fatty tissues. If you immerse yourself in a tub of warm ozonated water for 30 minutes once daily for two to three weeks, this will aid in removal of the toxins from your body. Ozone purifies the bath water by killing living viruses, bacteria, fungi, and parasites. It will also oxidize the water-insoluble toxins on the skin, turning them into water-soluble toxins. Once water soluble, they may be flushed from the system.

Here's how to do it. Purify the tapwater by running it through a KDF solid charcoal showerhead filter as you fill the tub. A KDF solid charcoal showerhead filter can remove up to 99% of the toxic substances found in tap water. Next, bubble ozone (a form of oxygen, SEE QUICK DEFINITION) into the water using an ultraviolet ozone generator and an ozone-diffusing bath bubbler. (Do not use an electric spark ozonating system because this produces more nitrates and other harmful chemical substances.) This converts the ozone that is accumulating in the air above the bubbling water back into oxygen so that it is not irritating to the lungs.

Bubble the ozone for 15 minutes before you get into the tub and also during your 30-minute soak. During this half-hour soak, scrub your entire skin surface with a loofa sponge or natural fiber brush three times (while in the water).

Adding ½ cup of Body Soak Gold to your bath water, and increasing this amount to one cup over two to three weeks, will usually produce a faster removal of toxins from the body than ozonated water alone. After you have used one full bottle of Body Soak Gold, you may gain additional detoxification benefit by switching to ¼ cup of Liquid Needles Foot Soak added to the bath water; over a period of several days, increase this amount to one cup for each 30-minute bath. Best results are obtained if both Soaks are added to KDF charcoal-filtered water.

Sixth, fortify yourself with nutrients. It is important to take at least 400 IU of vitamin E, 25,000 IU of beta carotene and/or mixed carotenoids, 2,000 mg vitamin C, and 100 mg of grape seed extract (pycnogenol) 30-40 minutes before your ozonated bath or 10-15 minutes after it.

Seventh, take one lozenge of superoxide dismutase (SOD) and 100 mg of L-glutathione powder. Dissolve both substances under your tongue before each bath; this enables them to be absorbed faster and more completely. These nutrients will facilitate toxin removal from your system. SOD is an antioxidant enzyme that protects the system against free-radical damage from chemicals or radiation. L-glutathione is a sulfur-containing peptide (made of amino acids, protein building blocks) and antioxidant essential to the body's toxic waste disposal system.

Ozone (O_3) is a less stable, more reactive form of oxygen, containing three oxygen atoms. This extra atom enables ozone to more readily oxidize other chemicals. In oxidation, the extra oxygen atom breaks off, leaving ordinary oxygen (O_2), thereby favorably increasing the oxygen content of body tissues or blood. Ozone is a commonly occurring natural substance. Medical-grade ozone is used as part of oxygen therapy to increase local oxygen supply to lesions, speed wound healing, reduce infections, and stimulate metabolic processes. Ozone may be administered intravenously or by injection, or applied topically in a water- or olive oil–based solution; it may also be taken orally or rectally as ozonated water.

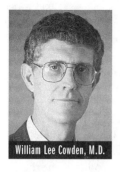

Many of the toxins that build up in the body (and especially the breasts) gather in the fatty tissues. If you immerse yourself in a tub of warm ozonated water for 30 minutes once daily for two to three weeks, this will aid in removal of the toxins from your body, says Dr. Cowden.

For **Body Soak Gold**, (containing water, sea minerals, and glycerin) and **Liquid Needles Foot Soak** (containing electrolytes from mineral particles in a clear solution), contact: Great Health USA, Inc., 1202 Executive Drive West, Richardson, TX 75081; tel: 972-480-8909; fax: 972-480-8807. For a source of **SOD** as **Opti-Guard**™ (Antioxidant/S.O.D. Enzyme Enhancer), contact: Optimal Nutrients, 1163 Chess Drive, Suite F, Foster City, CA 94404; tel: 800-966-8874 or 415-525-0112; fax: 415-349-1686.

⚠CAUTION⚠

Before beginning any parasite elimination program, consult a qualified health-care professional. This is especially important if you are pregnant.

For more about **parasites**, see Chapter 2: Breast Cancer, pp. 78-79, and Chapter 4: Chronic Fatigue Syndrome, pp. 170-172, 175-177.

How to Eliminate Parasites

Like other toxins, parasites can make it harder for the liver, kidneys, and intestines to detoxify and eliminate wastes from the body, so toxins build up in the blood and lymph system and are deposited in breast tissue where they form lumps, explains Dr. Cowden. If testing reveals that you have a parasitic infection, you may want to consider taking the following practical steps Dr. Cowden recommends to rid your system of parasites.

1) Cleanse the Intestines: Parasites tend to embed themselves in the intestinal wall, but over the course of several weeks, you can flush them out by using some of these natural substances (preferably in combination): psyllium husks, agar-agar, citrus pectin, papaya extract, pumpkin seeds, flaxseeds, comfrey root, beet root, and bentonite clay (take bentonite only in combination with another substance, such as psyllium).

You might also take extra vitamin C (minimum 2 g daily, but higher amounts up to individual bowel tolerance are more useful) to help flush out your intestines. Note, however, that vitamin C taken at the same time as wormwood (below) renders wormwood ineffective.

2) Do a Colon Irrigation: Irrigate the colon with 2-16 quarts of water via enema. To the water you may add black walnut tincture or extract, garlic juice, vinegar (two tablespoons per quart of water), blackstrap molasses (one tablespoon per quart of water), or organically grown coffee. Use filtered or distilled water for the enema; further sterilize it by boiling or ozonating it for 10-15 minutes before use, including before using it to prepare the coffee.

3) Prepare Your System: It is prudent to give your gallbladder and liver a week to prepare for the parasite program.

To flush the gallbladder of its toxins, take lime juice in warm water or Swedish Bitters before each meal. Eliminate all refined and natural sugars, meats, and dairy products during the parasite program; even better, start cutting back on them during this preparatory week. Take barberry bark capsules, dandelion, or a similar herbal extract to help cleanse the liver. The amount depends on health and the strength or composition of the specific substance or brand-name product used.

4) The Herbal Cleanout: Naturopathic physician Hulda Regehr Clark, N.D., Ph.D., recommends using a blend of three herbs to flush the parasites out of your system: black walnut hull tincture, wormwood capsules, and fresh ground cloves (to kill the parasites' eggs).

Small Intestine

Large Intestine

THE INTESTINES—BREEDING GROUND FOR NUMEROUS PROBLEMS. When the intestines are sluggish and clogged, toxins and waste products accumulate and begin to poison the body from within, contributing to many health problems, including breast lumps.

Natural Progesterone Therapy

Natural progesterone cream, applied to the skin, can have a beneficial effect on FBD, as it does on other women's health conditions involving excess estrogen. French researchers discovered that progesterone gel rubbed into the breasts relieved breast pain 95% of the time.[20] The healing agent of the cream is diosgenin, the active ingredient of the herb wild yam. It works by increasing circulating progesterone levels and thus balancing the effects of excess estrogen.

For more about **William Lee Cowden, M.D., detoxification,** and specifics of **Dr. Hulda Clark's antiparasite program,** see *Alternative Medicine Definitive Guide to Cancer* (Future Medicine Publishing, 1997; ISBN 1-887299-01-7); to order, call 800-333-HEAL.

The idea of supplementing with progesterone is not new. Researchers who developed synthetic estrogen replacement therapy for women in menopause (a popular brand is Premarin) later added a synthetic progesterone (called a progestin, a popular brand being Provera) to balance the cell-proliferation and breast-stimulating effects of the excess estrogen, which scientists believed increased breast cancer risk.

Progesterone Content of Selected Creams/Oils, As Reported By an Independent Laboratory

The following list of natural progesterone products and their progesterone content was compiled by Dr. John Lee, based on laboratory tests conducted for him by Aeron LifeCycles in San Leandro, California (reprinted by permission of John R. Lee, M.D.).

PRODUCT	COMPANY	LOCATION
1,000-1,500 mg progesterone per ounce:		
Progest-E Complex	Kenogen	Eugene, OR
700-800 mg progesterone per ounce		
ProCreme Plus	Health Products	Manassas, VA
Renewed Balance	American Image Mktg.	Nampa, ID
500-700 mg progesterone per ounce		
Femarone-17	Wise Essentials	Hallendale, FL
Pro-Oste-All	Sarati International	Los Fresnos, TX
400-500 mg progesterone per ounce		
Adam's Equalizer	HM Enterprises	Norcross, GA
Angel Care	Angel Care	Atlanta, GA
Bio Balance	Elan Vitale	Scottsdale, AZ
Edenn Cream	SNM	Norcross, GA
E'Pro & Estrol Balance	Sarati International	Los Fresnos, TX
Equilibrium	Equilibrium Labs	Boca Raton, FL
Fair Lady	Village Market	Fond du Lac, WI
Femarone-17	Wise Essentials	Minneapolis, MN
Fem-Gest	Bio-Nutritional Formulas	Mineola, NY
Feminique	Country Life	Hauppauge, NY
Gentle Changes	Easy Way, Int'l.	Indianapolis, IN
Happy PMS	HM Enterprises	Norcross, GA
Heaven Sent	Answered Prayers, Inc.	Malibu, CA
Kokoro Balance	Kokoro, LLC	Laguna Niguel, CA
NatraGest	Broadmoore Labs	Ventura, CA
Natural Balance	South Market Service	Atlanta, GA
Natural Woman	Products of Nature	Ridgefield, CT
Natural Woman's Formula	Ultra Balance	Savannah, GA
New Woman	Pinnacle Nut, Inc.	Tulsa, OK
Nugest 900	Nutraceutics Corp.	Deerfield Beach, FL
Marpe Wild Yam	Green Pastures	Flat Rock, NC
Osterderm	Bezwecken	Beavertown, OR
PharmWest	PharmWest	Marina Del Ray, CA

PRODUCT	COMPANY	LOCATION
PhytoGest	Karuna	Novato, CA
Pro-Alo	Health Watchers	Scottsdale, AZ
ProBalance	Springboard	Monterey, CA
Progessence	Young Living	Payson, UT
Pro-G	TriMedica	Scottsdale, AZ
Pro-Gest	Transitions for Health	Portland, OR
Progest-DP	Life Enhancement	Petaluma, CA
Progonal	Bezwecken	Beaverton, OR
Serenity	Health & Science	Crawfordville, FL
Ultimate Total Woman	New Science Nutrition	N. Lauderdale, FL
Wild Yam Cream	Enrich, International	Orem, UT

10-20 mg progesterone per ounce

Endocreme	Wuliton Labs	Palmyra, MO
EFX Wild Yam	Natural Efx, Inc.	Richardson, TX
Life Changes	MW Labs	Atlanta, GA
Novagest	Strata Dermatologics	Concord, CA
Nugestrone	Nutraceuticals	Boca Raton, FL
Phyto-Balance	Transitions for Health	Portland, OR
Progesterone Plus	Prof. Health Products	Sewickley, PA
Woman Wise	Jason Natural Cosmetics	Culver City, CA

Less than 5 mg progesterone per ounce

Born Again	Alvin Last, Inc.	Yonkers, NY
Dioscorea Cream	Saroyal Int'l., Inc.	Toronto, Canada
Nutrigest	NutriSupplies, Inc.	West Palm Beach, FL
Progerone	Nature's Nutrition	Vero Beach, FL
Progestone 10	Dixie Health, Inc.	Atlanta, GA
Progestone-HP	Dixie Health, Inc.	Atlanta, GA
Yamcon	Phillips Nutrition	Laguna Hills, CA

However, the side effects of Provera and the other progestins are so severe that many women stop hormone therapy within the first year. Natural progesterone cream, however, has no side effects.

Specifically for fibrocystic breasts, John R. Lee, M.D., a women's health expert in Sebastopol, California, recommends natural progesterone cream (usually 3% natural progesterone mixed with other substances, such as aloe vera). Applied directly to the breasts, it is absorbed transdermally (through the skin). This is an efficient method of progesterone supplementation and helps restore the correct estrogen-to-progesterone ratio.

"Using progesterone transdermally from day 15 of the monthly cycle to day 25 will usually cause breast cysts to disappear," Dr. Lee

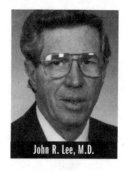

John R. Lee, M.D.

Dr. Lee recommends 3% natural progesterone mixed with aloe vera, applied directly to the breasts. This is an efficient method of progesterone supplementation and helps restore the correct estrogen-to-progesterone ratio, he says.

Natural progesterone cream is available at health food stores. One brand, ProGest, is available from Transitions for Health, 621 S.W. Alder St., Suite 900, Portland, OR 97205-3627; tel: 800-888-6814 or 503-226-1010; fax: 800-944-2495.

John R. Lee, M.D., who retired from private practice in 1989 and now is a consultant on hormone balancing, requests that people not contact him until they have read his book, *What Your Doctor May Not Tell You About Menopause*, (Warner Books, 1996). The book contains instructions for using natural progesterone cream, a complete osteoporosis prevention program, and the answers to many common questions. If people still have questions after reading the book, he can be reached at: BLL Publishing, P.O. Box 2068, Sebastopol, CA 95473; tel: 707-823-9350; fax: 707-829-8279.

states. The typical dosage for the cream is ⅛ to ½ teaspoon twice a day. Most physicians advise discontinuing usage for one to two days before the menstrual period is due to start. Discontinue use during menstruation, and begin again on day 15 (start counting from the first day of bleeding). Dr. Lee also recommends taking the following supplements with the natural progesterone cream regimen: vitamin E (600 IU at bedtime), magnesium (300 mg per day), and vitamin B6 (50 mg a day).[21]

Thyroid Support Therapy

As discussed in the section on causes of FBD, hypothyroidism can contribute to the disorder in a number of ways. The following case demonstrates the links between an underactive thyroid, toxic buildup, and breast lumps, and how thyroid glandular extracts can be used, along with other therapies, to reverse the condition.

Success Story: Thyroid Support Cures Fibrocystic Breasts

Five months before consulting Gary S. Ross, M.D., of San Francisco, California, Vicki, an aerobics instructor, noticed lumps in her breasts, around the same time she started a rigorous teaching schedule at a new health club which left her no time for regular meals or rest. Vicki, 24, came to Dr. Ross because the lumps had become increasingly tender in the week or two before her period. Vicki had not had the lumps biopsied to rule out any malignancy, preferring to try natural treatments first to see if they made a difference.

Vicki had a lifelong history of constipation and frequently used laxatives and enemas. In addition, she had noticed an increasing fatigue—mostly that she did not have the buoyancy in her daily life that she was used to enjoying. Her diet, since starting at the health club, consisted almost exclusively of muffins, breads, and coffee, because she didn't have time for anything else. Dr. Ross immediately advised Vicki to eliminate all caffeine—including coffee, tea, chocolate, and soft drinks—from her diet because, as mentioned previously, caffeine has been linked to FBD.

He also suggested she stop eating muffins and bread which are mucus-forming and tend to clog the digestive tract. Instead, he instructed Vicki to prepare snacks before work every morning, consisting of raw and steamed vegetables, along with a lunch of a chicken breast or fish and salad. During her short breaks, Vicki could munch on the vegetables instead of muffins and coffee.

Vicki's chronic constipation, as well as her fatigue and slightly dry skin, presented a classic pattern of an underactive thyroid gland, or hypothyroidism, but conventional blood tests had not shown any abnormalities in Vicki's thyroid hormone levels. Dr. Ross knew, however, that many cases of subclinical hypothyroidism are missed by conventional testing. He had Vicki perform a basal temperature test for three days during her menstrual period, which involved taking her underarm temperature first thing in the morning. As Dr. Ross suspected, Vicki's basal temperature average, at 97.2° F, was well below the normal range of 97.8° F to 98.2° F.

"It is crucial to correct this condition [hypothyroidism] in fibrocystic breast disease," Dr. Ross says. "When thyroid function is low, the body is unable to metabolize excessive amounts of congesting foods." Dr. Ross adds that the thyroid's hormones exert a catabolic, or cleansing effect, meaning that they burn up excess tissue (including tumors or lumps) and speed up the metabolism.

For more about **thyroid testing**, see Chapter 4: Chronic Fatigue Syndrome, pp. 182-183, and Chapter 5: Depression, pp. 218-220. For more about **basal temperature testing**, see Chapter 4: Chronic Fatigue Syndrome, p. 182.

To revive Vicki's thyroid function, Dr. Ross put her on a ¼ grain daily dose of Armour thyroid (a glandular extract, SEE QUICK DEFINITION, from a pig's thyroid; available only by prescription). He kept Vicki at that low dose for ten days, and then increased the dose by another ¼ grain, repeating the process until her energy was back to normal.

In addition, Dr. Ross prescribed the antioxidants (SEE QUICK DEFINITION) selenium and vitamins A, C, and E to help soothe and strengthen the cell walls of breast tissue inflamed by toxic congestion. To assist in detoxification, Vicki applied a castor oil pack (SEE QUICK DEFINITION) nightly on her liver and pancreas areas. Dr. Ross prefers this application, rather than on the breasts, in order to give more

To contact **Gary S. Ross, M.D.:** 500 Sutter Street, Suite 300, San Francisco, CA 94102; tel: 415-398-0555; fax: 415-398-6228.

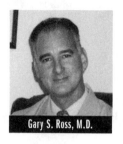

"It is crucial to correct hypothyroidism in fibrocystic breast disease," Dr. Ross says. "When thyroid function is low, the body is unable to metabolize excessive amounts of congesting foods."

Gary S. Ross, M.D.

QUICK DEFINITION

A **glandular extract** is a purified nutritional and therapeutic product derived from one of several animal glands including the adrenal, thymus, thyroid, ovaries, testes, pancreas, pineal, and pituitary. It is prescribed by a physician for a person whose corresponding gland is underfunctioning and not producing enough of its own hormone. The various glands are part of the endocrine system which, along with the nervous system, coordinates the functioning of all of the body's systems.

An **antioxidant** (meaning "against oxidation") is a natural biochemical substance that protects living cells against damage from harmful free radicals. Antioxidants work against the process of oxidation—the robbing of electrons from substances. If unblocked or left uncontrolled, oxidation can lead to cellular aging, degeneration, arthritis, heart disease, cancer, and other illnesses. Antioxidants in the body react readily with oxygen breakdown products and free radicals, and neutralize them before they can damage the body. Antioxidant nutrients include vitamins A, C, and E, beta carotene, selenium, coenzyme Q10, pycnogenol (grape seed extract), L-glutathione, superoxide dismutase, and bioflavonoids. Plant antioxidants include *Ginkgo biloba* and garlic. When antioxidants are taken in combination, the effect is stronger than when they are used individually.

support to the detoxifying and digestive work of these organs.

Within three to four weeks, Vicki's breast cysts and tenderness were reduced and she began to feel more energy. Her constipation also disappeared. In six weeks, Vicki was bubbling with new vitality and the lumps had shrunk to the point that they were almost undetectable.

Iodine Therapy

Given that many women with FBD have an iodine deficiency, iodine therapy may be an important part of treatment. As Dr. Tori Hudson explained previously, simply eating more iodine may not be enough to produce improvement in lumpy breasts (see pp. 32-33). She relies on supplemental iodine and has found the best form to be aqueous iodine (also called elemental or diatomic or molecular iodine). Aqueous iodine is "free" (not bound to proteins) elemental iodine dissolved in water. Dr. Hudson's typical dose, taken orally, is 3-6 mg daily.

In a study of 715 women with FBD given regular doses of oral aqueous iodine, the women experienced relief from pain and soreness within two to eight weeks. After four months, all of the women were cyst free and about 70% were completely pain free. By the end of one year, 95% of the women were completely pain free and had no more lumps or cysts. For the remaining 5%, who all had longstanding FBD, it took three years to reverse their condition.[22]

Another study of 1,365 women with FBD found that supplementation with oral molecular iodine (e.g., aqueous iodine) resulted in freedom from pain and the disappearance of cysts in 65% of the women, compared to 33% in the control group.[23] "Iodine appears to change the way estrogen binds to breast tissue," says Dr. Christiane Northrup, who uses a special iodine formula made for her clinic by a research chemist. [24]

Other forms of iodine therapy are Lugol's solution (SEE QUICK DEFINITION), potassium iodide (also called SSKI, for supersaturated potassium iodide), and caseinated iodine or iodaminol, which is iodine bound to the milk protein casein.[25]

David Derry, M.D., a family physician in Victoria, British Columbia, Canada, uses Lugol's solution for his patients with breast cysts and has treated more than 200 women with it since 1993. He reports a success rate of 100%, although the length of time to reverse the fibrocystic lumps varies among individuals. Dr. Derry typically prescribes five to ten drops of Lugol's solution taken once daily in a glass of orange juice.[26]

The history of iodine therapy dates back to the 1920s and 1930s, with the work of the late John Myers, M.D., a surgeon, gynecologist, and professor at Johns Hopkins University in Baltimore, Maryland. Dr. Myers experimented with using intravaginal iodine on female beagle dogs, a species which contracts fibrocystic breast disease. Dr. Myers achieved best results "painting" the dogs' vaginal areas with diatomic (e.g., aqueous) iodine and, immediately afterward, intravenously injecting the dogs with magnesium to potentiate the iodine.

Dr. Myers chose the vaginal area because of its proximity to the ovaries, which he believed would absorb the iodine and, because of the ovaries' reproductive connection with the breasts, heal the breast lumps. Oral iodine, he believed, was not as good because much of it would be absorbed first by the thyroid gland.[27]

Dr. Jonathan Wright, who studied with Dr. Myers in the late 1970s, has since adapted the intravaginal iodine treatment for his patients with FBD, particularly those with severe cases. First, he takes a baseline thyroid hormone blood test so he can monitor the patient to make sure the iodine is not inhibiting her thyroid function. Then he "paints" the iodine solution on the woman's vaginal walls.

Within five minutes, he gives the woman an intra-

CAUTION

If you have a hyperactive thyroid, iodine supplementation may not be advisable. Consult your physician.

To contact **Tori Hudson, N.D.**: A Woman's Time—Menopause Options and Natural Medicine, 2067 N.W. Lovejoy Street, Portland, OR 97209; tel: 503-222-2322; fax: 503-222-0276. Dr. Hudson's extensive protocol for cervical dysplasia and cervical cancer is featured in *Alternative Medicine Definitive Guide to Cancer* (Future Medicine Publishing, 1997; ISBN 1-887299-01-7); to order, call 800-333-HEAL.

QUICK DEFINITION

To prepare a **castor oil pack** for the abdomen, lightly heat enough castor oil to thoroughly wet but not soak a 10" x 12" flannel cloth. Immerse the flannel in the hot oil, then fold to make three to four layers and place against the skin. The oil will help to draw out toxins, release tension, and improve blood circulation, such as in the lower abdomen where such packs are often used for relief of menstrual cramps, or at joints to relieve pain. Place a heating pad or hot water bottle (wrapped in a towel) over the pack, then cover pack and bottle with another towel to retain heat. Keep in place for one to two hours; then store flannel wrapped in plastic in a refrigerator for later use. After the flannel has been used 20 times, discard it.

venous injection of 2 g of magnesium. Then, the patient is instructed to take daily oral supplements of: vitamin E (800 IU), an antioxidant and to aid hormone balance; selenium (200 mcg), an antioxidant and to help the action of the vitamin E; magnesium (300 mg) to further potentiate the iodine; and evening primrose oil (1 g to 2 g) to provide gamma-linolenic acid, helpful for reducing breast lumps.

The woman continues the daily supplements and returns for weekly intravaginal treatments until the FBD is gone. Sometimes, a softening of the lumps and lessening of the pain is immediate after the first intravaginal treatment, Dr. Wright says. In other cases, it takes several weeks. If the woman does not wish to receive the iodine intravaginally, Dr. Wright prescribes an ointment of 2 tsp Lugol's solution mixed with 2 tsp DMSO (SEE QUICK DEFINITION). The patient rubs the ointment on her breasts three times a week.

Nutritional Supplements

In addition to an iodine deficiency, the other nutrient that women with fibrocystic breast disease are often lacking is gamma-linolenic acid (GLA), an omega-6 essential fatty acid. When that is the case, supplemental GLA can produce significant improvements in painful FBD symptoms.

As excellent sources of GLA, Dr. Northrup recommends evening primrose, flaxseed, or black currant seed oils at a dosage of 500 mg, four times daily. Another option, mentioned earlier under dietary factors of FBD, is to add ground flaxseed to your food. Dr. Northrup suggests one tablespoon daily, sprinkled on soup, salad, or cereal, after grinding the seed in a coffee or nut grinder.[28]

Alternative medicine physicians also frequently recommend vitamin E for FBD because it helps balance estrogen excess and, as an antioxidant, helps repair inflamed breast tissue. Maria Perillo, N.D., of Nauset Health Associates in Orleans, Massachusetts, recommends 800 IU of vitamin E daily. She also suggests taking vitamin C (3,000 mg daily) and beta carotene (25,000-40,000 IU daily) as well.

Along with aqueous iodine as discussed in the previous section, Dr. Tori Hudson uses the following supplements and dosages in treating fibrocystic breast lumps:[29]

- Evening primrose oil: 1,500 mg daily
- Vitamin E: 800-1,200 IU daily
- Beta carotene: 150,000 IU daily
- SLF Forte: lipotropics to metabolize fatty deposits in the liver, contains choline, methionine, inositol, vitamins B6 and B12, beet powder, and dandelion; aids liver in detoxifying excess estrogen and other toxins; two tablets twice daily

Additional supplements, if needed, include:

- Choline (already included in SLF Forte for liver detoxification): 1 g daily
- Flaxseed oil: 2 tbsp per day
- Vitamin B complex: to reduce stress; ten times the RDA
- Methionine (already included in SLF Forte): 1 g daily

For **SLF Forte**, contact: NF Formulas, 9775 Southwest Commerce Circle, Suite C-5, Wilsonville, OR 97070; tel: 800-547-4892 or 503-682-9755; fax: 503-682-9529.

Traditional Chinese Medicine

A key cause of fibrocystic breasts discussed throughout this chapter is poor blood and lymph circulation. In addition to detoxification protocols, exercise on a mini-trampoline, supporting the thyroid, and improving diet and digestion, another effective alternative medicine therapy to free blocked or sluggish circulation is acupuncture, a central component of traditional Chinese medicine or TCM (see "A Glossary of Traditional Chinese Medicine Terms," p. 48).

In China, acupuncture is routinely used to treat fibrocystic breast disease, with great success. The effect of acupuncture is to improve and balance energy flow in the body which in turn improves the sluggish blood and lymph circulation that is so problematic with fibrocystic breasts. Traditional Chinese medicine often finds a liver involvement in FBD; that is, there is an imbalance in liver energy or the meridian which supplies energy to the organ. This interferes with the liver's function of processing and eliminating toxins and excess estrogen.

Acupuncture can restore the energy flow to the liver. When the liver is once again fully performing its detoxifying function, shrinkage of even large breast lumps can be the result. The following case, based on a report in *Acupuncture Case Histories From China*, exemplifies how TCM approaches the problem.[30]

A Glossary of Traditional Chinese Medicine Terms

Traditional Chinese medicine (TCM) originated in China over 5,000 years ago and is a comprehensive system of medical practice that heals the body according to the principles of nature and balance. A Chinese medicine physician considers the flow of vital energy (*qi*—pronounced CHEE) in a patient through close examination of the patient's pulse, tongue, body odor, voice tone and strength, and general demeanor, among other elements. Underlying imbalances and disharmony in the body are described in terminology analogous to the natural world (heat, cold, dryness, or dampness). The concept of balance, or the interrelationship of organs, is central to TCM. In TCM, imbalances are corrected through the use of acupuncture, moxibustion, herbal medicine, dietary therapy, massage, and therapeutic exercise.

Acupuncture is an integrated healing system developed by the Chinese over 5,000 years ago and introduced in the United States in the mid-1800s. The treatment is administered by an acupuncturist using hair-thin, stainless-steel needles, generally presterilized

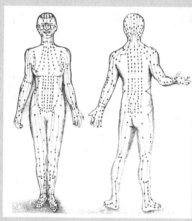

and disposable; these are lightly inserted into the skin at any of over 1,000 locations on the body's surface, known as acupoints. Acupoints are places where *qi* can be accessed by acupuncturists to reduce, enhance, or redirect its flow. Acupuncture is employed for a wide variety of conditions (the World Health Organization counts 104), including pain relief, asthma, migraines, and arthritis.

Acupuncture meridians are specific pathways in the human body for the flow of *qi*. In most cases, these energy pathways run up and down both sides of the body, and correspond to individual organs or organ systems, designated as Lung, Small Intestine, Heart, and others. There are 12 principal meridians and eight secondary channels.

In **moxibustion**, a dried herb called moxa (usually mugwort) is burned over the skin at a specific acupuncture point. The moxa may be attached to a special acupuncture needle or in a free-standing cone set on a slice of ginger; its slow burning provides a penetrating heat. The purpose is to warm the blood and *qi*, particularly when a patient's energy picture is cold or damp.

Success Story: Acupuncture Reduces Breast Cysts

Su Li, 45, went to her traditional Chinese medicine physician complaining of painful breast lumps in both breasts, a frequent occurrence over the previous two years. The pain radiated to her armpit and back, and was worse during menstruation or during emotional stress.

Su Li told the physician that she had frequent episodes in which her breasts swelled and her chest felt constricted, a sensation she tried to relieve by heaving deep sighs. She was also irritable, and complained of both forgetfulness and excessive dreaming during sleep. Further, Su Li had a bitter taste in her mouth and her throat felt dry, although she was not thirsty. Other significant symptoms were a small flow at urination, and a red, dry tongue with a thin, yellow coat. Her pulses were tight, thin, and rapid.

On examination, the physician found a mass of 1 cm by 2 cm in Su Li's right breast and a mass of 2 cm by 3 cm in her left breast. There was tenderness, but the lumps were fluid and moved freely when manipulated. Su Li was diagnosed with a "stagnation" of Liver energy or *qi* (pronounced CHEE), based on the symptoms of chest congestion, sighing, and emotional upset. This meant that the energy in the channels that nourish the liver was not circulating freely, so Su Li's liver was not being supplied with enough energy to do its job efficiently. As a result, it had became "stagnant" or sluggish.

Su Li also was diagnosed with what is called "deficient heat," meaning that her liver was working hard but inefficiently to overcome its lack of

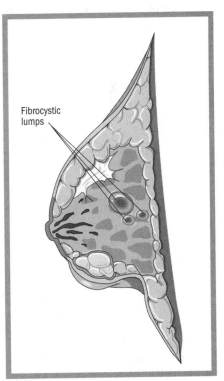

Fibrocystic lumps

THE FIBROCYSTIC BREAST. Lumps in the breast may take one of three forms: a) cyst (a fluid-filled round sac, painful to the touch, and short-lived); b) fibroadenoma (rubbery to the touch, oval, but not painful); and c) lipoma or fatty tumor (irregularly shaped, painless, and ranging in consistency from soft to firm.

49

energy. The effort created heat in Su Li's body, but it was not the productive heat energy of a healthy body; instead, it was a destructive, drying heat that depleted her body of fluids, coolness, and moistness, or what the Chinese call "yin" energy. The symptoms of the deficient heat were the bitter taste in the mouth, dry throat, scanty urination, red and dry tongue with a thin, yellow coat, and the tight, thin, rapid pulse.

The physician did an acupuncture treatment designed to promote healthy circulation in the liver's energy channels, thereby reducing the "stagnation" and restoring more "yin" energy to balance the deficient heat. The physician also treated points along the pathways around Su Li's breasts to improve circulation in that area. The treatment was done once daily throughout one menstrual cycle. Points were needled on the hands, feet, knees, chest, and shoulders.

After 15 treatments, Su Li's breast swelling and soreness were markedly reduced. However, the masses remained. The physician then added moxibustion (see Glossary, p. 48), a heat treatment involving burning of the herb mugwort near the skin. In Su Li's case, the burning dried herbs were placed on a stick held at a point just below the center of each breast. The stick was circulated around the point, not touching the skin, for 20 minutes until the skin became flushed.

After ten days of daily acupuncture and moxibustion treatments, the masses had shrunk to 0.5 cm by 0.7 cm in the right breast and 1 cm by 0.8 cm in the left breast. Daily treatment continued for another month, after which time both masses were gone. Treatment continued for one more week to consolidate the effect. A follow-up two years later showed the masses had not returned.[31]

Herbal Medicine

Milk thistle and dandelion have already been mentioned as herbs which can aid in the treatment of fibrocystic breast disease by supporting the liver in its detoxifying function. Dr. Kulhay cited *Phytolacca* as an anti-inflammatory herb which can help draw toxins from the breasts and break up lumps.

Herbalist Susun Weed of Woodstock, New York, also recommends dandelion, along with a number of other herbs, for FBD treatment. "When the breasts are lumpy, look to the liver," she says. To support liver function, Weed prescribes dandelion root tincture, 20-30 drops, taken up to four times daily. You can also apply the tincture (15-25 drops on a clean cloth) externally to the breasts, she says. (A tincture is the extracted essence of fresh plant material preserved in alcohol.)

Herbs can also address other causes underlying FBD. According to Weed, the following have hormonal balancing properties and thus can help restore the estrogen-progesterone ratio: a tincture of chastetree berry (*Vitex agnus-castus*), 60-90 drops daily; and an infusion of dried raspberry leaf (*Rubus idaeus*), one cup daily. (An infusion is a tea made from dried herbs steeped in boiled water for 30 minutes to several hours, depending on the part of the plant used.)

For dissolving breast lumps, you can drink up to a quart daily of the following in tea form, says Weed: red clover (*Trifolium pratense*, improves hormone balance), nettles (*Urtica dioica*, improves blood and lymphatic flow in the breasts), and violet (*Viola odorata*, slows abnormal cell proliferation). Tinctures of the following herbs also improve lymphatic flow: cleavers (*Galium aparine*, 20 drops daily), calendula (*Calendula officinalis*, 5-20 drops, three times daily), and burdock (*Articum lappa*, 30 drops, 3-8 times daily).[32]

Dr. Gary Ross recommends rubbing the breasts with peppermint oil to help stimulate the poor circulation associated with FBD. In addition to its stimulant effects, peppermint (*Mentha piperita*) is a pain-reliever and antispasmodic, which can help soothe sore and tender breasts.

Homeopathy

Homeopathy (SEE QUICK DEFINITION) is a powerful therapy because it addresses both the physical and emotional components of an illness. Judyth Reichenberg-Ullman, N.D., a prominent homeopathic physician in Seattle, Washington, has successfully treated FBD with homeopathy. The following case from her patient files demonstrates the multidimensional healing of homeopathic remedies and how the correct remedy for a particular individual can clear emotional blocks and cure fibrocystic breasts.

Success Story: FBD Reversed With Homeopathy

Jackie, 42, had fibrocystic breast disease along with multiple uterine fibroids (SEE QUICK DEFINITION). Her breasts were sore during the week before her period, and consuming caffeine or touching her breasts made the soreness worse. Other symptoms included premenstrual irritability, eczema, dandruff, gas, and tendinitis in her right elbow.

At the time Jackie consulted Dr. Reichenberg-Ullman,

For more information on **alternative treatments for uterine fibroids**, see *Alternative Medicine Guide to Women's Health 1* (Future Medicine Publishing, 1998; ISBN 1-887299-12-2); to order, call 800-333-HEAL.

she had just lost a sister to breast cancer and was terrified that she would develop it as well. There was other cancer in her family and Jackie was childless which she knew put her at greater risk of developing breast cancer. Jackie, who had a high need for control, was feeling powerless.

Dr. Reichenberg-Ullman looks at the complete physical, emotional, and psychological picture of the patient in order to determine the best single, constitutional remedy for this particular person. In Jackie's case, it was one dose of *Conium maculatum* 200C. On a physical level, *Conium* is indicated if the breast cysts are hard and painful, there are pains in the nipple, and there is itching inside the breast. Also, it is used if the pain is worse just before and during the menstrual period and if the woman has a feeling of wanting to press her breast hard with her hand.[33]

In less than two months, Jackie's breast tenderness was 90% better and her fear about breast cancer had lessened dramatically. Her other symptoms were improved as well. Eleven months after beginning treatment, Jackie required another dose of *Conium* 200C because she had antidoted the remedy by drinking a cup of decaffeinated coffee (both decaffeinated and regular coffee are known to antidote homeopathic remedies). Her symptoms had returned, but after taking a second remedy, she was doing fine.[34]

Today, one in eight women develop breast cancer, but the diagnosis doesn't have to be a death sentence. By determining the underlying factors— from toxic overload to nutritional deficiencies— which combined to produce your breast cancer and by addressing each one, you can reverse this disease. Through diet, detoxification, supplements, homeopathy, and traditional Chinese medicine, many women have successfully recovered, even from metastasized breast cancer.

2 Breast Cancer

THE INCIDENCE OF BREAST CANCER in the United States is rising steadily and dramatically. In the beginning of the 1900s, the disease was an uncommon occurrence,[1] but in 1968, one in 20 women were developing breast cancer and, today, it is one in eight.[2] From 1973 to 1987, the incidence in women between the ages of 30 and 34 tripled; in women 35 to 39 years old, the rate quadrupled. Every 15 minutes five new cases of breast cancer are diagnosed and at least one woman dies of the disease.[3] Breast cancer is now the leading cause of death in women between the ages of 40 and 45.[4] Despite $30 billion spent on research and treatment in the conventional medical establishment's "war on cancer," the death rate from breast cancer is no lower today than it was more than 50 years ago.[5]

Alternative Medicine Therapies for Breast Cancer

- Detoxification therapy
- Dietary recommendations
- Glandular extracts
- Herbal medicine
- Homeopathy
- Nutritional supplements
- Orthomolecular medicine
- Stress-management counseling
- Traditional Chinese medicine

These statistics are grim indeed and, as long as the standard breast cancer treatment continues to be restricted to chemotherapy, radiation, and/or surgery, it is likely they will only get more grim. While these conventional methods have saved some women's lives, they fail to address the root causes of a woman's breast cancer. This means that the factors that allowed the cancer to grow in the first place remain and can result in a recurrence. In a more comprehensive, whole-body approach to cancer, alternative medicine treats the underlying imbalances as well as the cancer.

In this chapter, you will learn about 33 factors—ranging from nutritional deficiencies and glandular malfunction to dental problems and environmental toxins—which weaken the body and contribute to the development of breast cancer. You will also see how leading alternative physicians have addressed the underlying causes and successfully treated the disease using therapies such as detoxification, homeopathy, nutritional supplements, and herbal and glandular anticancer agents, among many others. Some of the women in the case histories in this chapter used only alternative medicine to reverse their cancer; others combined alternative therapies with conventional medicine.

Regardless of the treatment plan you ultimately choose, the abiding message here is that every woman has the right to know that there are alternatives to chemotherapy, radiation, and surgery, and that a breast cancer diagnosis does not have to mean losing your breasts—or your life.

Success Story:
Metastasized Breast Cancer in Remission

Maria's case illustrates that, even when breast cancer has metastasized (spread to other parts of the body), complete recovery is possible. Here, the power of alternative medicine, in the form of dietary changes, oral and intravenous nutritional supplements, and natural anticancer substances, to reverse cancer is clearly demonstrated.

When Maria, 42, came to Michael B. Schachter, M.D., director of the Schachter Center for Complementary Medicine in Suffern, New York, in February 1994, she had been diagnosed with breast cancer which had spread to her lung, liver, and bones. The previous June, her doctors had found first a huge liver tumor, then bone cancer in her ribs and spine. Maria underwent extensive chemotherapy and radiation, but her condition only worsened.

When Dr. Schachter started treating her, he put Maria on his multifaceted cancer recovery program, beginning with a mostly vegetarian diet, ample fresh, raw vegetable juices, and moderate amounts of fish and range-grown chicken. She also began taking a long list of supplements, including high doses of vitamin C, coenzyme Q10, and pycnogenol (all antioxidants, SEE QUICK DEFINITION), amygdalin (laetrile or B17), and bovine cartilage (an antitumor agent), among others.

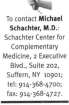

To contact **Michael Schachter, M.D.:** Schachter Center for Complementary Medicine, 2 Executive Blvd., Suite 202, Suffern, NY 10901; tel: 914-368-4700; fax: 914-368-4727.

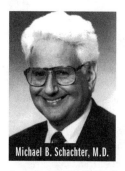

Michael B. Schachter, M.D.

"My goal is to help my cancer patients choose a treatment path that makes sense to them," says Dr. Schachter. **"However, I believe that, in many cases, patients who select only the alternative program and leave out the more** destructive elements of conventional treatment will do better."

QUICK
DEFINITION

An **antioxidant** (meaning "against oxidation") is a natural biochemical substance that protects living cells against damage from harmful free radicals. Antioxidants work against the process of oxidation—the robbing of electrons from substances. If unblocked or left uncontrolled, oxidation can lead to cellular aging, degeneration, arthritis, heart disease, cancer, and other illnesses. Antioxidants in the body react readily with oxygen breakdown products and free radicals, and neutralize them before they can damage the body. Antioxidant nutrients include vitamins A, C, and E, beta carotene, selenium, coenzyme Q10, pycnogenol (grape seed extract), L-glutathione, superoxide dismutase, and bioflavonoids. Plant antioxidants include *Ginkgo biloba* and garlic. When antioxidants are taken in combination, the effect is stronger than when they are used individually.

Two months after her first visit, Dr. Schachter put her on a vitamin C and amygdalin intravenous drip. Two days after this, feeling improved, Maria decided to cancel any further chemotherapy. By August, she was off all her pain medications and was regaining weight steadily. Blood tests proved she was making a major improvement and by September 1995, when Maria's metastasized cancer was in remission, she told Dr. Schachter that she was "feeling great" thanks to his program.

"My goal is to help my cancer patients choose a treatment path that makes sense to them, that they can follow with conviction and enthusiasm," says Dr. Schachter. "This may include some conventional treatment modalities as well as alternative treatments. However, I believe that, in many cases, patients who select only the alternative program and leave out the more destructive elements of conventional treatment will do better."

Success Story: Strengthening the Immune System and Avoiding Mastectomy

A strong focus of alternative medicine's approach to cancer treatment is to strengthen the immune system and thus allow the body's natural cancer-fighting abilities to resume full functioning. This was central to the successful outcome for Maria, above, and in the following case as well.

When she was 49, Rebecca, a switchboard supervisor, noted a lump in her left breast. When a needle-guided excision biopsy indicated a tumor was present, Rebecca's doctor planned a mastectomy for her. When she insisted that he perform a simple excision instead and he refused, Rebecca started looking for an alternative. She found it in Douglas Brodie, M.D., of Reno, Nevada.

This was bold on Rebecca's part because, first, the breast cancer was highly malignant, and second, both her mother and a cousin had died of breast cancer at an early age. Rebecca told Dr. Brodie that if she must have conventional treatment she wanted to at least build herself up in preparation. Along with the small cancerous mass in her

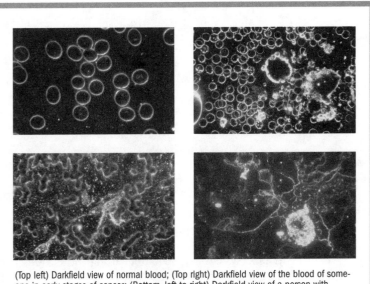

(Top left) Darkfield view of normal blood; (Top right) Darkfield view of the blood of someone in early stages of cancer; (Bottom, left to right) Darkfield view of a person with advanced cancer and another with very advanced cancer.

STUDYING LIVING BLOOD. Darkfield microscopy is a way of studying living whole blood cells under a specially adapted microscope that projects the dynamic image, magnified 1400 times, onto a video screen. With a darkfield light condenser, images of high contrast are projected, so that the object appears bright against a dark background. The skilled physician can detect early signs of illness in the form of microorganisms in the blood known to produce disease. Relevant technical features in the blood include color, variously shaped components such as spicules, long tubules, and roulous, and the size of certain immune cells. The amount of time the blood cell stays viable and alive indicates the overall health of the individual. Specifically, darkfield microscopy reveals distortions of red blood cells (which in turn indicate nutritional status), possible undesirable bacterial or fungal life forms, and blood ecology patterns indicative of health or illness.

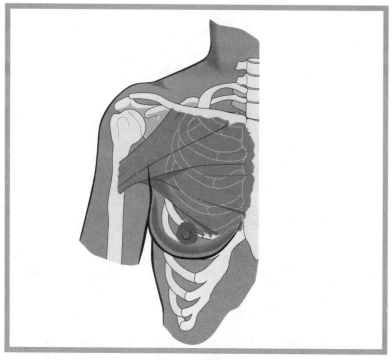

MUSCULATURE AND UNDERLYING SKELETAL STRUCTURE OF THE BREAST.

breast, her immune function was very poor, based on an analysis of her live blood cells with darkfield microscopy (see below).

A glandular extract is a purified nutritional and therapeutic product derived from one of several animal glands including the adrenal, thymus, thyroid, ovaries, testes, pancreas, pineal, and pituitary. It is prescribed by a physician for a person whose corresponding gland is underfunctioning and not producing enough of its own hormone. The various glands are part of the endocrine system which, along with the nervous system, coordinates the functioning of all of the body's systems.

Dr. Brodie started Rebecca on his program of immune system augmentation, using intravenous infusions of high doses of numerous nutritional substances, along with injections into the muscles of thymus peptides (complex amino acids). To complement the injections, Rebecca took oral supplements and glandular extracts (SEE QUICK DEFINITION). This phase took three weeks. During this time, Rebecca's immune system vitality improved from 20% of normal to 100%, as evidenced by white blood cell activity viewed through darkfield microscopy. Dr. Brodie sent her home with a self-care supplement program.

Rebecca managed to persuade her surgeon to perform a lumpectomy (surgery to remove just the tumor in the breast) in which he removed only 25% of her left breast where the tumor resided. He had wanted to cut the whole breast off and excise the lymph nodes as well. The surgical pathology indicated that this 25% portion actually contained no cancer at all. About ten weeks later, an AMAS test, which quite accurately measures levels of antibodies to cancer cells, came back normal, indicating no trace of cancer.

Eight months later, Rebecca saw Dr. Brodie again, reporting that stress from obstacles she was facing in her life had weakened her system. Tests indicated she had no return of cancer but that her immune system had dropped in vitality. Dr. Brodie put her on a seven-day intravenous supplementation program and gave her stress-management counseling. In one week, her immune system had regained its vitality. Back home, once she dealt with the personal stress in her life, her mood, energy level, and sense of well-being rapidly improved. Two years after her initial visit with Dr. Brodie, Rebecca told him that all her cancer markers

For more about
AMAS, see this chapter, pp. 92-94

To contact **Douglas Brodie, M.D.:** 309 Kirman Avenue #2, Reno, NV 89502; tel: 702-324-7071; fax: 702-324-7639.

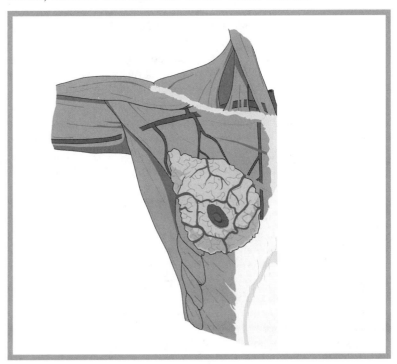

BLOOD SUPPLY TO THE BREAST.

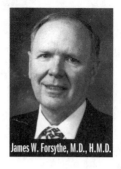

James W. Forsythe, M.D., H.M.D.

"Here is a woman with a Stage IV cancer who didn't take the prescribed radiation and chemotherapy. She did not have what we call a complete cancer surgery, yet she is doing beautifully, extremely well," reports Dr. Forsythe.

To contact **James W. Forsythe, M.D., H.M.D.**: Cancer Screening and Treatment Center of Nevada, Hematology Oncology Ltd., 75 Pringle Way, Suite 909, Reno, NV 89502; tel: 702-329-5000; fax: 702-329-6219.

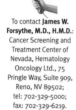

QUICK DEFINITION

A **cancer marker** refers to any of a variety of blood tests which measure the level of a protein material or other chemical produced by cancer cells. These numbers become elevated in the presence of a cancer or tumor. There are different cancer markers for different kinds of cancer; CEA (carcinoembryonic antigen) test for colon cancer, AFP (alpha-fetoprotein) test for liver cancer (primary hepatocellular carcinoma), PSA (prostate specific antigen) for prostate cancer, CA (carcinoma) 15-3 or 27.29 for breast cancer, and CA 125 for ovarian cancer, to name a few.

(SEE QUICK DEFINITION) were normal and that she was in an "excellent state of mind and health."

Success Story: Taking Charge of Her Healing

Unlike Rebecca, the woman in the next case went the conventional route of cancer treatment before she realized that she needed a safer, more effective approach. Jane, 65, a highly successful realtor, investor, and developer, was diagnosed with Stage IV (SEE QUICK DEFINITION) breast cancer which had metastasized from her left breast to her bones. She underwent a lumpectomy. At the same time, she refused radiation, but accepted chemotherapy and had two cycles of Cytoxan, methotrexate, and 5-FU. Based on research she conducted herself, Jane decided that she did not want any more chemotherapy; she believed it was doing her body more harm than good.

Jane went to James W. Forsythe, M.D., H.M.D., director of the Cancer Screening and Treatment Center of Nevada, in Reno. "She was feeling awful, very tired and weak, having some hair loss and nausea, and decided she wanted to go on her own," says Dr. Forsythe, who helped her design a program that included the following vitamins, minerals, herbs, and other substances:

■ Germanium: a superantioxidant trace mineral; 150 mg every 12 hours

■ DHEA: an immune stimulant and hormone vital to the production of other hormones; 25 mg daily

■ Bovine (or shark) cartilage: for antitumor activity; 4-12 g daily in

powder or 500-mg capsules

■ Thymus glandular extract: to enhance the immune system, specifically T cells; 200 mg, three times daily

■ Evening primrose oil: a botanical high in essential fatty acids, for antioxidant support; one gelatin capsule every 12 hours

■ Red clover: for herbal anticancer support; 300 mg every eight hours

■ Vitamin C: an antioxidant; 2.5 g every six hours

■ Garlic (non-odorous) capsules: for immune support and anticancer activity; three capsules every eight hours

■ Glucosamine (a molecule of glucose and an amine): for bone pain relief and bone repair; 500 mg every eight hours

■ Calcium citrate: for bone growth and prevention of osteoporosis; 500 mg every eight hours

■ Armour natural thyroid glandular extract: to enhance metabolism and speed healing; two grains daily

■ Chlorella: a blue-green algae, to aid in detoxification; three capsules daily

■ Pau d'arco: for herbal antitumor support; 200 mg daily

■ Essiac tea: a combination of herbs used to treat cancer, for herbal antitumor support; three cups daily

■ Glutathione: an amino acid complex, for immune support; 500 mg daily

Staging, in cancer terminology, is a relative index of how much cancer exists in the body, its size, its location, and the containment or metastasis of the growth. Stage I, the earliest, most curable stage, shows only local tumor involvement. Stage II indicates some spreading of cancer to the surrounding tissues and perhaps to nearby lymph nodes. Stage III involves metastasis to distant lymph nodes. Stage IV, the most advanced and least easily cured, means the cancer has spread to distant organs.

Jane began this program immediately after discontinuing chemotherapy and remained on it faithfully for 3½ years, says Dr. Forsythe. Her cancer markers, which had been elevated before, became normal. "Here is a woman with a Stage IV cancer who didn't take the prescribed radiation and chemotherapy. She did not have what we call a complete cancer surgery, yet she is doing beautifully, extremely well," reports Dr. Forsythe. "Jane is a very assertive person who runs her own business. She really took charge of her disease and did the healing her own way. She's been very successful."

The preceding three case histories illustrate the dramatic potential of alternative medicine to reverse the breast cancer process and restore a woman's health. Later, you will see how alternative medicine can strengthen the body to better withstand the toxic and traumatic actions of conventional breast cancer treatment, including diminishing the side effects of chemotherapy and radiation.

The alternative medicine approach to breast cancer treatment focuses on strengthening the weakened systems of the body and cor-

Multiple factors, both internal and external, ranging from environmental toxins and food additives to chronic stress and genetic predisposition, together weaken the body and tax its systems until they finally overwhelm the body's defenses and manifest as disease.

recting imbalances in order to liberate the body's natural healing abilities. To prevent a recurrence of the condition that allowed cancer to flourish, it is important to identify and eliminate the internal and external factors that produced the imbalances and weaknesses. The following section presents 33 such factors, beginning with those in the world around us and progressing to the most deeply rooted influences within the body.

33 Factors Linked to Cancer

The alternative medicine view of what causes cancer diverges from the widely held conventional research focus on a single precipitating cause. Rather, alternative medicine points to multiple factors, both internal and external, which, in combination, contribute over time to a disease process in a given individual. These factors—ranging from environmental toxins and food additives to chronic stress and genetic predisposition—together weaken the body and tax its systems until they finally overwhelm the body's defenses and manifest as disease.

Alternative medicine physicians design treatment plans that address the multiple causes, eliminating them and/or rectifying any imbalances they have created. As a result, you and your alternative medicine practitioner will look at some health issues that your conventional physician may not see as relevant to your cancer. These may include poor nutrition, a toxic bowel or liver, an underactive thyroid gland, stressful emotional history, or chemicals in your drinking water, to name just a few.

Keep in mind as you read through the 33 factors that it is the *combined* burden of these factors which place a person at high risk for cancer, and every individual is different. One person may have ten of these elements present and not develop cancer, while another may have only five and that is sufficient to create a climate in which cancer can grow in that particular person. However, it is good cancer *prevention* to do your best to eliminate or address any of these factors which are present in your life. Certainly, if you already have breast cancer, such action should be central to your treatment plan.

Sunlight

Solar radiation, particularly ultraviolet-B and ultraviolet-C radiation, is a common carcinogen, accounting for over 400,000 skin cancers of the overall 1 million new cases of skin cancer occurring annually in the United States. Today, even more ultraviolet radiation is present in sunlight because the ozone hole in the Earth's upper atmosphere has expanded, weakening the Earth's natural shield against it.

Chronic Electromagnetic Field Exposure

According to an Environmental Protection Agency study, there is growing evidence of a link between exposure to electromagnetic fields (EMFs)—which are generated by electrical currents—and cancer. While EMFs are part of nature and in fact are radiated by the human body and its individual organs, the quality and intensity of the energy can either support or destroy health. As a rule, EMFs generated by human-made technological devices or installations tend to be much more harmful than naturally occurring EMFs.

We are surrounded by EMFs, produced by electrical wiring in homes and offices, televisions, computers and video terminals,

33 Factors That Contribute to Cancer

- Sunlight
- Chronic electromagnetic field exposure
- Geopathic stress
- Sick building syndrome
- Ionizing radiation
- Nuclear radiation
- Pesticide/herbicide residues
- Industrial toxins
- Polluted water
- Chlorinated water
- Fluoridated water
- Tobacco and smoking
- Hormone therapies
- Immune-suppressive drugs
- Irradiated foods
- Food additives
- Mercury toxicity
- Dental factors
- Nerve interference fields
- Diet and nutritional deficiencies
- Chronic stress
- Toxic emotions
- Depressed thyroid action
- Intestinal toxicity and digestive impairment
- Parasites
- Viruses
- Blocked detoxification pathways
- Free-radical overload
- Cellular oxygen deficiency
- Cellular terrain
- Oncogenes
- Genetic predisposition
- Miasm

Magnetic radiations from the Earth, presumably connected with geological fractures and subterranean water veins, have been associated with an increased risk of cancer in communities situated near these geopathic, or pathogenic, influences.

For more on the **33 causes of cancer**, see *Alternative Medicine Definitive Guide to Cancer* (Future Medicine Publishing, 1997; ISBN 1-887299-01-7); to order, call 800-333-HEAL.

microwave ovens, overhead lights, and electrical poles. "Only a few farsighted individuals have given much thought to the fact that the new electromagnetic environment created by 20th-century technology may be exerting subtle, yet very important effects upon human biology," says John Zimmerman, Ph.D., president of the Bio-Electro Magnetics Institute. EMFs affect enzymes related to growth regulation, gene expression, and cell division and multiplication—all of which can exert a major influence on cancer tumor growth.

Geopathic Stress

Magnetic radiations from the Earth, presumably connected with geological fractures and subterranean water veins, have been associated with an increased risk of cancer in communities situated near these geopathic, or pathogenic, influences. According to some experts, the cause of geopathic stress may be localized magnetic anomalies—unusual, sudden changes and quirks that can upset delicate human physiological balance and thereby create health problems.

In 1971, the theory of geopathic stress was supported by research showing that water flowing underground, especially subterranean streams that cross, produces measurable increases in magnetic anomalies; these conditions also increase electrical conductivity in the air and soil. While the changes are small, they are still capable of contributing to the development of serious illness, including cancer. One large-scale study by the U.S. government reported that geopathic stress may be a factor in between 40% and 50% of all human cancers and account for between 60% and 90% of all cancers attributed to environmental radiation.[6]

Sick Building Syndrome

In the early eighties, physicians began using the term "sick building syndrome" (SBS) to refer to a host of symptoms produced by low-grade toxic environmental conditions found in living, work, or office spaces. SBS symptoms are numerous: mucous membrane irritation of

75% of Breast Cancer Caused by Radiation

‟ Our estimate is that about three-quarters of the current annual incidence of breast cancer in the U.S. is being caused by earlier ionizing radiation, primarily from medical sources," states John W. Gofman, M.D., Ph.D., the director of the Committee for Nuclear Responsibility, Inc., professor emeritus in the Department of Molecular and Cell Biology at the University of California at Berkeley, and the author of 100 scientific papers and several notable books on radiation and health.

Given that 182,000 new cases of female breast cancer occurred in 1995, this means that approximately 136,500 breast cancers might have been linked with diagnostic (mammograms) and therapeutic radiation sources. Even if Dr. Gofman's risk estimate is overstated, reducing it by two-thirds still leaves over 45,000 new breast cancer cases that would result annually from unnecessary exposure to medical sources of radiation.

The shocking conclusion from Dr. Gofman's research is that mammograms, used to detect breast cancer, are actually causing it. However, this may be good news in disguise because it means potentially 75% of breast cancer could be prevented by avoiding or minimizing exposure to the ionizing radiation from mammography, X rays, and other non-nuclear medical sources such as radiation therapy. Each reduction in breast irradiation today can prevent a possible future breast cancer from developing, says Gofman.[7]

Dr. Gofman documents the assurances given by doctors to patients regarding the safety and efficacy of relatively high doses of radiation in medicine, now proven to be erroneous. A new series of safety "assurances" are currently in circulation for low doses of radiation, but these are little better than wishful thinking, according to Dr. Gofman, who asserts that "all doses matter."

After investigating the effects of low-level ionizing radiation for 30 years, Gofman concludes that the longer the radiation exposure, the smaller the dose needed to do damage. The onset of cancer is often a delayed effect, says Dr. Gofman; individuals may live for ten years following irradiation before a cancer develops. Then new radiation exposures act as a "multiplier" upon the rate at which spontaneous cancers ordinarily occur which, in turn increases with age, Dr. Gofman warns.

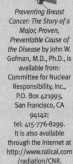

Preventing Breast Cancer: The Story of a Major, Proven, Preventable Cause of the Disease by John W. Gofman, M.D., Ph.D., is available from: Committee for Nuclear Responsibility, Inc., P.O. Box 421993, San Francisco, CA 94142; tel: 415-776-8299. It is also available through the Internet at http://www.ratical.com /radiation/CNR.

the eyes, nose, and throat, chest tightness, skin complaints, headaches, fatigue, lethargy, coughing, asthma, wheezing, chronic nasal stuffiness, temporary weight loss, infections, and emotional irritability. All of these depress the immune system, rendering the individual susceptible to long-term chronic illness and potentially to a cancer process.

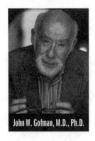

John W. Gofman, M.D., Ph.D.

"Our estimate is that about three-quarters of the current annual incidence of breast cancer in the U.S. is being caused by earlier ionizing radiation, primarily from medical sources," states Dr. Gofman.

"Indoor air pollution in residences, offices, schools, and other buildings, is widely recognized as a serious environmental risk to human health," explains Michael Hodgson, M.D., M.P.H., of the School of Medicine, University of Connecticut Health Center in Farmington. In most cases, problems with a building's engineering, construction, and ventilation system are the causes. Other sources of indoor toxic pollution include volatile organic compounds released by particleboard desks, furniture, carpets, glues, paints, office machine toners, and perfumes. In addition, the carcinogenic effects of certain indoor air pollutants, such as asbestos, environmental tobacco smoke, radon, and formaldehyde, are well described in the clinical literature and are now considered cancer risk factors.

Ionizing Radiation

Ionizing radiation consists of high-energy rays that are capable of ripping the electrons from matter, causing genetic mutations that can lead to cancer. This is the type of radiation used in X-ray technology, which may explain why radiologists (people who take many X rays each day) have historically had higher incidences of cancer, as have other workers exposed to low-dose radiation. In fact, medical X rays may cause about 75% of breast cancer (see "75% of Breast Cancer Caused by Radiation," p. 65). In addition to medical X rays, ionizing radiation also emanates from such common household items as fluorescent lights, computer monitors, and television screens.

Nuclear Radiation

Working or living in the proximity of nuclear power plants presents a cancer risk. Among the hazards are the small amounts of radioactive gases released daily from nuclear reactors. Although these radioactive gas emissions enter the atmosphere at levels deemed "permissible" by the U.S. Department of Energy, evidence suggests that low-level radioactive pollution may pose a significant cancer risk.

According to one study, workers who were exposed daily to low-

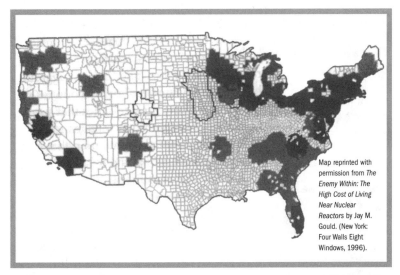

Map reprinted with permission from *The Enemy Within: The High Cost of Living Near Nuclear Reactors* by Jay M. Gould. (New York: Four Walls Eight Windows, 1996).

NUCLEAR COUNTIES. Of the country's 3,053 counties, nearly half, or 1,231, are situated within 100 miles of nuclear reactor sites. The darker areas on the map indicate "nuclear counties" and represent the highest risk areas.

level ionizing radiation had a much higher risk of cancer, particularly leukemia.[8] In the United Kingdom, a higher rate of leukemia has been reported in children living near a nuclear facility. Finally, the incidence of childhood thyroid cancer has increased 100 times in those areas of Ukraine, Belarus, and Russia most acutely exposed to the Chernobyl nuclear accident in April 1986, according to a United Nations report.

The dangers of nuclear radiation are not limited to those who work in or live close to a reactor, however. Low-level radioactive pollution returns to us in rainfall which then accumulates in the soil to contaminate the food chain. Chronic exposure to nuclear fission products through the diet and drinking water "may be the single largest factor in the increased incidence of most forms of malignancies" since 1945, according to Ernest Sternglass, Ph.D., a professor of radiation physics at the University of Pittsburgh. The prime carriers for fission products were municipal water and air and, to a lesser extent, fresh milk and dairy products.

Pesticide/Herbicide Residues

The potential of pesticides, alone and in combination, to cause and promote cancer should be of grave concern to all physicians and public health officials. Clear evidence has linked long-term exposure to pesticides with cancer, prompting a consortium of 75 Environmental Protection Agency experts to rank pesticide residues among the top three environmentally derived cancer risks.

"Many cancer-causing pesticides found in the environment and in food tend to accumulate in fatty tissues, whether in fish, cattle, fowl, or people," explains Samuel Epstein, M.D., professor of Occupational and Environmental Medicine at the University of Illinois School of Public Health. This slow, gradual process—called bioaccumulation—will continue as long as we continue to be exposed to pesticides.

Unfortunately, the use of these poisons is not being curtailed; rather, it has increased tenfold since the introduction of DDT in the 1940s. In the past 50 years, some 15,000 chemical compounds and more than 35,000 different formulations have come into use as pesticides worldwide. Many of those banned in the U.S. (including DDT) are sold to Third World countries, where they enter food products, such as coffee, fruits, and vegetables, which are then imported into the U.S. In addition to agricultural pesticides, home and garden herbicides represent another major source of toxicity. Indoor pesticides, such as no-pest strips, termite pesticides, home pesticide bombs, and flea collars for pets, have been implicated in certain forms of cancer, especially brain cancer in children.

High Rate of Breast Cancer in California

White women in the San Francisco Bay Area of California have the world's highest rate of breast cancer—104 cases per 100,000 women. This is double the rate for women in general in Europe, and five times higher than for women in general in Japan, reports the International Agency for Research on Cancer.

In 1983, the Bay Area also led the world in estrogen prescriptions for women. Yet as two-thirds of women who get breast cancer have no known risk factors, experts are querying whether exposure to radiation, pesticides, and chlorine-based chemicals may be contributing factors. California leads the U.S. with 17,800 new breast cancer cases and 4,400 mortalities every year. It also tops the list of America's toxic-waste sites, with 258, nearly 100 more than second place Alaska and almost 200 more than third place Maryland.[9]

Industrial Toxins

A great number of highly toxic chemicals, materials, and heavy metals are released by industrial processes. These toxins later find their way into human tissue, where they have negative health effects, including cancer. By 1980, the Environmental Protection Agency had detected over 400 toxic chemicals in human tissue.

In 1997, the National Academy of Sciences stated that the average American ingests 40 mg of pesticides per year from food sources alone and carries about one-tenth of a gram permanently stored in body fat. In addition, a variety of industrial by-products mimic the activity of estrogen once inside the human body, creating havoc in hormonal balance; these estrogen-mimicking chemicals are believed to contribute to breast cancer.

The claim that environmental chemicals can cause or promote cancer is supported by the fact that the distribution of toxic-waste dump sites closely correlates with the sites where the highest rates of breast cancer mortality have been registered, according to *Scientific American* (October 1995).

Polluted Water

Polluted water can raise the risk of developing cancer. Tap water from municipal sources is increasingly becoming a health hazard in the U.S. One out of every four public water systems has violated federal standards for tap water.[11] It is not only pesticides and agricultural runoff that contaminate public drinking water: according to the Environmental Protection Agency, the tap water of 30 million Americans contains potentially dangerous levels of lead. Tap water can contain many different contaminants, including radioactive particles, heavy metals (such as lead and copper), gasoline solvents, industrial wastes, chemical residues, disinfectant by-products, and solid particulates such as asbestos.

Breast Cancer Incidence and Industrial Toxins

As breast cancer incidence rises at 1.3% annually in the U.S. and Canada, researchers have found that women with the highest levels of the industrial toxins DDE and PCBs in their fat, tissues, and blood were two to three times more likely to develop cancer, according to the *Canadian Medical Association Journal* (April 1996). Women with the highest blood levels of DDT had four times the breast cancer risk of women with the least exposure.[10]

A survey of 100 municipal water systems and suppliers found significant levels of cancer-causing arsenic, radon, and chlorine by-products, reported the Natural Resources Defense Council in October 1995. An estimated 19 million Americans drink water with radon levels higher than federal safety standards. The answer isn't as easy as switching to bottled water, however. Approximately 70% of the toxins from water that enter the body do so through the skin during baths and showers.

Chlorinated Water

Disinfecting drinking water with chlorine is standard practice throughout the U.S. While there is little doubt that adding chlorine-type compounds to drinking water protects the public from several kinds of harmful bacteria, including *Salmonella* and *Vibrio cholera*, chlorine can also form cancer-causing agents when it interacts with other compounds present in drinking water.

New evidence indicates that chlorinated water increases the risk of cancer for the roughly 200 million Americans who drink it. According to a Norwegian study, consuming chlorinated water is associated with a 20% to 40% increase in the incidence of colon and rectal cancer. In addition, people who drink chlorinated water over long periods of time also increase their risk of developing bladder cancer by as much as 21%.[14]

As with other forms of pollution found in the water, it is not only drinking chlorinated water that is hazardous. The amount inhaled or absorbed through the skin during a typical shower may be six times higher than that absorbed from chlorinated drinking water, states *International Health News*. This exposure can be cut by 30% or more by using a bathroom fan, keeping the window open while showering, or running the water through an activated carbon filter.

Israel Proves the Pesticide-Cancer Link

In 1978, Israel banned toxic chemicals such as DDT and PCBs which had been directly linked with breast cancer in a 1976 study.[12] Over the next ten years, the rate of breast cancer deaths in Israel declined sharply, with a 30% drop in mortality for women under 44 years old, and an 8% overall decline, despite an increase in other cancer risks such as dietary factors and alcohol consumption. Meanwhile, worldwide death rates from breast cancer had increased by 4%.[13]

Fluoridated Water

Fluoride, a poison second in toxicity only to arsenic, has routinely been added to public drinking water and toothpaste since the 1950s, despite mounting evidence of its multiple health hazards. According to scientific research, fluoride in drinking water can *produce* cancer, transforming normal human cells into cancerous ones.

The National Academy of Sciences has found that fluorine (a component of fluoride) slows down vitally important DNA repair activity as mediated by enzymes that normally correct for possible flaws or mutations in the genetic material. These biological effects can be induced by fluoride present even in concentrations as low as one part per million, the official "safe" dosage set by the U.S. Public Health Service. In addition, fluoride can increase the cancer-producing potential of other cancer-causing chemicals.

Dean Burk, Ph.D., chief chemist emeritus of the National Cancer Institute, estimates that fluoride causes more cancer than any other chemical. Dr. Burk compared the cancer death rates of the largest fluoridated and nonfluoridated cities. These death rates were similar prior to 1953 when the use of fluoride was introduced, then increased markedly among fluoridated cities. According to Burk's estimates, fluoride caused about 61,000 cases of cancer in 1995 and is likely to cause 90,000 cancer cases by 2015.[16]

Tobacco and Smoking

About 30% of cancer deaths in the U.S. can be attributed to tobacco smoke, making it "the single most lethal carcinogen in the U.S.," according to researchers at the Harvard Center for Cancer Prevention, in Cambridge, Massachusetts. Over 2,000 chemical compounds are generated by tobacco smoke, and many of them are poisons.[17] Carbon monoxide is released during smoking, reducing the amount of oxygen to the brain, lungs, and heart. Nicotine is not only addictive, but also acts as a cancer promoter, making it easier for cancer cells of all types to spread throughout the body. Tar, the leading cancer-causing

Breast Cancer "Treatment" Can Cause Cancer in Other Organs

Women who take tamoxifen to prevent their breast cancer from recurring may be putting themselves at risk for developing another type of cancer. The synthetic hormone drug, which is typically prescribed after breast cancer surgery to block the regrowth of remaining cancer cells, has been linked with increased risk of endometrial (uterine lining) cancer.

In a study of 98 women who were diagnosed with endometrial cancer at least three months after a diagnosis of primary (first-time) breast cancer, researchers at the Netherlands Cancer Institute found that women who took tamoxifen for over two years more than doubled their chances of developing endometrial cancer.[15]

In addition, women who used the drug for longer periods of time or at higher dosages proportionally increased their cancer risk. Previous studies put the risk at six times higher for tamoxifen users, and tests involving laboratory rats have linked the drug with liver cancer as well. Other side effects of the drug, as listed in the *Physicians' Desk Reference*, include vomiting, vaginal discharge, hot flashes, nausea, and skin problems.

chemical found in tobacco smoke, contains carcinogenic hydrocarbons and other toxic substances, as well as some radioactive compounds.[18]

Hormone Therapies

Hormone therapies which increase the levels of estrogen (SEE QUICK DEFINITION) relative to progesterone (SEE QUICK DEFINITION) in women have been linked to some forms of cancer. In particular, prolonged use of oral contraceptives and hormone replacement therapy (HRT) for postmenopausal women have been associated with an increased risk of breast and endometrial cancer.

Regarding oral contraceptives, research pointed to serious cancer risks as early as the late 1960s. One study indicated that women who took the pill for more than four years were twice as likely as nonusers to develop breast cancer by age 50.[19] Another study found that women taking birth control pills had a 300% higher incidence of cervical dysplasia, usually benign changes in the shape of the cervix which, nonetheless, can be early indicators of possible later cancer.

The link between hormone replacement for menopausal women and endometrial and breast cancer was first firmly established in 1989, when Swedish researchers reported that postmenopausal women between the ages of 55 and 59 taking estrogen replacement therapy for five years or more had a 40% higher risk of developing breast cancer; among women between the ages of 60 and 64, the risk was 70% higher.[20] The risk of developing endometrial cancer while taking hormone replacement therapy also increases, both with age and with length of HRT use.

Immune-Suppressive Drugs

The widespread, habitual, and chronic use of a great number of conventional drugs, antibiotics, and even vaccinations can have a seriously suppressive effect on the immune system, acting in concert with all the other factors at play to prepare the system for a cancer process. Drugs such as aspirin, acetaminophen, and ibuprofen taken for aches and colds, and glucocorticosteroids such as cortisone, decrease antibody production and suppress immune vitality.

Antibiotics can directly hinder immune activity and increase the intestinal overgrowth of the yeast *Candida albicans*, which then can suppress the immune system. Research suggests that vaccinations can also suppress the immune system, in some cases for up to two weeks after inoculation. Finally, cytotoxic agents or chemotherapy drugs used to *stop* cancerous growths have powerful immune-suppressive effects, rendering the individual even more susceptible to new, secondary cancers.

Irradiated Foods

The intent of food irradiation is to kill insects, bacteria, molds, and fungi and thus to extend shelf life, but the results might be dangerous to consumers. The process of irradiation leads to the formation of toxic substances, such as benzene and formaldehyde, and other toxic chemical by-products that have been associated with cancer risk.

For example, food irradiation may increase the levels of aflatoxin, a deadly carcinogen; it may allow the *botulinum* toxin (which causes botulism food poisoning) to remain undetected in irradiated foods; over time it may induce some microorganisms to mutate, giving rise to new, dangerous species. In fact, much about the harmful effects of food irradiation is still not fully understood. The FDA estimates that 10% of the chemicals in irradiated foods are not found in normal (nonirradiated) foods and are unknown to science.[21]

Food Additives

Of the 3,000 chemical additives introduced into the American food supply every year, only a small fraction have been tested for their effects on humans (most are tested on animals). Among the most common are aspartame, saccharin, and cyclamates, artificial sweeteners that have been linked to greater incidences of cancer;[22] butylated hydroxytoluene, a food preservative which may contribute to liver cancer; and tannic acid, present in wines and fruits and linked to liver cancer. Aflatoxins, which are found in milk, cereals, peanuts, and corn, have been associated with liver, stomach, and kidney cancer.[23] Other food additives that may increase the risk of certain kinds of cancer include blue dye No. 2, propyl gallate, and red dye No. 3.[24]

Mercury Toxicity

Mercury, a toxic heavy metal which often comprises up to 50% of "sil-

Cytotoxic agents or chemotherapy drugs used to stop cancerous growths have powerful immune-suppressive effects, rendering the individual even more susceptible to new, secondary cancers.

ver" dental fillings, is a noted carcinogen. Like other heavy metals, mercury has been shown to cause damage to the lining of arteries and nerve bundles (ganglia), thereby contributing to cancer. In addition, heavy metals act as free radicals—highly reactive, charged particles that can cause damage to body tissues if inhaled or absorbed. The International Academy of Oral Medicine and Toxicology (IAOMT) cites evidence indicating that dental mercury amalgams are a major contributor to immune dysfunction and free-radical pathologies, including cancer, kidney dysfunction, and cardiovascular disease.[25]

"If amalgam fillings are present, your circulatory system is constantly being exposed to the damaging effects of this heavy metal and free radical," explains Daniel F. Royal, D.O., medical director of the Royal Center of Advanced Medicine, in Las Vegas, Nevada. The cumulative weakening effect these toxic "insults" have on the body makes it more vulnerable to cancer initiation.

Dental Factors

Alternative medicine health practitioners familiar with the principles of biological dentistry have long noted a link between dental problems and degenerative illness. According to Colorado dentist Hal Huggins, D.D.S., "Dental problems such as cavities, infections, toxic or allergy-producing filling material, root canal, and misalignment of the teeth or jaw can have far-reaching effects throughout the body." When a tooth is inflamed or infected, it can block the energy flow along one or more of the body's acupuncture meridians, causing the deterioration of a corresponding organ or tissue and, in time, leading to cancer. In effect, a problem in the tooth can focus its energy imbalance elsewhere in the body, a phenomenon known as "dental focus."

For information on **testing for mercury toxicity**, see Chapter 4: Chronic Fatigue Syndrome, p. 184.

Nerve Interference Fields

Dysfunctions and imbalances in the autonomic nervous system (ANS, SEE QUICK DEFINITION) can contribute to a cancer process. Most cases of chronic illness involve changes in the ANS, upsets in the electrical activity of ganglia (nerve bundles), according to Dietrich Klinghardt, M.D., Ph.D. The source of this electrical confusion is called an "interference field" or focus, and can be caused by

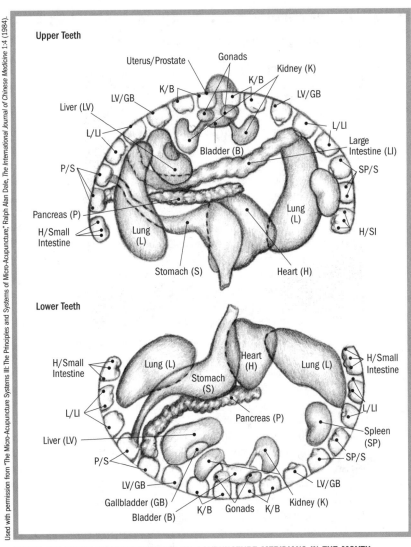

Upper Teeth

Uterus/Prostate — Gonads — Kidney (K)
K/B — K/B
LV/GB — LV/GB
Liver (LV)
L/LI — L/LI
Large Intestine (LI)
Bladder (B)
P/S — SP/S
Pancreas (P)
H/Small Intestine — Lung (L) — Lung (L) — H/SI
Stomach (S) — Heart (H)

Lower Teeth

H/Small Intestine — Lung (L) — Heart (H) — Lung (L) — H/Small Intestine
Stomach (S)
L/LI — L/LI
Pancreas (P)
Liver (LV) — Spleen (SP)
P/S — SP/S
LV/GB — LV/GB
Gallbladder (GB) — Kidney (K)
Bladder (B) — K/B — Gonads — K/B

ORGAN AND TOOTH CORRESPONDENCES ON ACUPUNCTURE MERIDIANS IN THE MOUTH.

skin scars from old accidents or surgeries; nerve bundles (called ganglia) made toxic from an accumulation of mercury, parasite toxins, solvents, and many other substances; restriction in blood flow to the ANS from strokes or carbon monoxide poisoning; and general trauma to the ANS from events such as gunshot wounds, surgical injury, or skull fracture.

High intake of animal protein, fats (especially animal fats), and refined carbohydrates and sugar is associated with an increased risk of breast cancer.

For information on **testing your nutritional status**, see Chapter 4: Chronic Fatigue Syndrome, pp. 190-192.

Diet and Nutritional Deficiencies

According to the National Academy of Sciences, 60% of all cancers in women and 40% of all cancers in men may be due to dietary and nutritional factors. The National Research Council's extensive 1982 report *Diet, Nutrition, and Cancer* provided strong evidence that much of the increase in cancer incidence may be related to typical U.S. dietary practices, among other factors.[26]

The rise of degenerative disease has paralleled the adoption of an overly refined and adulterated, high-protein, high-fat diet over the past 100 years. After World War II, the U.S. population shifted away from regular consumption of whole grains and fresh vegetables, and instead increased its consumption of less wholesome, overly refined foods. This new, so-called affluent diet is high in fat, which can more readily concentrate such chemicals as pesticides, preservatives, and industrial pollutants. High intake of animal protein, fats (especially animal fats), and refined carbohydrates and sugar is associated with an increased risk of breast cancer.[27]

Chronic Stress

Numerous studies have linked stress and its related psychological components to susceptibility to cancer. Adults who have recently lost a loved one, or been widowed, divorced, or separated, tend to have the highest cancer rates.[28] In addition, a basic inability to cope with stress has been regarded as a key risk factor in developing breast cancer.[29] Conversely, how people deal with illness, especially cancer, also has a dramatic impact on their recovery process.[30]

Unrelieved, chronic stress increases cancer risk by gradually weakening, even suppressing, the immune system. Stress can also lead to hormonal imbalances which, in turn, interfere with immune function. Under emotional distress, the brain may signal the adrenal glands to produce chemicals called corticosteroids, hormones which weaken the immune response.

Cancer-related (neoplastic) processes are accelerated in the presence of these chemicals as well as other stress hormones like prolactin. In other words, chronic stress manifests in the body in increased adrenaline levels, hormonal changes, and decreased immune function, creating an environment in the body which may increase the risk of serious disease, including cancer.

Toxic Emotions

Since the 1970s, research in the field of psychoneuroimmunology (PNI) has documented direct links between emotions and biochemical events in the body. Noted women's health expert Christiane Northrup, M.D., of Yarmouth, Maine, coined the term "toxic emotions" to indicate the powerful, strongly held, and often unconsciously active beliefs and emotions which help generate symptoms that keep illnesses in place. In the view of Dr. Northrup as well as other alternative practitioners working with cancer patients, beliefs and emotions can be legitimate toxins, contributing to an overall weakening of the immune system.

Although scientists have long debated the role of repressed emotions in cancer, at least three studies offer compelling evidence validating that role. In each of these studies, people were followed over time to determine their rates of disease in relation to various behaviors or exposures. Taken together, the results indicate a link between cancer resistance and emotional expression or suppression.[31]

Depressed Thyroid Action

An underactive or dysfunctional thyroid gland (a key endocrine gland located in the neck) may contribute to a cancer process. Broda O. Barnes, M.D., a doctor who specialized in treating patients with hypothyroidism (underfunctioning thyroid), observed in his clinical practice evidence to suggest a relationship between low thyroid activity and cancer. Research has tended to support Dr. Barnes' clinical observations.[32]

In 1954, studies by Dr. J.G.C. Spencer from Bristol, England, showed that there was a consistently higher incidence of cancer in areas of 15 countries and four continents where goiter (enlargement of the thyroid gland caused by hypothyroidism among other causes) was more prevalent among the population than in the non-goiter areas of the same localities. Dr. Barnes noted that Austria, a country with a high incidence of goiter, also had the highest incidence of cancer of any country reporting

For more about the **thyroid**, see Chapter 1: Fibrocystic Breast Disease, pp. 30-31, Chapter 4: Chronic Fatigue Syndrome, pp. 180-183, and Chapter 5: Depression, pp. 217-223.

Noted women's health expert Christiane Northrup, M.D., coined the term "toxic emotions" to indicate the powerful, strongly held, and often unconsciously active beliefs and emotions which help generate symptoms that keep illnesses in place.

malignancies at the time, further supporting the link between hypothyroidism and cancer.

Intestinal Toxicity and Digestive Impairment

Many illnesses, such as a number of cancers, most allergies, infections, liver diseases, acne, psoriasis, and asthma, start in the intestines. When the intestines become clogged and diseased by what and how we eat and by how poorly we eliminate waste material, the bowel becomes toxic. This creates toxicity for the entire body, resulting in an inability to absorb the nutrients necessary for health.

Around 1900, most people in the U.S. had a brief intestinal transit time (meaning it took only about 15-20 hours from the time food entered the mouth until it was excreted as feces.) Today, many people have a seriously delayed transit time of 50-70 hours—more time for stool to putrefy, for harmful microorganisms to flourish, and for toxins to develop and poison the tissues.

Mucus-producing foods such as dairy products, eggs, and meat contribute to slowing transit time. As a sticky mucoid lining builds up in the intestines as a result of eating these foods along with white flour products, it not only blocks the absorption of essential nutrients into the bloodstream but also produces a hiding place for bacteria, fungi, yeast, and parasites which are harmful to human health.

An overgrowth of these organisms creates a situation called dysbiosis (an imbalance in intestinal microflora), in which the contents of the intestines putrefy and harmful chemicals are generated. The resulting body-wide toxicity overloads the lymphatic system which can no longer drain and filter poisons efficiently. The inevitable result is illness.

Parasites

The possible presence of parasites in the body, mostly in the intestines, is a little appreciated but major health problem. While people assume they are vulnerable to parasites only if they travel in tropical areas, the fact is that anyone can get them (and many probably already have) from merely staying at home. Wherever they are contracted, the damage parasites cause can be extensive. They can destroy cells faster than they can be regenerated; they can release toxins that damage tissues, resulting in pain and inflammation; and, over time, they can depress, even exhaust, the immune system. Of the dozens of specific parasites of concern to human health, the major groupings include microscopic Protozoa, roundworms, pinworms, hookworms (Nematoda), tapeworms (Cestoda), and flukes (Trematoda).[33]

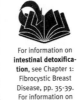

For information on **intestinal detoxification**, see Chapter 1: Fibrocystic Breast Disease, pp. 35-39. For information on **testing for parasites** and **intestinal overgrowth**, see Chapter 4: Chronic Fatigue Syndrome, pp. 171-172.

According to naturopathic physician Hulda Regehr Clark, Ph.D., N.D., who practices in Tijuana, Mexico, a single parasite—the fluke, a flatworm called *Fasciolopsis buskii*—may be responsible for cancer. While under healthy conditions the body is able to destroy flukes before they have completed their growth cycle, the presence of the solvent propyl alcohol (found in rubbing alcohol, commercial breakfast cereals, carbonated beverages, decaffeinated coffee, white sugar, and many cosmetics and toiletries) makes the immune system unable to destroy the flukes.

The pressure of a growing fluke population in the intestines causes the release of a special cell growth factor called orth-phosphotyrosine, which marks the beginning of the cancer process, states Dr. Clark. Two studies in the *Annual Review of Biochemistry* (1985, 1988) confirm that this chemical is a reliable cancer marker for different kinds of malignancies. In her best-selling *The Cure for All Cancers*, Dr. Clark presents 100 case histories illustrating the role of parasites and propyl alcohol in cancer.[34]

Viruses

According to some researchers, up to 15% of the world's cancer deaths are attributable to the activities of viruses, bacteria, or parasites. Among the cancer-producing viruses that work through a host's DNA-synthesizing and protein-building mechanisms are human papilloma viruses type 16 and 18 (which are sexually transmitted) associated with cervical cancer, among others, and the hepatitis B virus, associated with liver cancers. Epstein-Barr virus, which produces mononucleosis, is also carcinogenic.[35]

Blocked Detoxification Pathways

In a healthy individual, the body's normal detoxification systems, especially the liver, are generally able to eliminate toxins and thereby prevent illness. To prevent cancer, the liver's detoxification system must be working optimally, says Joseph Pizzorno, N.D., a naturo-pathic physician and educator based in Seattle, Washington. When the liver is not functioning well, it is unable to process and eliminate the multiplicity of carcinogens entering the body. "High levels of exposure to carcinogens coupled with sluggish detoxification enzymes significantly increase our suscepti-bility to cancer," says Dr. Pizzorno.

Free-Radical Overload

A free radical is an unstable molecule with an unpaired electron that steals an electron from another molecule, producing harmful effects on the body. Free radicals are generated by energy production and fat metabolism, from the immune response by white blood cells, and by the liver's own detoxification process. However, uncon-trolled free-radical production plays a major role in the development of at least 100 degenerative conditions, including cancer.

What makes the difference between normal function-ing of the immune system, which includes the deactivation of free radicals, and the initiation of a potential cancer process is the amount of antioxidants available in the sys-tem. An antioxidant (SEE QUICK DEFINITION) is a natural biochemical substance that protects living cells against damage from harmful free radicals. "When free-radical production exceeds the ability of the neutralizing systems, progressive cellular damage occurs," says Joseph Pizzorno, N.D. When this damage becomes chronic, the next step may be cancer.

Cellular Oxygen Deficiency

One of the most provocative theories of cancer causation was originally put forth by two-time Nobel laureate, Dr. Otto Warburg. He was a German biochemist who won his first Nobel Prize in 1931 for the discovery that oxygen deficiency and cell fermentation are part of the cancer process. According to Dr. Warburg's theory, when cells are deprived of oxygen, they can revert to their "primitive" state, deriving energy not from oxygen, as normal plant and animal cells do, but rather from the fermentation of blood sugar.

Blood sugar (glucose) breaks down into lactic acid,

which causes an imbalance in the body's acid/base ratio, or pH level (SEE QUICK DEFINITION); as the acidity of the body rises, it becomes even more difficult for the cells to use oxygen normally. "All normal cells have an absolute requirement for oxygen," stated Dr. Warburg, "but cancer cells can live without oxygen—a rule *without any exceptions.*"

One possible reason for the dramatic increase in cancer rates over the past century, according to Dr. Warburg's theory, may be the decreasing levels of oxygen and the increasing levels of carbon monoxide in urban air. Carbon monoxide (CO) has a higher affinity for hemoglobin (which transports oxygen to the cells) than does oxygen; for this reason, when we breathe in CO, our hemoglobin binds more CO and less oxygen.

By contrast, according to this same oxygen deficiency theory, cancer cells cannot exist in an oxygen-rich environment. Humans can become oxygen deficient through several routes, including long-term exposure to air pollution (tobacco smoke, auto exhaust, factory emissions), devitalized foods (overcooked, processed, preserved, all of which deplete oxygen), shallow breathing, and inadequate exercise.

Cellular Terrain

The term "cellular terrain," first coined by European practitioners of what is called biological medicine, refers to the general vitality, activity, and biochemical condition of the cells in the body. When the cell becomes imbalanced, conditions are set for infection, illness, and chronic diseases such as cancer, explains Thomas Rau, M.D., medical director of Parcelsus Clinic in Switzerland.

"As we see it," says Dr. Rau, "sickness is not *caused* by bacteria, but the bacteria comes *with* the sickness. Bacteria, viruses, or fungi can only develop if they have the suitable cellular conditions." Outside influences, such as faulty diet, inadequate nutrition, exposure to carcinogens, chronic organ toxicity, stress, or trauma provide the impetus to throw the cells out of balance, says Dr. Rau. Once imbalanced, disease processes can take root, potentially leading to cancer.

Oncogenes

The predominant emphasis in conventional cancer research today is to find individual genes capable of causing, initiating, or triggering cancer growth. First identified in the 1970s, these causal genes are referred to as oncogenes (meaning the gene that starts the *onkos*, or tumor mass; SEE QUICK DEFINITION). Oncogenes are believed to

To prevent cancer, the liver's detoxification system must be working optimally, says Joseph Pizzorno, N.D. When the liver is not functioning well, it is unable to process and eliminate the multiplicity of carcinogens entering the body.

transform normal cells into cancer cells. Researchers now believe that about 20% of all human cancers are partly brought about by oncogene mutations.

In healthy people, the activities of oncogenes are counterbalanced by tumor suppressor genes, also called anti-oncogenes. Under normal conditions, these genes act to prevent uncontrolled cell growth that could lead to tumors. However, oncogene mutations (technically, when the inactive, neutral proto-oncogene becomes a fully active, carcinogenic oncogene) inactivate the tumor suppressor genes so that, paradoxically, they actually contribute to tumor growth. Additional factors that can inactivate tumor suppressor genes include other DNA changes, chemical carcinogens, and electromagnetic energy.

Genetic Predisposition

The theory of gene causation for cancer inevitably leads researchers into speculations about inherited cancers—genetic configurations or mutations that might predict, if not guarantee, that a given individual will develop a particular form of cancer. The term "family cancer syndrome" is now used to describe the tendency of particular cancers (such as breast, colon, or ovarian) to show up in succeeding generations of the same family.

For example, many scientists now believe that the following inherited cancers may be linked to mutations in certain related tumor suppressor genes: melanoma and pancreatic cancer (MTS1, p16); breast and ovarian cancer (BRCA1); breast cancer (BRCA2); colon and uterine cancer (MSH2, MLH1, PMS1, PMS2); and brain sarcomas (p53). Inheritance of "flawed" genes probably accounts for about 5% of all cancers in the U.S.[36]

Miasm

More than 200 years ago, German physician Samuel Hahnemann, the founder of homeopathy, used the term "miasm" to indicate a particular predisposition to chronic disease. Just as cellular terrain underlies or precedes the appearance of actual cancer tumors, so do Hahnemann's miasms precede activities of the oncogenes. In other words, Hahnemann's concept of miasms accurately prefigures today's description of oncogenes. A miasm represents an *energy residue* of an illness from a previous generation, while an oncogene (inherited genetic mutation) represents a *molecular residue* of an illness from a previous generation.

According to Hahnemann, three miasms underlie all chronic illness, and these parallel broad stages in the history of the human experience with primary disease states. The *Psoric* miasm is the earliest and thus the most fundamental layer. In fact, according to this theory, the *Psoric* miasm is the foundation of sickness underlying all the diseases experienced by humans—cancer, diabetes, and arthritis as well as serious mental disorders such as epilepsy and schizophrenia. The *Syphilitic* miasm came next in the history of human diseases and derives from syphilis. The *Sycotic* miasm, the third layer, arose as a residue of gonorrhea. In recent years, homeopaths have added a *Cancer* miasm to Hahnemann's original three; the *Cancer* miasm is a combination of the effects (or taints) of the *Psoric*, *Syphilitic*, and *Sycotic* miasms.

Detecting Breast Cancer

An understanding of the causal factors of cancer makes it evident that many details of daily life—from the food you eat to the water you drink—can create an internal climate optimal for the development of breast cancer. Catching the cancer process in its earliest stages increases the likelihood that it can be halted and reversed.

In this section, we discuss breast cancer screening methods. Breast self-examination is the simplest and, if practiced consistently, can result in detection of abnormal lumps. Mammography (breast X ray) is conventional medicine's standard screening method for already-formed cancerous masses. Unfortunately, it is entirely inadequate and, since it relies on radiation, can actually contribute to cancer. However, two relatively new tests—thermography and AMAS—provide a superior option. In addition to being safer, more accurate, less invasive, and less expensive than mammograms, these tests can detect cancer far earlier than their conventional counterpart.

Breast Self-Examination

Given the rising incidence of breast cancer and the fact that early

Delayed Childbearing Increases Breast Cancer Risk

A study tracking over 16,000 women has identified a mother's age at the birth of her first child as a factor in evaluating breast cancer risk. For every year a woman waits to have a child, researchers noted a 3.5% increase in breast cancer risk. In addition, age at each birth after the first could be an independent risk factor; every year that passes between the first birth and all subsequent births was associated with a 0.9% increase in risk.

Women who have their first child at an early age may actually enjoy some degree of protection from breast cancer. According to the study, a woman may reduce her risk of breast cancer if she gives birth before age 35. By contrast, women who wait until after age 35 to carry a pregnancy to term increase their cancer risk.[37]

detection is one of the primary strategies for successful treatment, it is imperative that women conduct monthly breast self-examinations. One study found that self-examination was responsible for a greater percentage of cancer discoveries than mammograms. A 1996 survey of 281 women by Breast Cancer Action in San Francisco, California, revealed that of the 226 women (of whom 70% were 40-59 years old) who had breast cancer, 44% discovered this through breast self-examination, 37% through mammograms, and 8% through a physician's exam.

A breast self-examination must be done each month at the same time in your menstrual cycle, in the same physical positions, and using the same sequence of steps. Some lumps are easier to find when lying down, and others are more apparent when sitting or standing, so it is advisable to do an examination in several positions. Using the flat part of the fingertips, feel each area of the breast, systematically moving around it (following one or both of the patterns in the illustration on p. 85). Note any changes; some women draw a sketch each time to record what they feel. Becoming familiar with the composition of your breasts is central to effective breast examination because it makes detection of abnormalities easier.

What's Wrong With Mammography?

Although mammography is the most widely employed screening method for breast cancer, there are a number of compelling arguments for adopting other methods in its place. Current research within conventional medicine itself provides five strong reasons why the use of mammogram screening for detection of breast cancer ought to be reconsidered. They are: increased cancer risk, high rate of false

HOW TO PERFORM A BREAST SELF-EXAM. This exam should be conducted once a month (for pre-menopausal women, just after your period). Start by standing in front of a mirror and looking carefully at each breast and the chest muscle area above it. (1) Look for anything out of the ordinary, such as puckering, dimpling, or scaling skin, nipple discharge or retraction, lumps, or asymmetry of breasts. (2) Raise your arms or clasp them behind your head and check for the same in this position. (3) Do the same check with your hands on your waist, pulling your shoulders and elbows slightly forward. (4) Feel for lumps in the lymph node area, from your breast into your armpit. (5) Squeeze each nipple to check for discharge. (6) Some women prefer to do this stage of the breast exam standing up, perhaps in the shower using soapy water so the fingers will glide more easily. In either case, with your right arm behind your head, examine your right breast with the fingers of your left hand. Using the pads of three or four fingers to press firmly into the breast, feel for lumps and cover the entire breast by following the patterns shown here. Some women prefer the radiating pattern (6a), thoroughly examining the breast by moving outward from the nipple in straight lines. Others prefer the circular pattern (6b), starting from the nipple and moving outward around the breast or vice versa. Repeat on the left breast. If you notice anything abnormal or something you're not sure about at any point in the exam, consult your physician.

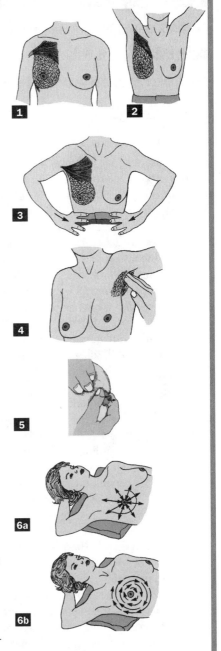

Mammography (breast X ray) is conventional medicine's standard screening method for already-formed cancerous masses. Unfortunately, it is entirely inadequate and, since it relies on radiation, can actually contribute to cancer.

positives, high rate of false negatives, distortion caused by estrogen, and high cost.

Mammograms Add to Cancer Risk—Perhaps most damning, mammography exposes the breast to damaging radiation. As noted previously, Dr. Gofman spent 30 years studying the effects of low-dose radiation on humans. Dr. Gofman's findings are worth repeating: He estimates that 75% of breast cancer could be prevented by *avoiding* or *minimizing* exposure to the ionizing radiation from mammography, X rays, and other medical sources.

Other research has shown that, since mammographic screening was introduced in 1983, the incidence of a form of breast cancer called ductal carcinoma *in situ* (DCIS), which represents 12% of all breast cancer cases, has increased by 328%, and 200% of this increase is due to the use of mammography. For women under 50, the increase in DCIS diagnoses rose 4000% during this same period.[38]

For more about **radiation and Dr. Gofman's findings,** see this chapter, p. 66, and "75% of Breast Cancer Caused by Radiation, p. 65. For more about **fibrocystic breast disease,** see Chapter 1: Fibrocystic Breast Disease.

In addition to exposing a woman to harmful radiation, the mammography procedure may help spread an existing mass of cancer cells.[39] During a mammogram, considerable pressure must be placed on the woman's breast, as the breast is squeezed between two flat plastic surfaces. According to Lorraine Day, M.D., a pathologist and former breast cancer patient, this compression could cause existing cancer cells to move (metastasize) from the breast tissue. Even if cancer is not present in the breast, mammogram screening is uncomfortable and even painful.

High Rate of False Positives—Mammography's high rate of false-positive test results wastes money and creates unnecessary emotional trauma. A Swedish study of 60,000 women, 40-64 years old, who were screened for breast cancer, revealed that of the 726 actually referred to oncologists for treatment, 70% were found to be cancer free.[40]

According to the British medical journal *The Lancet*, of the 5% of mammograms that suggest further testing, up to 93% are false positives. *The Lancet* report further noted that because the great majority of positive screenings are false positives, these inaccurate results lead to many unnecessary biopsies and other invasive surgical procedures.[41] In fact, 70% to 80% of all positive mammograms do not, on biopsy, show any presence of cancer.[42] According to some estimates, 90% of these "callbacks" result from unclear readings due to dense, overlying breast tissue.[43]

Similarly, fibrocystic breast tissue can be mistaken for tumors and lead to unnecessary biopsies. Perhaps 25% to 30% of women have fibrocystic lumps in their breasts; conventional doctors, worrying about malpractice suits for failing to diagnose cancer, can construe every fibrocystic lump as cancerous and order a rash of biopsies. The biopsy itself is injurious to healthy breast tissue. Breast augmentation (silicone or saline implants) also obscures a fair amount of otherwise imageable breast tissue. In addition, the mammography procedure itself can potentially damage the implants, producing leakage.

High Rate of False Negatives—Mammography also produces a high rate of false-negative test results. While false positives cause unnecessary distress and intervention, false negatives can be fatal. The breast tissue of women under 40 years old is generally denser than in older women, making it more difficult to detect tumors via mammography. In addition, tumors grow more quickly in women in this age group, so they may develop between screenings.[44]

As for women between the ages of 40 and 49, even the National Cancer Institute notes that there is a high rate of "missed tumors" in this age category; that is, 40% false-negative test results. Despite these findings, the American Cancer Society still recommends a mammogram every two years for women aged 40 to 49.[45]

Estrogen Distorts Breast X Rays—Estrogen therapy confuses mammogram results. According to a study of 8,800 postmenopausal women, aged 50 and older, the use of estrogen replacement therapy (ERT) leads to a 71% increased likelihood of receiving a false-positive result on mammogram screening, according to Mary B. Laya, M.D., M.P.H., study leader at the University of Washington at Seattle, who published the results in the *Journal of the National Cancer Institute* in 1996. Dr. Laya also found that women on ERT were more likely to get false-readings. It should be noted that women over 50 are the primary target of conventional medicine's recommendation of yearly mammography screening.

Mammograms are costly and can directly endanger a woman's health. Faulty test results further endanger her health, exact a heavy emotional toll, and can lead to expensive and unnecessary tests.

High Cost—In addition to the expenses accrued as a consequence of faulty mammogram results, mammograms themselves are costly (from $50-$120). Given their lack of accuracy, this level of expenditure is a doubtful investment.[46]

In summary, mammograms are costly and can directly endanger a woman's health. Faulty test results further endanger her health, exact a heavy emotional toll, and can lead to expensive and unnecesssary tests. A study reported in *The Lancet* (July 1995) concludes that breast cancer screening via mammography for women under 50 years old is inappropriate due to the low accuracy level.

According to the *Lancet* study, of the 5% of mammograms that suggest further testing, up to 93% are false-positives, meaning that follow-up biopsies do not indicate cancer. The study further states that, in general, "The benefit is marginal, the harm caused is substantial, and the costs incurred are enormous, [so] we suggest that public funding for breast cancer screening [mammography] in any age group is not justifiable."[47]

Thermography: Safe and Accurate Imaging

A nontoxic, highly accurate, and inexpensive form of diagnostic imaging does exist and has been used by progressive physicians in the U.S. and Europe since 1962. Called thermography, it's based on infrared heat emissions from targeted regions of the body. As the body's cells go through their energy conversion processes, called metabolism, they emit heat. Thermography is able to register these heat emssions, display them on a computer monitor, and thereby provide a diagnostic window into the functional physiologic status of a given body area, such as the female breast.

For breast cancer, thermography offers a *very early* warning system, often able to pinpoint a cancer process five years before it would be detectable by mammography. Most breast tumors have been growing slowly for up to 20 years before they are found by typical diagnostic techniques. Thermography can detect cancers when they are at a *minute* physical stage of development, when it is still relatively easy to halt and reverse the progression of the cancer.

THERMOGRAPHIC BREAST IMAGES.

1) **TH2 Category.** This patient demonstrates benign (non-cancerous) fibrocystic disease. The light grey bands represent blood vessels, while the darker areas suggest the presence of benign growths. Because cancer cells are energy inefficient, giving off more heat than healthy cells, the darker shading of these growths indicates that cancer is probably not the cause. It is common for women to develop growths or abnormalities in the breast, but most do not result in cancer.

2) **TH3 Category.** Warning signs: the light bands (blood vessels) form an irregular, complicated pattern throughout the breast, widening and narrowing erratically. This pattern may suggest metabolic processes which are "out of control," a key characteristic of cancer cells. After a few months, this patient will return for a follow-up evaluation of this possibly cancerous situation.

3) **TH5 Category.** The cancer can be identified by the light area in the top portion of the right breast. Warning signs: the "hot" spot is concentrated in one place, indicating a localized growth; the difference in shading occurs in only one breast, suggesting that this is not a routine abnormality.

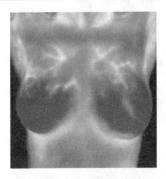

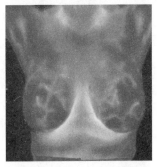

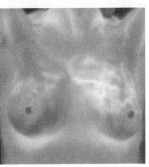

More Breast-Friendly Than Mammography—Philip Hoekstra, Ph.D., of Thermoscan, in Huntingdon Woods, Michigan, is a pioneer in the use of thermography. Dr. Hoekstra's clinic has screened more than 50,000 women since 1971, at a typical cost of $55 for imaging and interpretation. The average mammogram, in contrast, can cost between $50 and $120. While a price differential of about $50 may

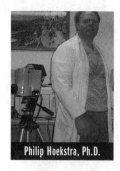

Philip Hoekstra, Ph.D.

While mammography tends to lose effectiveness with dense breast tissue, thermography is not dependent upon varied tissue densities. For this reason, Dr. Hoekstra says thermography is especially useful for screening younger women (who typically have denser breast tissue).

seem insignificant when compared with the escalating costs of health care in this country, the risks associated with low-dose radiation exposure from mammograms (discussed in detail above) *in addition* to their extra cost makes thermography the obvious choice for breast cancer screening.

The procedure is simple and noninvasive, says Dr. Hoekstra. The woman stands bare chested about ten feet from the device; the imaging takes only a matter of minutes, as results are displayed instantaneously on the monitor; and generally the data can be rapidly interpreted with the assistance of sophisticated image analyzing software. No rays of any kind enter the patient's body; there is no pain or compressing of the breasts as in a mammogram. Thermography is thus a breast-friendly procedure, and its widespread use could save many women from the development of breast cancer and/or highly traumatic surgery and radiation treatments later.

Dr. Hoekstra points to the errors, false negatives, and radiation exposure dangers of mammograms, as discussed above. "Mammography is not an acceptable way of screening breasts, but it's tolerated perhaps because it is a major source of steady income for radiologists," Dr. Hoekstra says. "They have come to covet mammography and want no competition from other approaches." He believes that once women start making demands on their physicians for a *different* imaging approach, thermography can become the preferred initial screening method. Then mammography will be used only as needed to pinpoint the precise location of breast tumors.

While mammography tends to lose effectiveness with dense breast tissue, thermography is not dependent upon varied tissue densities. For this reason, Dr. Hoekstra says thermography is especially useful for screening younger women (who typically have denser breast tissue). Dr. Hoekstra adds that thermography is 86% to 96% accurate for indicating cancer in premenopausal women. When there is a mistake with thermography, it is almost never a false negative, but rather a false positive. That means the trained thermography technician's interpretation of the thermography imaging led the technician to suspect a cancer process when in fact there was none.

Breasts That Glow in Infrared—From the viewpoint of thermography, the body is like a walking beacon—we glow in infrared. The glow is based on heat emissions from our tissues as they convert (metabolize) food into energy and as the energy is picked up by the blood circulation. Our circulatory system acts as a giant radiator to distribute and equalize body heat derived from metabolism. The thermographic image shows us areas of diminished energy flow.

During a typical thermography session, the subject stands in front of the heat-sensitive thermography camera while the operator takes a set of computerized pictures of the body's internal heat patterns. The subject then places both hands in cold water as a "challenge" to the nervous system. This sudden exposure to cold causes healthy blood vessels to constrict as an adaptive response intended to cool the skin. Blood vessels associated with cancerous growths, however, lack a smooth muscle layer and therefore cannot constrict. When a second set of pictures is taken, any cancerous area of the breast will scan as higher in temperature than the surrounding tissue, due to the relatively greater amount of blood flow (hypervascularity) in the area.

In addition to hypervascularity of blood vessels, cancerous growths tend to give off more infrared energy. That's because cancer itself is by definition an uncontrolled growth; it can't use its energy as efficiently as other cells in the body. This lack of energy efficiency in a cancerous growth, added to the inflammation of surrounding tissues—a result of the body's natural immune reaction against a cancerous mass—helps to emphasize the difference in infrared energy between cancer cells and healthy cells and thereby to accurately pinpoint the tumor process. The inflammation itself, produced by breast tissue injury from the tumor, gives off excess heat.

The thermography diagnosis is then based on a comparison of the "pre-challenge" and "post-challenge" pictures, taken before and after the cold water treatment. The thermography technicians normally expect to see body temperature go down by about 0.25° C after the challenge to the system. If it stays essentially the same or actually goes up—this means there is no cold water–induced constriction—then the alarm bells go off and the technician starts suspecting cancer. Often with cancerous tissue, the blood flow increases as a result of the cold water challenge and the blood vessels in that area register thermo-

According to Dr. Hoekstra's estimates, and those of independent clinical studies, thermography screening has an accuracy rate of between 86% and 96%, compared to the 40% to 60% accuracy rate of traditional mammography.

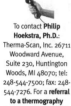

To contact **Philip Hoekstra, Ph.D.**: Therma-Scan, Inc. 26711 Woodward Avenue, Suite 230, Huntington Woods, MI 48070; tel: 248-544-7500; fax: 248-544-7276. For a **referral to a thermography technician** in your area, contact: American Association of Thermology, 2740 Chain Bridge Road, Vienna, VA 22181; tel: 703-938-6140; fax: 703-938-1482.

graphically as emitting more energy and a lighter image.

Through thermography, the technicians can tell if a blood vessel is unusually large, has a complex structure, or has a high degree of blood flow. If the energy flow pattern (vascularity) in one breast is higher than in the other breast (usually by at least 1.5° C), this is a warning sign. Typically, five irregularities are screened as indicators of a cancer process, but generally if even two of these are present, then there is about a 96% certainty of cancer, says Dr. Hoekstra.

Depending on the results of the thermography test, subjects are classified into the following categories, according to the system of interpretation developed at the Pasteur Institute in Paris, France, in 1976. Specifically these categories are: TH1, there are no abnormal features; TH2, some unusual metabolic activity is present, but probably due to causes such as hormonal imbalance; TH3, abnormalities are present in metabolic function, but the results are inconclusive; TH4, abnormalities are found which are possibly cancerous, but it's too soon to diagnose with certainty (approximately 38% of TH4 patients develop cancer within five years); and TH5, metabolic abnormalities suggest a very high probability (about 96%) of cancer. Usually thermography technicans request that TH3 patients return for a follow-up within 90 to 120 days.

According to Dr. Hoekstra's estimates, and those of independent clinical studies, thermography screening has an accuracy rate of between 86% and 96%, compared to the 40% to 60% accuracy rate of traditional mammography. At present, there are perhaps 1,000 thermography devices in the U.S. for providing this detailed, clinically valuable information.

AMAS: 95% Accurate Cancer Screening

Until recently, there was no single blood test that could reliably and accurately indicate whether cancer was present, either in an initial diagnosis or when monitoring a recurrence. Many oncologists and cancer specialists use blood tests called cancer markers which detect substances present in abnormal amounts in the blood of a person with cancer.

But cancer markers can be unreliable for a variety of reasons. Some fail to indicate the presence of the new, previously undetected cancers and show only whether known cancers are shrinking or expanding. Others register levels of substances that could be produced by diseases other than cancer. Still others are not sensitive enough to pick up cancers in a certain percentage of patients.

However, thanks to the efforts of Harvard-trained biochemist and physician Sam Bogoch, M.D., Ph.D., we now have a reliable blood test for cancer. Dr. Bogoch labored for 20 years before finally uncovering the secret to detecting all forms of cancer in its earliest stages. The test he developed, called AMAS (anti-malignin antibody screen), analyzes a sample of blood to reveal whether antibodies to cancer are present.

The test is called an immunoassay, which means it measures the amount present of a specific antibody (SEE QUICK DEFINITION), in this case, anti-malignin. This is an antibody that acts against the inner protein layer of a cancer cell, called malignin. According to Dr. Bogoch, AMAS is 95% accurate on the first test, and 99% when repeated; the test can detect cancer up to 19 months before conventional medical tests can find it. "If there are any cancers that don't respond to the [AMAS] test, we haven't found them yet," says Dr. Bogoch.

Although it was approved by the FDA in 1977, it was not until late 1994 that the clinical trials with 4,278 patients were completed, validating the test's effectiveness. Now the patented, FDA-approved AMAS is available to doctors worldwide through Dr. Bogoch's Oncolab.

AMAS screens for the earliest signs of all types of cancer and, unlike mammography which does not distinguish between benign and malignant growth, AMAS detects malignant growth only. If the AMAS is positive, a mammogram or ultrasound may be performed to ascertain the location of the tumor for surgical purposes and a needle biopsy may be recommended. If two consecutive AMAS tests are negative, however, then a mammogram is unwarranted.

AMAS can also monitor the results of any treatment or assess the degree of remission. This means it can objective-

QUICK DEFINITION

An **antibody** is a protein molecule containing about 20,000 atoms, made from amino acids by B lymphocyte cells in the lymph tissue and set in motion by the immune system against a specific foreign protein, or antigen. An antibody is also referred to as an immunoglobulin and may be found in the blood, lymph, colostrum, saliva, and the gastrointestinal and urinary tracts, usually within three days after the first encounter with an antigen. The antibody binds tightly with the antigen as a preliminary for removing it from the system or destroying it.

For more information on **AMAS**, contact: Oncolab, 36 The Fenway, Boston, MA 02215; tel: 800-922-8378; fax: 617-536-0657. The test costs $135 (follow-up, $85) and can be ordered by any physician who is licensed to order clinical laboratory tests.

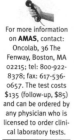

For more on **AMAS** and breast cancer, see *Alternative Medicine Definitive Guide to Cancer* (Future Medicine Publishing, 1997; ISBN 1-887299-01-7); to order, call 800-333-HEAL.

ly measure the effect of alternative cancer treatments in removing cancer from the body. It also means lives can be saved because approximately 35% of people who die from cancer could be saved with an earlier diagnosis followed by prompt treatment.

When the last malignant cancer cells are destroyed in the body, the anti-malignin antibody levels return to normal, providing evidence that the cancer has been reversed. A study by Bogoch involving 1,175 breast cancer patients proved that clinical remission, whether after one or 30 months, is directly correlated with normal AMAS levels. In addition, the test has been extensively evaluated with respect to early detection of breast cancer.[48]

With AMAS, mammography is no longer needed as a primary screening tool. Even for women older than 49 (the age group in which mammography claims its best results), monthly breast self-examinations and an annual AMAS can do far more in detecting breast cancer than mammography. AMAS will spare many women unnecessary grief and, along with thermography, will hopefully soon replace mammography as the standard screening test.

More Alternative Medicine Therapies for Breast Cancer

By now in this chapter, you know that if you do discover you have breast cancer, you have many more options than the terrifying ones offered by conventional medicine. In addition to the therapies covered in the earlier case histories, there are a range of other alternative medicine modalities that have been successfully used in the treatment of breast cancer. These include homeopathy, traditional Chinese medicine, orthomolecular medicine, detoxification therapy, and several little-known, but highly effective oral supplements.

Homeopathy and Traditional Chinese Medicine

Homeopathic physician and co-author of *Alternative Medicine Definitive Guide to Cancer*, W. John Diamond, M.D., of Reno, Nevada, uses a combination of homeopathy (SEE QUICK DEFINITION) and traditional Chinese medicine (SEE QUICK DEFINITION) to treat breast cancer. With these methods, he is able to address what he views as the four components of disease. According to Dr. Diamond, a positive treatment outcome is unlikely unless these components are attended to in the treatment plan.

Here, **Dr. Diamond** explains the four components and offers a case history to illustrate the effectiveness of homeopathy and traditional Chinese medicine in treating breast cancer:

Treating the Four Components of Cancer

I do not treat cancer so much as I treat patients who have cancer as a prime physical manifestation. This is the essential distinction between an orthodox approach to cancer treatment, which seeks to destroy the tumor, and the approach of the alternative physician, who treats the patient and enables the patient's system to destroy the tumor. To accomplish this task, I try to empower the patient at all levels of being, knowing that one's state of health is the ability of the body/mind to balance out the stresses that confront one every day.

If the stresses and our body's response are evenly balanced, then we are in a state of homeostasis or good health. If the stresses are too strong or our response is too weak, then we are in an imbalance which can lead to illness and disease. The disease can be subclinical and hidden at first, not showing any symptoms, but if it continues, it will eventually manifest as physical symptoms. It may start with a disorder of the body's biochemistry, then the cells, organs, and finally the whole body begins to self-destruct and produce a cancer.

From this simple explanation of our biology we can show that every disease, including cancer, has four major components to it: emotional/mental, biochemical, structural, and energetic.

Emotional/Mental–Emotional/mental factors are the most important and the least addressed by conventional medicine. As children, sometimes even as babies or in the womb, we are wounded by circumstances (parental attitudes, relationships with siblings, and the overall family environment).

To survive, we produce a response—many call it a wall—to maintain emotional and biological balance and

QUICK DEFINITION

Homeopathy was founded in the early 1800s by German physician Samuel Hahnemann. Today, an estimated 500 million people worldwide receive homeopathic treatment; in Britain, homeopathy enjoys royal patronage. Homeopathy is now practiced according to two differing concepts. In classical homeopathy, only one single-component remedy is prescribed at a time, in a potency specifically adjusted to the patient; the physician waits to see the results before prescribing anything further. In complex homeopathy, typified by *Hepar compositum*, a prescription involves multiple substances given at the same time, usually in low potencies.

Traditional Chinese medicine (TCM) originated in China over 5,000 years ago and is a comprehensive system of medical practice that heals the body according to the principles of nature and balance. A Chinese medicine physician considers the flow of vital energy (*qi*) in a patient through close examination of the patient's pulse, tongue, body odor, voice tone and strength, and general demeanor, among other elements. Underlying imbalances and disharmony in the body are described in terminology analogous to the natural world (heat, cold, dryness, or dampness). The concept of balance, or the interrelationship of organs, is central to TCM. In TCM, imbalances are corrected through the use of acupuncture, moxibustion, herbal medicine, dietary therapy, massage, and therapeutic exercise.

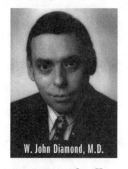

W. John Diamond, M.D.

"I do not treat cancer so much as I treat patients who have cancer as a prime physical manifestation. I try to empower the patient at all levels of being, knowing that one's state of health is the ability of the body/mind to balance out the stresses that confront one every day," says Dr. Diamond.

To contact **W. John Diamond, M.D.**: Triad Medical Center, 4600 Kietzke Lane, M-242, Reno, NV 89502; tel: 702-829-2277; fax: 702-829-2365.

W. John Diamond, M.D., is co-author of *Alternative Medicine Definitive Guide to Cancer* (Future Medicine Publishing, 1997, ISBN 1-887299-01-7); to order, call 800-333-HEAL.

protect ourselves. For example, if you were always told by your father that you were no good and would never amount to much, your response could either be to become passive, believing the lie and fulfilling the dire prophecy, or you could become active, an overachiever, always trying to prove your father wrong.

Either way, you will have trouble later in life as you continue responding to this old imprint—producing a mask of behavior behind which you hide your potential and destiny. In the case of the passive responder, repressed emotions, if not vented or expressed, will seek physical expression, such as functional bowel disease, fibromyalgia, or even cancer. In the case of the over-responder, the tendency is to burn out because they never get the approval they seek no matter how well they perform. Heart attack and ulcer are the typical physical expressions. Against either scenario, the physician's role is to help patients become aware of the issues and patterns and aid them in changing these patterns to produce emotional balance.

The emotional balance that we seek may be accelerated and simplified by counseling, hypnosis, classical homeopathy, or time and experience. Homeopathy can energetically change the emotional patterns adopted in childhood which have contributed most to the eventual manifestation of cancer. If we change these patterns early enough in the course of cancer, there is a real chance of reversing this process. Homeopathy can also be used to help clear the emotions of fear, hopelessness, and depression that can accompany the diagnosis of cancer.

Once emotional balance is obtained, the organism no longer needs to manifest symptoms in a physical way to reach balance, and the person may then go on to evolve still further. The essence of existence, one might suggest from a homeopathic viewpoint, is to evolve beyond childhood trauma and our primitive protective responses to an understanding, acceptance, and, finally, resolution of the tensions imposed by early emotions and feelings.

After all, if everything in life were the same or if it were perfect, there would be nothing to struggle against and no improvement would be possible. Illness also can be seen from this philosophical viewpoint. It is the struggle to balance the opposites that leads to our advancement—these are natural laws.

Biochemical—The biochemical component can be detected by sophisticated analyses of metabolic and energy pathways, as well as hormonal, heavy metal, cellular terrain, detoxification, and vitamin/mineral status. This information enables the physician to best advise the patient regarding appropriate nutritional supplementation, therapeutic dietary changes, and/or hormonal and glandular support. Detoxification of organs and the lymphatic and gastrointestinal systems can be accomplished through diet, supplements, and homeopathy.

Structural—The structural component relates to the musculoskeletal system of the body, as disease often has a muscular or pain factor. Consider the tension headache or migraine which are expressed as a spasm of the trapezius and temporalis muscles connecting the neck and head. We treat the myofascial (muscles and the fascia or fibers enclosing the muscles) and skeletal systems with acupuncture, chiropractic, osteopathy, craniosacral therapy, trigger point therapy (also known as myotherapy), and neural therapy, among others.

Energetic—The energetic component is usually the most difficult to understand—on the part of doctors and patients alike. It relates to the electrical and electromagnetic energy that flows through the body in the various energy pathways, known to acupuncturists as "meridians." Disturbances of these electrical energy channels cause internal organ dysfunction and decrease the overall function of our immune system.

We treat and balance this system with acupuncture, Chinese herbs, and homeopathy. The acupuncturist "reads" the patient's pulse at the wrist—up to 28 different energy qualities can be read—and thereby determines which energy pathways are out of balance. Based on this information, the acupuncturist places acupuncture needles at selected points on the body to correct the energy conditions.

Acupuncture can be used both as a preventive measure as well as a curative art. Done regularly, it can keep the immune system and all organs operating at maximum efficiency.

Acupuncture can be used both as a preventive measure as well as a curative art. Done regularly, it can keep the immune system and all organs operating at maximum efficiency. Chinese herbs have been shown to affect the energy meridians much like acupuncture and are often used to augment the activity of acupuncture and to prolong its effects.

In addition to the applications of homeopathy and traditional Chinese medicine as discussed in the context of the four components involved in cancer, acupuncture can also be used to improve energy levels and strengthen the immune system, to create a sense of well-being, and to symptomatically treat the side effects of radiation and chemotherapy and cancer-associated pain.

Homeopathy is also helpful to decrease the nausea and side effects of chemotherapy and radiation. Chinese herbs can be used as antivirals and energy and immune boosters, as well as support for stressed organs during chemotherapy and radiation. These herbs are especially useful in aiding the bone marrow to produce new immune cells. Chinese ointments are used to lessen the skin burns and pain caused by radiation therapy.

The following case of Andrea demonstrates the multiple causal nature of cancer and how homeopathy, acupuncture, and Chinese herbs can work together in its treatment.

Success Story: Reversing Metastasized Breast Cancer

Andrea, 58, came to me for treatment of what had been diagnosed as intraductal carcinoma of the left breast. She had undergone a radical mastectomy, which revealed cancer in three lymph nodes, and had completed eight courses of chemotherapy (involving the drugs Cytoxan, 5-FU, and methotrexate). After this, Andrea was disease free for six years; testing then showed metastases to her bones and liver.

Andrea was treated with tamoxifen (an estrogen-blocking drug found to be of some benefit in treating breast cancer) for eight weeks, but it produced no positive effect and it increased the size of the liver metastases; her oncologist next started her on a different chemotherapy formula. At this point, she came to me. Andrea wanted to take control of her disease and use support measures to help her with the nausea and lethargy from the chemotherapy.

During my initial interview with Andrea, she told me she had been exposed to diazinon and other pesticides as a child. As far as her dental history went, Andrea had had a root canal filling removed from a tooth, and she had received extensive dental care (such as crowns and treatment for gingivitis). She had experienced dizziness and facial pain (neuralgia) and earache on the left side of her head just prior to the cancer recurrence.

Electrodermal screening (see p. 100) revealed inflammations of the lymph channels, teeth, nerve points, and several acupuncture meridians that passed through her feet, including Liver, Stomach, Gallbladder, and Kidney. Electrodermal screening of nosodes (SEE QUICK DEFINITION) showed resonance with tooth infection, pesticides, and Coxsackie virus.

The positive resonance of tooth infection, pesticides, and Coxsackie virus indicates that these factors are disturbing the energy balance of the organism. Specifically, they are producing the abnormal readings of acupuncture meridians or energy lines in Andrea's body. For these conditions, application of homeopathic nosodes will correct the energetic imbalance and restore the immune system to a more efficient and functioning entity. If left untreated, however, these imbalances could hinder Andrea's ability to fight the cancer.

I gave Andrea liver and lymphatic detoxification formulas in the form of Hepeel drops for the liver and Lymphomyosot drops for the lymphatic detoxification. Both were given for two weeks in the dose of ten drops taken three times daily, sublingually (under the tongue) for faster absorption. I gave Andrea these two remedies together with homeopathic nosodes to clear the energy taints of the tooth infection and residual pesticides. Andrea also took homeopathic *Carcinocin* 200C twice weekly for four weeks; this is a homeopathic preparation made from cancerous tissue cells that is effective in removing the energy preconditions underlying cancer.

Next I gave Andrea a single dose one month later of *Causticum* 200C. This is a homeopathic "polycrest," which means a remedy with widespread biological effects. It was originally formulated by Samuel Hahnemann, the 19th-century German founder of homeopathy, as a solution of slaked lime and potassium sulfate.

Among other symptoms, Andrea's left-sided facial neuralgia was an indicator of the appropriateness of this reme-

A homeopathic **nosode** is a super-diluted remedy made as an energy imprint from a disease product, such as bacteria, tuberculosis, measles, bowel infection, influenza, and about 200 other substances. The nosode, which contains no physical trace of the disease, stimulates the body to remove all "taints" or residues it holds of a particular disease, whether it was inherited or contracted. Only qualified homeopaths may administer a nosode.

For more about **tamoxifen**, see "Breast Cancer 'Treatment' Can Cause Cancer in Other Organs," p. 71. For more about **dental factors in cancer**, see p. 74.

Electrodermal Screening

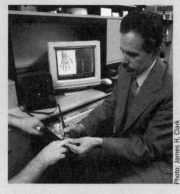

Electrodermal screening is a form of computerized information gathering which is based on physics, not chemistry. A blunt, noninvasive electric probe is placed at specific points on the patient's hands, face, or feet, corresponding to acupuncture points at the beginning or end of energy meridians. Minute electrical discharges from these points serve as information signals about the condition of the body's organs and systems, useful for the physician in evaluation and developing a treatment plan.

dy. Andrea also received three acupuncture treatments for muscle spasm related to her liver imbalance and for chronic nausea. She elected to use her own Western herbs including echinacea (an immune booster), silymarin (for liver support), and pycnogenol (an antioxidant from Maritime pine bark) which she obtained over the counter from a health food store.

During the course of treatment, Andrea had an episode of Coxsackie myalgia (involving pain in the voluntary muscles of the chest wall) for which I prescribed the nosode and a homeopathic antiviral. Specifically, I treated her with injectable Engystol, a good general homeopathic viral infection remedy, along with the nosode for Coxsackie virus. Around the same time, I treated Andrea's sinusitis with Chinese herbs, relying on a classical Chinese combination called Purearia "N" Formula; this included ephedra, ligusticum, glycyrrhiza, and magnolia. A year after her last course of chemotherapy, Andrea was re-evaluated by her oncologist; no evidence of liver or bone metastases was found and she remains disease free. ∎

Success Story: Orthomolecular Medicine Reverses a "Terminal" Sentence

When Martha learned she had a large tumor and two smaller tumors in her left breast, she refused surgery and chemotherapy. The tumors continued to grow. She tried a variety of dietary treatments, including the raw foods diet (the Living Diet) designed by Ann Wigmore, Ph.D., N.D., of Boston, Massachusetts. For three months she felt well, but her tumors showed no sign of reversal. Five months later, when Martha consulted Abram Hoffer, M.D., Ph.D., of Victoria, British Columbia, Canada, a pioneer of orthomolecular medicine (SEE QUICK DEFINITION), she was extremely ill and emaciated, weighing only 85 pounds.

Conventional physicians considered Martha to be a "terminal" case and expected her to die within two weeks. "One doctor refused to give her another appointment in a week, telling her she would be dead before then," says Dr. Hoffer. "I could see how he could arrive at this decision, but I could not comprehend his unwillingness to provide her any support." Under Dr. Hoffer's guidance, Martha began taking vitamin C (4 g, sodium ascorbate) three times a day. One month later, she consulted a naturopath, who recommended organ extracts and vitamins in small doses, as well as large doses of vitamin A (1 million IU per day), and Martha took these as well.

After three months on this program, Martha began to gain weight. However, more metastases were found and she was told her prognosis was still very bleak. She might live six months at best. In an attempt to slow the still progressing cancer, Martha received an experimental preparation of intravenous collagen (a connective tissue that helps hold bone together) for two weeks, after which she took it orally. Only one month later, having gained a few pounds, Martha felt upbeat and more energetic. For the next few months, she received vitamin C in both the oral and intravenous forms. Nevertheless, the cancer ulcerated, meaning it rose and broke out on the skin of her breasts.

Several months later, and a little under one year since being diagnosed, Martha's hair fell out and her liver became enlarged. She was still on high doses of vitamin A. Fluid had entered her lungs and abdomen, and she was declared anemic. Dr. Hoffer immediately had her discontinue the vitamin A and within a month her hair began to grow back. Martha's liver was still enlarged.

Yet after another three months, Martha was showing clear signs of recovery. Her energy levels were substantially higher, she weighed 102 pounds, her liver tests were improved, and her hair was growing. The breast pains she had experienced were gone. After another six months, with her condition not showing any further signs of substantial

QUICK DEFINITION

Orthomolecular medicine is the use of nontoxic nutritional therapies, such as vitamins, minerals, amino acids and other such substances, to treat people with various health conditions. The term "orthomolecular" was coined in 1968 by Nobel Prize-winner Linus Pauling, Ph.D., to describe an approach to medicine that uses naturally occurring substances normally present in the body. Ortho means "correct to normal." In addition to giving nutrition a prime role in treatment programs, orthomolecular physicians subscribe to a principle called biochemical individuality, meaning that each individual is nutritionally unique and requires variations in nutrient intake to function optimally. Orthomolecular physicians tend to avoid using drug treatments, counsel patients to reduce exposure to environmental pollution and food adulterations and encourage patients to cultivate hope about their medical condition.

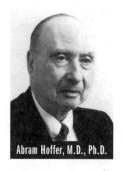

Abram Hoffer, M.D., Ph.D.

Dr. Hoffer says that his nontoxic treatments do not interfere with conventional treatments, but reinforce or complement them. "By reducing side effects and boosting my patients' regenerative abilities, my approach simply *completes* their treatment program."

To contact **Abram Hoffer, M.D., Ph.D.**: 2727 Quadra, Suite 3, Victoria, British Columbia, V8T 4E5 Canada; tel: 250-386-8756; fax: 250-386-5828.

For more about **Dr. Hoffer's cancer protocols**, see *Alternative Medicine Definitive Guide to Cancer* (Future Medicine Publishing, 1997; ISBN 1-887299-01-7); to order, call 800-333-HEAL.

improvement, following Dr. Hoffer's recommendation, Martha opted for chemotherapy without radiation.

The results were immediately apparent. The tumor began to recede, new skin began to cover up the previous ulceration (lesion) on her breast, and the painful swelling that had affected her arm for months was gone. "She experienced very little nausea or discomfort during the chemotherapy treatment, probably because of the nutritional program we placed her on," says Dr. Hoffer.

After about 15 months on Dr. Hoffer's orthomolecular program, Martha could no longer tolerate vitamin C, so Dr. Hoffer placed her on bioflavonoids (vitamin C helpers) instead, at a dosage of 1 g taken three times daily. After a month, the lesion on her breast was healing well, with only one small sign of cancer on the surface. After three more months, Martha's hair was continuing to grow back, she weighed 111 pounds, and the tissue on her breast had returned to normal. There was no sign of cancer upon visual examination and palpation. By all indications, says Dr. Hoffer, Martha was in remission.

Dr. Hoffer says that his nontoxic treatments do not interfere with conventional treatments, but reinforce or complement them. "By reducing side effects and boosting my patients' regenerative abilities, my approach simply *completes* their treatment program. The combination of nutritional therapy plus standard approaches is a highly promising, comprehensive approach to cancer treatment. Patients who follow this combined approach for at least two months have a significantly better outcome than patients on the standard therapy alone."

As you can see, alternative medicine brought Martha back from a death sentence. Her case also illustrates how alternative therapies can be successfully combined with conventional medicine to reduce side effects and to give the body the strength it needs to undergo such toxic treatments as chemotherapy.

Detoxification Therapy

A number of the 33 factors which contribute to cancer, as listed previously, involve the accumulation of toxins in the body. In fact, many alternative medicine physicians view cancer as a disease of toxic overload. As the body is unable to keep up with processing and eliminating the flood of toxins, fatty tissue such as that found in the breast is targeted as a storage place for these poisonous invaders.

This may partially explain the rise of breast cancer in the 20th century. In treating breast cancer, then, detoxifying the body can be an important part of the treatment program. (See Chapter 1: Fibrocystic Breast Disease, pp. 35-39, for details of detoxification therapy for breast health.)

Oral Supplements for Breast Cancer Treatment

As evidenced in the case histories throughout this chapter, nutritional, botanical, and other natural oral supplements can be vital components in breast cancer treatment, both to rebuild a depleted system and to attack the cancer itself. This section discusses lesser known, but highly useful supplements. First, essential oils taken orally along with volcanic clay comprise an unusual protocol developed by a radiation oncologist. Next, the specific value of coenzyme Q10 (mentioned in Dr. Schachter's case early in the chapter) for breast cancer treatment is explained. Lastly, Béres Drops, a powerful formula of trace elements and minerals, has been shown to strengthen the immune systems of breast cancer patients, as well as reduce the side effects of chemotherapy and radiation.

Essential Oils and Volcanic Clay

Victor Marcial-Vega, M.D., of Coconut Grove, Florida, was formerly in practice as a radiation oncologist. Now he employs a holistic approach to cancer treatment and has developed some unique therapies. Here, **Dr. Marcial-Vega** discusses essential oils given orally and an unusual "medicinal" clay, illustrating their success in treating breast cancer with a case history from his medical files:

Essential plant oils can bring relief for a wide range of conditions, including urinary tract infections, high blood pressure, trauma, dental infections, bleeding gums, and, with the help of a medicinal earth, appendicitis, hemorrhoids, candidiasis, and even breast cancer. Known

If You Are Having Surgery, Read This

If surgery for breast cancer is medically unavoidable, choosing the time in a woman's menstrual cycle for the operation can make a crucial difference in its success. A study of 289 pre-menopausal women undergoing mastectomy or lumpectomy revealed that those who had the surgery between days 18 and 20 of their cycle fared the best, with a 76% better survival rate (up to 18 years of follow-up) than women having surgery during days three to 12 of their cycle.[49] In addition, matching surgery to menstrual cycles doubles the survival rate for cancers involving the lymph nodes. The difference is progesterone. Its levels increase steadily as the menstrual cycle progresses, but especially after ovulation until about day 23. The optimum level of progesterone in relation to surgery was placed at four nanograms/ml, the level occurring between days 18 and 20.

as aromatherapy oils (SEE QUICK DEFINITION), essential plant oils can be taken orally, not just used on the skin or for inhalation as aromas.

However, this needs to be done under the guidance of a qualified health-care practitioner and the quality of the oil is an important consideration. Quality is an issue because essential plant oils function as potent antioxidants (SEE QUICK DEFINITION). The shelf life of a good aromatherapy oil can be at least 30 years, which means it doesn't spoil or lose its essence—it is preserved against the negative effects of oxygen, or oxidation. Protecting against these effects is the job of antioxidants such as vitamins A, C, and E, yet too often vitamin pills begin to smell rotten after a few months. In this state, their antioxidant effect is lost. There is nothing alive there to keep oxygen from doing its damage; in effect, they're dead nutrients.

This line of thinking has led me to experiment with using aromatherapy oils *orally*, as vitamins, remedies, and medications. There is an essence of life in these plant oils that keeps the oxidation at bay—a quality that acts as an antioxidant. You might think of the oil as the blood of the plant: without it, the plant is dead. This is why in my practice the antioxidant activity determines whether a substance is alive or not. Unfortunately, many aromatherapy oils are not pure but carry contaminants that can act as mild poisons or produce unpleasant side effects if taken orally. Some oils may be pure, but they are not of the highest quality. For example, if they are prepared from dry rather than fresh herbs (that still contain the vital oils intact), they are most likely to be incomplete.

Through my research, I've found that you will have no problems taking essential plant oils orally if they are pure. But like any other powerful organic substance, such as enzymes or blue-green algae, you must introduce essential plants into your system slowly with proper monitoring. In addition to taking selected aromatherapy oils orally myself, I have administered them in this way to over 200 patients and have had no evidence of toxicity resulting from oral use. As I mentioned above, essential oils can be used to treat even serious medical conditions, especially when they are given in complement with another substance I have developed, variously called volcanic clay, VMV product, or hemorr-cream.

Volcanic clay—a form of "medicinal earth"—is a natural and organic food supplement made of clay from volcanic lake areas and mixed with 18 herbal root extracts from Amazonian rain forest plants. I developed this preparation to supply essential and trace minerals as well as several vitamins in a completely natural and organic form. The approach is based on the concept that using the same organic elements that make up the cells of the human body will renew those cells by restructuring the whole organism. I always say I do not "cure" anyone. But if we give the body what it needs, all the essential building blocks, there is no disease that can withstand this.

For oral use, I mix $^1/_2$ teaspoon of the volcanic clay with a small amount of water in a vial, shaking it thoroughly. It is best to use a plastic or wood (but not metal) teaspoon as the high mineral content of the clay can corrode metal. Then the patient mixes the solution with her saliva, and swallows. Alternatively, the clay may be mixed with one tablespoon of unsweetened organic yogurt. To ensure full absorption, no food is eaten for 30 minutes after taking the clay. You will probably find that your bowels move more often and, if the odor was strong previously, these smells begin to disappear.

Approximately 85% of people taking the clay daily in this fashion will experience an energy surge within three to five days, due to the enhanced nutrition delivered to the body by the clay. If this causes insomnia, decrease the amount or frequency of clay taken. The product may be taken up to three times daily—more in

QUICK DEFINITION

Aromatherapy uses the essential oils extracted from plants and herbs to treat conditions ranging from infections and skin disorders to immune deficiencies and stress. The volatile constituents of the plant oils (its essence) are extracted through a process of steam distillation or cold-pressing. Although the term "aromatherapy" would seem to suggest an exclusive role for the aroma in the healing process, the oils also exert much of their therapeutic effect through their pharmacological properties and their small molecular size, making them one of the few therapeutic agents to easily penetrate bodily tissues. The benefits of essential oils can be obtained through inhalation, external application, or ingestion. The term aromatherapy was coined in 1937 by the French chemist Rene-Maurice Gattefosse, who observed the healing effect of lavender oil on burns.

An **antioxidant** (meaning "against oxidation") is a natural biochemical substance that protects living cells against damage from harmful free radicals. Antioxidants work against the process of oxidation—the robbing of electrons from substances. If unblocked or left uncontrolled, oxidation can lead to cellular aging, degeneration, arthritis, heart disease, cancer, and other illnesses. Antioxidants in the body react readily with oxygen breakdown products and free radicals, and neutralize them before they can damage the body. Antioxidant nutrients include vitamins A, C, and E, beta carotene, selenium, coenzyme Q10, pycnogenol (grape seed extract), L-glutathione, superoxide dismutase, and bioflavonoids. Plant antioxidants include *Ginkgo biloba* and garlic. When antioxidants are taken in combination, the effect is stronger than when they are used individually.

105

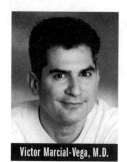

Victor Marcial-Vega, M.D.

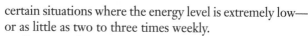

"Through my research, I've found that you will have no problems taking essential plant oils orally if they are pure. But like any other powerful organic substance, such as enzymes or blue-green algae, you must introduce essential plants into your system slowly with proper monitoring," says Dr. Marcial-Vega.

To contact **Victor Marcial-Vega, M.D.**: 4037 Poinciana Avenue, Miami, FL 33133; tel: 305-442-1233; fax: 305-445-4504. For information about the **aromatherapy oils and volcanic clay**, contact: Phyto Medicine Company, 6701 Sunset Drive, Suite 100, Miami, FL 33143; tel: 305-662-6396; fax: 305-667-5619.

For more information about **Dr. Marcial-Vega's approach to cancer**, see *Alternative Medicine Definitive Guide to Cancer* (Future Medicine Publishing, 1997; ISBN 1-887299-01-7); to order, call 800-333-HEAL.

certain situations where the energy level is extremely low—or as little as two to three times weekly.

Increasingly, I concentrate on finding the freshest, purest, and *simplest* way to deal with disease, to have my patients take fewer but more powerful supplements. Eventually, I would like them to have to take only one substance. The closest I've come to this is the combination of aromatherapy oils and volcanic clay. The oils deliver nutrients that dissolve in fat while the clay with minerals delivers nutrients that dissolve in water. This is how the body's nutrition is divided, between fat-soluble and water-soluble nutrients. If you can deliver both through the diet, you are providing the body with everything it needs to be healthy.

Success Story: Shrinking a Breast Tumor With Clay and Oils

Ellen, 76, had a breast cancer eight inches across that was eroding her chest wall and spreading to her lymph nodes and lungs. She had endured this condition for over two years and refused all conventional treatments. Under my supervision, she started applying a mixture of lavender and orange essential oils to her breast and taking one drop of orange oil orally with meals, increasing it in a few days to two drops, then after a week, to three drops. After a month, I added one drop of lavender oil to the orange, to be taken orally.

Ellen also took a small amount of the volcanic clay orally twice daily. In addition, I instructed her to take aloe vera (one tablet daily), green tea (two cups daily), Essiac herbs (three ounces, three times daily), and one drop of peppermint essential oil added to the orange and lavender taken with each meal to reduce the parasites in her system.

After two months on this program, Ellen's tumor had shrunk by 50%. When she discontinued the clay for two weeks, the tumor started to grow again; she resumed the clay and the tumor continued regressing, as before. Ellen tells me she is feeling "fantastic." After having lost 20 pounds—cancer patients almost always lose too much weight—she is now gaining back her weight and her skin color is improving. ■

Coenzyme Q10

Coenzyme Q10, also known as ubiquinone, is one of a family of brightly colored substances, called quinones, which are widely distributed in nature because they are essential for generating energy in living things that use oxygen. It is called a "coenzyme" because it enhances the activity of other enzymes. CoQ10 is found in fairly high concentrations in fish (especially sardines), soybean and grapeseed oils, sesame seeds, pistachios, walnuts, and spinach.[50] The body produces its own coQ10, but production usually declines with aging.

CoQ10 plays an important part in the body's antioxidant system. Taking coQ10 supplements has been proven to help in conditions such as breast cancer and a weakened immune system, among others. In studies reported by Karl Folkers, M.D., who is now retired but was formerly of Merck Research Laboratories, based in West Point, Pennsylvania, breast cancer patients who took 300-400 mg daily of coQ10 found their tumors completely regressed.[51]

In one study, 90 mg of coQ10 were given daily to 32 breast cancer patients for two years. All patients survived and six had partial remissions. In all cases, the tumor size had stabilized. One of the partial responders then received a high dose of 390 mg of coQ10 per day; within three months her tumor had disappeared. The researchers then gave 300 mg of coQ10 per day to a second partial responder; after three months, all traces of her cancer were gone.

One of the researchers commented that in treating almost 7,000 cases of breast cancer during a 35-year period, he had "never seen a spontaneous complete regression of a 1.5 cm to 2 cm breast tumor, and [had] never seen a comparable regression on any conventional antitumor therapy."[52] Other research substantiates the view that supplementation with coQ10 can cause complete regression of tumors in advanced breast cancer, including one patient with numerous metastases to the liver.[53]

Animal studies have shown that even at high doses, coQ10 has no toxic side effects and is safe as a nutritional supplement. Generally, it

Even if you believe you are eating a balanced diet rich in essential nutrients, you may still be lacking the trace elements and minerals crucial to good health.

For information about **coenzyme Q10** (as capsules), contact: Prolongevity Ltd., P.O. Box 229120, Hollywood, FL 33022; tel: 800-544-4440.

takes four to eight weeks for coQ10 to build up a peak concentration in the body and to produce noticeable effects. CoQ10 is best absorbed as a supplement when it's prepared dissolved in oil rather than as a powdered capsule. In fact, one of the leading authorities on the substance states that the body cannot absorb coQ10 unless it is made fat soluble. Chewable wafers of coQ10, combined with fatty acids, work well. While coQ10 is not yet generally prescribed by physicians in the U.S., in Japan it is among the most widely used of drugs.[54]

Béres Drops

If your body lacks sufficient levels of a variety of trace elements and minerals, clinical evidence suggests you may be vulnerable to numerous health problems, including general immune system weakness and cancer. Even if you believe you are eating a balanced diet rich in essential nutrients, you may still be lacking the trace elements and minerals crucial to good health.

To remedy this problem, Hungarian physician Dr. József Béres put together 20 trace elements in a single dietary supplement called Béres Drops Plus to be taken orally every day. Dr. Béres' idea was to formulate the minerals and trace elements in their "lowest reduced state to limit the production of free radicals" and as a low-level supplement to ensure better absorption.

The product "contains the trace elements in physiologically necessary amounts and proportions so that it maintains the optimal trace element level even if dietary supply is insufficient," states Dr. Béres. The elements include EDTA, L-tartaric acid, succinic acid, molybdenum, manganese, and vanadium. Europeans evidently thought Dr. Béres was on to something because an estimated three million bottles of his drops were sold in their first three months on the market.

Numerous European clinical studies (at least 30 technical papers) indicate that Béres Drops Plus can aid the immune system in its efforts to deal with a variety of diseases including breast cancer. The drops can also work as an adjunct to other treatments and help reduce the negative impact of certain treatments such as chemotherapy and radiation. A Hungarian study (1991) evaluated the effect of the drops on the physical and psychological status of patients with gynecological

Will Your Chemotherapy Work? A Test Can Tell You

In the event you decide to include chemotherapy in your breast cancer treatment program, a new lab test can help you determine the most effective chemotherapy drug for your particular cancerous tissues. In addition, the test, called the "Ex Vivo Apoptotic Assay," can identify the smallest dosage that will be sufficient to kill your specific cancer. Lower dosages can reduce the severity of chemotherapy's notoriously awful side effects. Without this test, chemotherapy prescription is a process of trial and error as doctors try to determine what kind and dosage of chemotherapy will work best.

The test, developed by Robert A. Nagourney, M.D., involves placing a biopsied piece of your own cancer tissue in a test tube with a concentration of one of more than 70 drugs available in chemotherapy regimens. The mixture sits for 72 to 96 hours to allow the cancer to "grow," after which time the physician can determine which drugs caused the most cell death. The test tube simulation provides a reasonable picture of the likely effect of the drug on the body of that individual. Generally, the assay's ability to predict outcomes was scored at 19 out of 21 in a test published in the *Journal of Hematology Blood Transfusion* in 1990.

The process, because it is tailored for each individual, is said to improve the outcome of chemotherapy by about two to three times. Also, the patient doesn't have to endure a battery of different drugs—and their side effects—in the hopes that one will work. Let's say your physician tells you that the use of Adriamycin (a chemotherapy drug) induces remissions in 38% of women with breast cancer. How can you tell in advance if you're part of the 38% for whom it works or the 62% for whom it has no effect? "We can now painlessly determine things in a test tube for a patient that they would only be able to find out if they went through the treatments," Dr. Nagourney says. "This is crucial since I've never seen a correctly administered chemotherapy for an 'average' patient."

Based on their cumulative results, Dr. Nagourney's team has compiled a bell-shaped data curve that shows the range of sensitivity and resistance to different drugs among individuals with the same kinds of cancer. From this he now knows that out of 100 women with breast cancer, perhaps 35 will have cancer cell death taking 0.15 mcg/ml of doxorubicin, while 25 will require only 0.05 mcg/ml, and still others will need 1.0 mcg/ml.

In addition to about 70 chemotherapy drugs, given singly or in combination, the assay can test botanical substances such as betulinic acid (from white birch bark), Alvium (a 12-herb formula), antineoplastons, interferons, or theoretically any substance capable of killing cancer cells.

Robert Nagourney, M.D., a board-certified oncologist, hematologist, and pharmacology professor, is founder and medical director of Rational Therapeutics, of Long Beach, California, which provides the test. For more information about the **Ex Vivo Apoptotic Assay**, contact: Rational Therapeutics Cancer Evaluation Center, 360 Elm Avenue, Long Beach, CA 90807; tel: 310-989-6455; fax: 310-989-6454; website: http://www.Rational-T.com. The Assay generally costs $2,000 for lab studies and $3,500 with a consultation with Dr. Nagourney.

and breast cancers. After three weeks, 60% of cancer patients reported an improvement in their condition and 63% said their appetite was stronger. After six months on the program, 54% of the patients had gained body weight.[55]

For general, everyday supplementation, the product is easy to use: simply dribble 18 drops into a glass of water and drink once daily. The product comes in 1.1-fluid-ounce bottles which provide about thirty 18-drop servings. The company recommends that users supplement their daily dose of drops with at least 100 mg of vitamin C.

3

One of the most prevalent myths about osteoporosis is that it is an inevitable fact of aging. The truth is that it is a disease of Western civilization that often can be prevented or reversed by dietary and lifestyle changes, nutritional supplements, and natural hormone therapies. Another common myth is that osteoporosis is caused by estrogen deficiency. In fact, the disease is caused by multiple and far-reaching factors.

Osteoporosis

BONES ARE LIVING TISSUES that grow and develop throughout childhood and adolescence. In a person's twenties, bone mass increases by 15%. Every bone is composed of a combination of compact tissue and spongy tissue, with the amount and proportion in continual flux. Some bones are so dense that they appear solid, while others are primarily a complex webbing of bone tissue.

While bones reach their basic form by the time we are adults, they are constantly changing in composition throughout our lives, undergoing normal "remodeling" in 90-day cycles. For the first ten days, there is bone loss (called bone resorption) during which osteo-clast cells detect older or slightly damaged bone matter and slowly dissolve it, leaving behind a space. For the next 80 days, bone rebuilding takes place, with osteoblast cells moving into the space and forming new bone matter to fill it. With osteoclast/osteoblast equilibrium, bone mass remains stable. When the equilibrium shifts, bone mass is altered.

Bone, like all living tissue, requires adequate nutrition for proper growth; specifically, sufficient levels of calcium, phosphorous, magnesium, manganese, zinc, copper, and silicon, plus vitamins A, C, and K. Further, vitamin D is necessary to help ensure proper absorption and utilization of calcium.

Physical stress on a bone caused by gravitational pull and the contraction of

Causes of Osteoporosis

- Poor calcium absorption
- Nutritional deficiencies
- Hormonal imbalance
- Hyperthyroidism
- Conventional drugs
- Low body fat
- Lack of exercise
- Cigarette smoking
- High alcohol intake
- Fluoride
- Environmental toxins and heavy metals

muscle stimulates bone growth. An arm placed in a cast for a week or two will lose bone mass, as will the bones of astronauts in the gravity-free atmosphere of space flight. It is the positive impact of some physical stress which makes weight-bearing exercise so important in maintaining bone health.

Hormones direct bone-building action. In females, estrogen (SEE QUICK DEFINITION) exerts some control over the osteoclast after puberty, suppressing excessive bone loss, while progesterone (SEE QUICK DEFINITION) stimulates the osteoblast. In males, these functions are mediated by testosterone. For both sexes, the thyroid hormone calcitonin helps maintain proper levels of serum calcium while enhancing bone formation (although calcitonin is not required for bone formation, according to John R. Lee, M.D., of Sebastopol, California). Assuming a woman has no thyroid hormone imbalance, bone growth should continue normally as long as adequate levels of estrogen, progesterone, and nutrients are maintained and lifestyle risk factors such as smoking and heavy drinking are avoided.

> ### Alternative Medicine Therapies for Osteoporosis
>
> - Ayurvedic medicine
> - Enzyme therapy
> - Herbal medicine
> - Homeopathy
> - Lifestyle changes
> - Exercise program
> - Dietary recommendations
> - Natural progesterone therapy
> - Nutritional supplements
> - Traditional Chinese medicine

In the United States, bone loss in the years before menopause occurs at the rate of about 1% annually, accelerating to 3% to 5% per year during menopause, and then dropping back to 1% to 1.5% yearly after that.[1] Contrary to popular belief, the hormonal factor in escalating bone loss during menopause is not due to decreased estrogen, but to lower levels of progesterone, according to Dr. Lee. Natural progesterone therapy can prevent this bone loss, he reports.

For more about **synthetic hormones**, see "Read This Before You Agree to HRT," pp. 134-135. For more about **progesterone**, see this chapter, pp. 147-149, and Chapter 1: Fibrocystic Breast Disease, pp. 39-42. For a list of **products**, see Chapter 1: Fibrocystic Breast Disease, pp. 40-41.

While an estimated 25 million American women (including one-third of all postmenopausal women) have osteoporosis, 80% of them are unaware that they are suffering from the disease.[2] The loss of bone mass and thinning of the bones which characterize osteoporosis may not be detected until the later stages when the risk of fractures increases and a broken bone calls attention to the condition.

Estrogen is a female "sex" hormone produced mainly in the ovaries (some in the fat cells) which regulates the menstrual cycle. Estrogen is important for adolescent sexual development, prepares the uterus for receiving the fertilized egg by stimulating the uterine lining to grow, and affects all the body's cells; its levels decline after menopause. Estrogen slows down bone loss, which leads to osteoporosis, and it can help reverse the incidence of heart attacks; estrogen also improves skin tone, reduces vaginal dryness, and can act as an antiaging factor. For the first ten to 14 days in a woman's cycle, the uterus is mainly under the influence of estrogen. Estrogen levels begin to climb right before menstruation, from about days seven to 14, and peak at ovulation. There are three natural types of estrogen: estradiol (produced directly in the ovary); estrone (produced from estradiol); and estriol (formed in smaller amounts in the ovary). Estradiol is the most potent of the three. It prepares the uterus for the implantation of a fertilized egg, and also helps mature and maintain the sex characteristics of the female organs.

Progesterone is a female "sex" hormone (produced in the *corpus luteum* of the ovaries) which prepares the uterus for a fertilized egg and then stops the cell proliferation in the uterus if pregnancy does not occur. When estrogen is high, during days seven to 14 of a woman's cycle, the level of progesterone is at its lowest. Its levels climb to a peak from around days 14 to 24, and then dramatically drop off again just before the start of menstruation. When the cells stop producing progesterone, it's a signal to the uterus to let go of all the new cells produced during the month and to start afresh. In a sense, menstruation is progesterone withdrawal. Starting around age 35, a woman's progesterone production begins to decline.

While people commonly associate easily broken bones with osteoporosis, many may not realize just how serious the disease is. A woman's risk of developing osteoporosis is higher than the combined risks of developing uterine, ovarian, and breast cancers, and osteoporosis is the fourth leading cause of death in American women.[3]

The statistics on osteoporosis-related fractures are equally shocking. One of every two women in the United States will suffer such a fracture after the age of 50.[4] About 1.5 million fractures every year are attributable to osteoporosis; of those, over 538,000 are of spinal vertebrae, more than 300,000 are of the hip, and over 200,000 are in the wrist.[5] The collapse of spinal vertebrae can lead to a loss of height, one of the identifying signs of osteoporosis. After a few vertebrae collapse, the spine can become rounded, forming what is colloquially known as a "dowager's hump," often accompanied by continuous back pain.

Men also develop osteoporosis, but the number of female sufferers is much higher for several reasons: 1) the hormonal changes of menopause are one of the causes of osteoporosis; 2) women's bones are usually thinner and smaller to begin with; and 3) women traditionally do not get as much vigorous, weight-bearing exercise as men do (such exercise is a strong preventive of osteoporosis).

Let's get the concept of osteoporosis clear before proceeding. Osteoporosis is generally regarded as a metabolic bone disorder. The rate of bone loss (resorption) speeds up while the rate of making new bone tissue slows down. Levels of calcium and phosphate salts decline so that the bones (osteo) become porous, brittle, and susceptible to fracture for lack of new bone tissue to replace the old tissue that's been removed.

In a sense, you end up with, literally, less bone (or skeletal mass) in your body and the bone you have is more fragile and subject to fracture. You may not even know you have sustained single or multiple minor bone fractures at first; then back pain or a sudden collapse of a bone while in use lets you know.

A Brief Look at Bone Cells

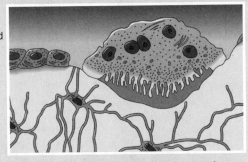

Bones are living tissue in which three types of specialized cells are responsible for building, modeling, and taking apart bone tissue on a regular basis. The bulk of the active bone modeling process takes place in the haversian canals within the bones; both osteoblasts and osteoclasts are found in abundance in these canals.

Osteoblasts, a cell type that helps form bone tissue, are especially active in the early development of the skeleton. They secrete substances that form osteoid, a precursor of bone before calcium is added; osteoblasts also influence the availability of both calcium and phosphate which are necessary for bone formation.

Osteoclasts are much larger specialized cells responsible for destroying, absorbing, and removing old bone tissue as part of the natural remodeling process continuously under way in bones. Minerals such as calcium are removed as part of this bone loss (resorption) process.

Osteocytes are regarded as nonactive osteoblasts residing within bone and are believed to play a part in mobilizing minerals needed for bone processes.

Scientists estimate that during a lifetime, women lose about 50% of trabecular bone (the network of osseous tissue within bone) and 30% of cortical bone (the compact bone of the shaft of the bone that surrounds the marrow), and that about 30% of all Caucasian women who have passed menopause experience bone fractures due to osteoporosis.[6]

Conventional wisdom regards the loss of bone mass as an inevitable part of aging. In actuality, osteoporosis, like coronary heart disease, is a "disease of Western civilization created by our lifestyles," according to Susan E. Brown, Ph.D., director of the Osteoporosis Education Project, in Syracuse, New York. Some gradual decline in bone mass is a natural fact of aging in all cultures, but in non-Westernized societies it rarely progresses to the point of causing easy fractures, states Dr. Brown. Nature has designed our bones to last a lifetime, and that includes after menopause, she says.[7]

Osteoporosis is viewed as a disease of postmenopausal women

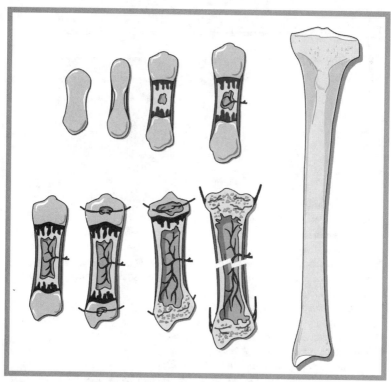

STAGES OF BONE DEVELOPMENT. Adult bones go through a regular, continuous 90-day cycle of remodeling as new bone cells are created and old bones are removed. Bone loss, called resorption, usually takes ten days, while bone rebuilding occupies up to 80 days. When these phases remain in equilibrium, bone mass remains stable, but if the balance shifts, osteoporosis may result.

because menopausal drops in estrogen and progesterone can contribute to bone mass loss and the consequent fractures generally occur later in life. In fact, during the first five to ten years of menopause, a woman may lose 10% to 15% of her cortical bone and 25% to 30% of her trabecular bone.[8] However, osteoporosis can begin in a woman as young as age 35 if her lifestyle includes such factors as chronic stress, cigarette smoking, lack of exercise, and a poor diet. Contrary to popular belief, even if a woman's estrogen levels stay high and she consumes adequate calcium, she can still develop osteoporosis because these lifestyle practices promote the disease.

"What we are now witnessing is a generation of women who've been sedentary, smoked cigarettes, and consumed unprecedented quantities of protein, sugar, and coffee—all well-known risk factors for osteoporosis," says naturopathic physician Linda Showler, N.D.[9]

Women who diet or exercise to the extreme, keeping themselves excessively thin, also put themselves at risk of developing osteoporosis long before menopause. They do not have enough body fat to maintain a normal menstrual period which is essential for bone health.

A hysterectomy (removal of the uterus) is another risk factor of early osteoporosis, even if the ovaries are still intact. "This is because anywhere between 16% and 57% of all women who undergo uterus removal suffer from premature loss of ovarian function with its associated rapid bone loss," explains Dr. Brown.[10] Unfortunately, this surgery, a conventional medical solution for uterine fibroids and endometriosis, is all too common among premenopausal women. Every year in the U.S., 750,000 women undergo hysterectomies (many including ovary removal);[11] about 90% of these are unnecessary and many are performed on women in their twenties and thirties who have no children, according to surgeon Vicki Hufnagel, M.D., of Beverly Hills, California.[12]

Obviously, women in the U.S. and other Western nations would be wise to implement osteoporosis prevention long before they approach menopause. This chapter provides the details to enable you to start taking these steps today. If you already have osteoporo-

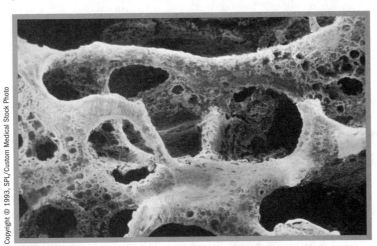

OSTEOPOROTIC BONE. Osteoporosis is generally regarded as a metabolic bone disorder. The rate of bone loss (resorption) speeds up while the rate of making new bone tissue slows down. Levels of calcium and phosphate salts decline so that the bones (osteo) become porous, brittle, and susceptible to fracture for lack of new bone tissue to replace the old tissue that's been removed.

The U.S. has the highest rate of osteoporotic fractures in the world. In addition to the personal trauma, the cost of the disease to the health-care system is estimated at $18 billion a year, of which 80% is attributed to hip fractures. The cost to each person who has a hip fracture is approximately $35,000.

sis, this chapter tells you how you can stop the progression of the disease and actually reverse existing bone loss.

Before we look at case studies illustrating how this is done, let's consider the conventional medical approach to osteoporosis. Little is offered in the way of prevention other than the recommendation to get more calcium to make up for a supposed deficiency which, as you will learn later in the chapter, is often not the problem. After menopause, the conventional medical approach to osteoporosis is to give all women synthetic estrogen replacement therapy and, again, to push calcium supplements. Besides the fact that this prescription ignores all the other causal factors of osteoporosis, synthetic estrogen has been linked to breast cancer. "You might end up trading a broken wrist for breast cancer," says Susan Love, M.D., director of the Santa Barbara Breast Cancer Institute, in California.[13]

Another conventional treatment for osteoporosis is bisphosphonates, drugs designed to decrease bone loss. A popular one is Fosamax (alendronate) which has been touted as a replacement for estrogen without its cancer-causing potential. However, other side effects, including ulcers of the esophagus if the drug isn't taken correctly, have been reported with Fosamax. Earlier bisphosphonates resulted in substandard, spongy bone formation if the drugs were taken continuously, but Fosamax is supposed to avoid that problem, reports Dr. Love.[14]

For more about **synthetic hormones**, see "Read This Before You Agree to HRT," pp. 134-135. For more about **natural progesterone**, see this chapter, pp. 147-149, and Chapter 1: Fibrocystic Breast Disease, pp. 39-42. For a list of **products**, see Chapter 1: Fibrocystic Breast Disease, pp. 40-41.

If you still think conventional medical treatments are worth the risk, consider the statistics. The U.S. has the highest rate of osteoporotic fractures in the world.[15] In addition to the personal trauma, the cost of the disease to the health-care system is estimated at $18 billion a year, of which 80% is attributed to hip fractures. The cost to each person who has a hip fracture is approximately $35,000.[16] Given these figures, it is difficult to conclude that the conventional medical approach to osteoporosis is working for anyone but those reaping the financial rewards.

As with other health conditions in this book, the more effective approach, both in terms of cost and successful outcome, is to look at the *total* causal picture of osteoporosis and identify all of the factors that are contributing to the condition. With that information, an alternative medicine physician can then design an anti-osteoporosis program which addresses the individual needs of a woman of any age.

The following three case histories demonstrate how different alternative medicine therapies can be used to meet these varying needs. In the first case, natural progesterone was the answer for not only correcting the hormonal imbalance that was causing Elsie's osteoporosis, but also restoring nearly 40% of her lost bone mass. The success of the therapy for this 72-year-old woman demonstrates that you can benefit from osteoporosis treatment even at an advanced age.

Success Story: Natural Progesterone Reverses Osteoporosis

Elsie, 72, was a woman who had always prided herself on her younger-looking appearance. A vegetarian and natural health enthusiast, she had paid special attention to her diet all her life. Elsie decided in her forties, when she went through menopause, not to go on the hormone replacement therapy recommended by conventional doctors. Instead, Elsie relied on a positive attitude and the program of good nutrition she already had in place. This worked well for many years, and Else had no apparent health problems, staying youthful and vibrant.

However, Elsie awoke one morning to severe back pain. She had not done anything out of the ordinary the day before nor injured herself. Elsie immediately went to her conventional doctor who diagnosed a spontaneous compression fracture in one of her spinal vertebrae. A bone mineral density test (a common screening method for osteoporosis) revealed that Elsie had already lost between 40% and 50% of her bone mass. Her doctor advised her to start taking synthetic estrogen or a drug called Fosamax.

Resistant to both, Elsie instead contacted John R. Lee, M.D., who suggested topical application of natural progesterone cream (from diosgenin, the active component in wild yam). Transdermal (through the skin) absorption is an effective way to deliver proges-

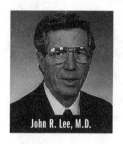

John R. Lee, M.D.

In a study of his osteoporosis patients, Dr. Lee found that natural progesterone contributed to an increase in bone mass without the side effects associated with synthetic progesterone.

For **Pro-Gest®**, one brand of natural progesterone cream, contact: Transitions for Health, 621 Southwest Alder, Suite 900, Portland, OR 97205; tel: 800-888-6814 or 503-226-1010; fax: 800-944-0168 or 503-226-6455.

John R. Lee, M.D., who retired from private practice in 1989 and is now a consultant on hormone balancing, requests that people not contact him until they have read his book, *What Your Doctor May Not Tell You About Menopause* (Warner Books, 1996). The book contains instructions for using natural progesterone cream, a complete osteoporosis prevention program, and the answers to many common questions. If people still have questions after reading the book, he can be reached at: BLL Publishing, P.O. Box 2068, Sebastopol, CA 95473; tel: 707-823-9350; fax: 707-829-8279.

terone to the body, Dr. Lee reports. In a study of his osteoporosis patients, he found that natural progesterone contributed to an increase in bone mass without the side effects associated with synthetic progesterone (progestins). In contrast to estrogen, which prevents a loss of existing bone mass but does not create new bone, natural progesterone actually builds bone, explains Dr. Lee.

Despite considerable opposition from her conventional doctor and two family members (including her husband) who were also physicians, Elsie started using the natural progesterone cream, rubbing ¼ teaspoon at bedtime into soft tissue areas, such as her belly and the inside of her thighs, for three weeks out of every month. After six weeks on the cream, the constant pain from her vertebral fracture completely disappeared, indicating that the bone had healed, says Dr. Lee. The pain never returned.

In addition to the pain indicator, hard data provided evidence that Elsie's osteoporosis was not only halted, but reversing. Elsie's husband had had her take a baseline bone mineral density test before starting the progesterone cream, then follow-up tests at periodic intervals after commencing usage. At 18 months, Elsie had gained back 18% of her bone mineral density. Encouraged, she continued on the program. At 28 months, the test revealed that she had gained back 32% of her bone mineral density, and after four years, it was 38.9%.

Dr. Lee reports that Elsie's story is only one of many similar accounts he has received since he began recommending natural progesterone cream. He points to the rapid (six-week) healing time for Elsie's compression fracture, noting that some women suffer pain from vertebral fractures for as long as a year before the bone heals and the pain goes away. "Compression fractures all heal eventually, but with progesterone, they heal more quickly because the osteoblasts start making new bone," Dr. Lee adds. As for Elsie, she is very pleased. "Her doctors wrote me a very nice note saying, had they not seen it, they would never have believed it," says Dr. Lee. "Her radiologist wrote to say he's never seen anything like it."

Like Elsie, the woman in the following case history also discovered she had osteoporosis when she sought medical help for back pain. In her case, acupuncture and Chinese herbs healed her vertebral fracture in six weeks and reversed a significant amount of her bone density loss.

Success Story: Traditional Chinese Medicine Restores Bone Density

Sela, 51 and menopausal, was suffering from moderate yet constant back pain, a classic osteoporosis symptom usually due to a compression fracture of a spinal vertebra. X rays confirmed an osteoporosis diagnosis and also showed a 30% bone density loss. Due to cultural beliefs of her Persian heritage, Sela did not want to take the hormone replacement therapy prescribed by her conventional physician.

She sought the help of Maoshing Ni, D.O.M., Ph.D., L.Ac., president of Yo San University of Traditional Chinese Medicine, in Santa Monica, California. After taking an extensive medical and personal history, Dr. Ni used the traditional Chinese medicine (TCM, see glossary, p. 122) diagnostic techniques of reading the wrist pulses and evaluating the qualities of the tongue to determine the health and functional status of Sela's organs.

Based on the results of the exam, Dr. Ni diagnosed a deficiency in Sela's kidney *jing* (vital essence) and kidney yang (warm, masculine, and active energy). In Chinese medicine, the kidney is the organ system that governs the reproductive forces and the life force energy a person has at birth. TCM physicians view menopause as the result of a decline in kidney energies, as reflected by the hormonal changes.

Kidney energies are naturally depleted by the aging process, but additionally by stress, overwork, childbearing, excessive sexual activity, and intense fear. In Sela's case, she and her family had been forced to flee an oppressive regime in the Middle East, leaving all their possessions behind. They eventually settled in the United States. "They lost everything," says Dr. Ni. "I think the fear element

A Glossary of Traditional Chinese Medicine Terms

Traditional Chinese medicine (TCM) originated in China over 5,000 years ago and is a comprehensive system of medical practice that heals the body according to the principles of nature and balance. A Chinese medicine physician considers the flow of vital energy (*qi*—pronounced CHEE) in a patient through close examination of the patient's pulse, tongue, body odor, voice tone and strength, and general demeanor, among other elements. Underlying imbalances and disharmony in the body are described in terminology analogous to the natural world (heat, cold, dryness, or dampness). The concept of balance, or the interrelationship of organs, is central to TCM. In TCM, imbalances are corrected through the use of acupuncture, moxibustion, herbal medicine, dietary therapy, massage, and therapeutic exercise.

Acupuncture is an integrated healing system developed by the Chinese over 5,000 years ago and introduced in the United States in the mid-1800s. The treatment is administered by an acupuncturist using hair-thin, stainless-steel needles, generally presterilized and disposable; these are lightly inserted into the skin at any of over 1,000 locations on the body's surface, known as acupoints. Acupoints are places where *qi* can be accessed by acupuncturists to reduce, enhance, or redirect its flow. Acupuncture is employed for a wide variety of conditions (the World Health Organization counts 104), including pain relief, asthma, migraines, and arthritis.

Acupuncture meridians are specific pathways in the human body for the flow of *qi*. In most cases, these energy pathways run up and down both sides of the body, and correspond to individual organs or organ systems, designated as Lung, Small Intestine, Heart, and others. There are 12 principal meridians and eight secondary channels. Numerous points of heightened energy, or *qi*, exist on the body's surface along the meridians and are called acupoints. There are more than 1,000 acupoints, each of which is potentially a place for acupuncture treatment.

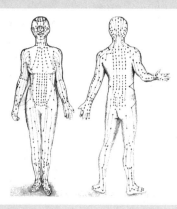

had an effect in depleting Sela's kidney energies."

Dr. Ni also diagnosed Sela with a "stagnation" or obstruction of both blood energy and *qi* (see TCM glossary), the life force energy that circulates throughout the body and nourishes the internal organs. The "stagnation" meant that Sela's energies were not flowing smoothly and were blocked in certain channels, known as acupuncture meridians (see TCM glossary). The energy blockage and "stagnation" were causing Sela's back pain.

Dr. Ni began a twice-weekly acupuncture treatment program with Sela, designed to unblock the "stagnated" energy channels associated with Sela's kidneys and bladder. He inserted acupuncture needles in points on her back as well as on her hands and feet. Dr. Ni also prescribed a Chinese herbal tea consisting of ²/₃ ounce of each of the following "raw" or unprocessed herbs: eucommia, to strengthen kidney yang energy; dipsaci, to strengthen and repair bones; and *dong quai*, to strengthen kidney energy, regulate hormones, and "tonify" or nourish Sela's blood.

To contact **Maoshing Ni, D.O.M., Ph.D., L.Ac.**: Tao of Wellness, 1131 Wilshire Blvd., Suite 300, Santa Monica, CA 90401; tel: 310-917-2200; fax: 310-917-2267. To purchase **Chinese herbs**, contact: Health Concerns, 8001 Capwell Drive, Oakland, CA 94621; tel: 800-233-9355 or 510-639-0280; fax: 510-639-9140. Mayway Corporation, 1338 Mandela Parkway, Oakland, CA 94607; tel: 510-208-3113; fax: 510-208-3069.

Sela drank two cups of the tea daily. To prepare it, she put the total of two ounces of the herbs in a saucepan with five cups of water. She boiled the mixture for an hour, letting the water boil down to four cups, then removed the herbal material and discarded it. Sela made a fresh batch of tea every two days.

After six weeks on this treatment program, Sela's back pain disappeared, indicating that her vertebral compression fracture had healed. She had another series of X rays and her radiologist informed her that there was a 50% increase in her bone density. In addition, blood tests showed that Sela's estrogen and progesterone levels, which had been deficient prior to the TCM therapy, had returned to normal.

Sela reduced her acupuncture treatments to once weekly and continued with the daily herbal tea for the next three months. By the end of that period, her further improvement was dramatic enough to allow her to resume a normal and happy lifestyle.

While the cases of Elsie and Sela demonstrate effective treatment of osteoporosis, the next case illustrates how alternative medicine can be used as preventive intervention when signs and symptoms point to a high risk of developing the disease.

Success Story: Preventing Osteoporosis

As Joan, 47, approached menopause, she began to develop health problems. She often felt nervous and irritable, and each monthly period was preceded by severe premenstrual syndrome (PMS, SEE QUICK DEFINITION). She also suffered from occasional heart palpitations, muscle cramping and fatigue whenever she exercised, and muscle strength far below average for a woman of her age.

Joan consulted Maile Pouls, Ph.D., a clinical nutritionist and director of the Health Enhancement Center, in Santa Cruz, California. Based on Joan's symptoms, Dr. Pouls suspected that she was at risk of developing osteoporosis. In particular, the muscle cramping, heart palpitations, and irritability suggested severe deficiencies in calcium and magnesium, key bone nutrients. In addition to being needed for building bone mass, these two minerals have calming properties that relax the muscles and the nervous system. Deficiencies in one or both can cause symptoms of muscular and nervous tension.

If Joan was, in fact, lacking calcium, her bones were probably beginning to thin. "It is common knowledge that when the body's chemistry becomes deficient in calcium, the body will pull calcium from the bones in an attempt to balance this deficiency," Dr. Pouls explains. "This leads to osteoporosis." Additionally, Joan's inability to exercise was compounding her risk. For bones to stay strong, they need to be stimulated by weight-bearing activities, such as running, hiking, or weight-lifting.

Dr. Pouls ran a urine analysis on Joan to confirm her diagnosis and to test for other nutritional deficiencies. "A urine analysis clearly shows the relatedness between chemistry imbalances, nutritional deficiencies, and multiple symptoms which can be related to the same imbalances or deficiencies," Dr. Pouls states.

The test confirmed that Joan indeed had low levels of calcium and magnesium and further revealed a deficiency in amino acids (SEE QUICK DEFINITION) as well. As these protein building blocks are essential for healthy muscle tissue, the amino acid deficiency explained why Joan was too tired and weak to exercise—her muscles had no strength to sustain physical activity.

The urine analysis also indicated that Joan's pH level

QUICK DEFINITION

Premenstrual syndrome (PMS) symptoms include bloating, cramping, achiness, headaches, short temper, irritability, sudden mood swings, depression, frustration, breast tenderness, crying spells, and abdominal discomfort. Typically, these symptoms are most intense from 1-2 days before a woman's period to onset of bleeding. Estrogen (a key female hormone) is at its lowest during these two days, and as low estrogen is known to coincide with low endorphins (pleasure-inducing chemicals in the brain), some researchers associate onset of PMS with falling estrogen levels. Others maintain, however, that it is the ratio of estrogen to progesterone (another female hormone) that dictates which women suffer from PMS. While estrogen levels do fall shortly before menstruation, they may still remain high in comparison to progesterone, a condition known as estrogen dominance. For this reason, many alternative physicians prescribe natural progesterone to treat PMS. An estimated 5% of American women have such severe PMS symptoms that they are incapacitated for a few days every month.

(SEE QUICK DEFINITION) was far too alkaline, a condition which prevents adequate digestion of proteins. This in turn interferes with absorption of calcium and magnesium. "What moves these minerals across the tissue wall is protein and amino acids," says Dr. Pouls. "Joan was not digesting her protein, so not only were her calcium and magnesium levels low to begin with, but she also didn't have the amino acids to effectively use what little of these minerals she had."

To start building Joan's amino acid reserve, Dr. Pouls prescribed Aminoplex, an amino acid complex (760 mg, two capsules twice daily). Dr. Pouls also recommended that Joan begin taking two capsules of Enzyme #21 at mealtimes. This enzyme (SEE QUICK DEFINITION) formula was to improve her digestion, thereby addressing Joan's pH imbalance. As her digestion improved, her pH levels would return to a normal range, permitting optimal assimilation of proteins.

Finally, to directly address Joan's calcium deficiency, Dr. Pouls prescribed Calcium Plus (one capsule, four times daily), a nutritional supplement containing high doses of magnesium and calcium. In addition, Joan took trace minerals (20 drops daily of Concentrated Mineral Drops Complex in a quart of water). The trace minerals were to treat Joan's heart palpitations and muscle cramping and to improve her bone strength.

With this program, Joan's nervousness and irritability subsided. Within a few weeks, she began to feel more energy and was able to start exercising. Her premenstrual discomfort and menstrual cramps disappeared as well.

With Joan's biochemistry stabilized, Dr. Pouls ran a blood test to check hormone levels. Joan was slightly low in both estrogen and progesterone, but not enough to warrant treatment. Dr. Pouls emphasizes, however, the importance of monitoring these hormones. "It is essential for women

QUICK DEFINITION

Amino acids are the basic building blocks of the 40,000 different proteins in the body, including enzymes, hormones, and the key brain chemical messenger molecules called neurotransmitters. Eight amino acids cannot be made by the body and must be obtained through the diet; others are produced in the body but not always in sufficient amounts. The body's main "amino acid pool" consists of: alanine, arginine, aspargine, aspartic acid, carnitine, citrulline, cysteine, cystine, GABA, glutamic acid, glutamine, glycine, histidine, isoleucine, leucine, lysine, methionine, ornithine, phenylalanine, proline, serine, taurine, threonine, tryptophan, tyrosine, and valine.

The term **pH**, which means "potential hydrogen," represents a scale for the relative acidity or alkalinity of a solution. Acidity is measured as a pH of 0.1 to 6.9, alkalinity is 7.1 to 14, and neutral pH is 7.0. The numbers refer to how many hydrogen atoms are present compared to an ideal or standard solution. Normally, blood is slightly alkaline, at 7.35 to 7.45; urine pH can range from 4.8 to 8.0, but is usually somewhat acidic, with a normal reading between 5.0 and 6.0.

QUICK DEFINITION

Enzymes are specialized living proteins fundamental to all living processes in the body, necessary for every chemical reaction and the normal activity of our organs, tissues, fluids, and cells. Enzymes are essential for the production of energy required to run cellular functions. There are hundreds of thousands of these Nature's "workers." Enzymes enable the body to digest and assimilate food. There are special enzymes for digesting proteins, carbohydrates, fats, and plant fibers. Specifically, protease digests proteins, amylase digests carbohydrates, lipase digests fats, cellulase digests fiber, and disaccharidase digests sugars. Enzymes also assist in clearing the body of toxins and cellular debris.

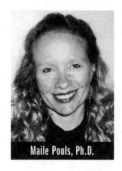

Maile Pouls, Ph.D.

"It is essential for women approaching menopause to have their hormone levels evaluated," Dr. Pouls says. "It has been shown that low estrogen and progesterone levels contribute to osteoporosis, and therefore natural hormone replacement is crucial."

To contact **Maile Pouls, Ph.D.**: Health Enhancement Center, 517 Liberty Street, Santa Cruz, CA 95060; tel: 408-423-7554; fax: 408-425-2222. For **Calcium Plus**: Rainbow Light, P.O. Box 600, Santa Cruz, CA 95061; tel: 800-635-1233 or 408-429-9089; fax: 408-429-0189. For **Concentrated Mineral Drops Complex**, qualified health practitioners may contact: BioNativus, a division of Trace Minerals Research, 1996 W. 330 Street, Ogden UT 84401; tel: 888-628-4887 or 801-731-6051. For **Aminoplex**: Tyson Nutraceuticals Inc., 12832 South Chadron Avenue, Hawthorne, CA 90250-5525; tel: 800-318-9766 or 310-675-1080; fax: 310-675-4187. For **Enzyme #21**: NESS (Nutritional Enzyme Support System), 100 Northwest Business Park Lane, Riverside, MO 64150; tel: 800-637-7893 or 816-746-0110; fax: 800-844-1957.

approaching menopause to have their hormone levels evaluated," Dr. Pouls says. "It has been shown that low estrogen and progesterone levels contribute to osteoporosis, and therefore natural hormone replacement is crucial."

Over the next few months, Joan's muscle strength improved, along with her physical stamina during exercise. "Joan's increased amino acids reserves supported increased muscular endurance," says Dr. Pouls. "These amino acids, in their role as 'carriers' of calcium across the cell walls, along with the calcium, magnesium, and trace minerals, will be her best defenses against osteoporosis."

Joan's case clearly demonstrates the interlinked functioning of nutrients and how a deficiency in one can create a chain reaction that can lead all the way to osteoporosis if nothing is done to correct the imbalances. Fortunately for Joan, she sought help before the osteoporosis process was fully under way. As with any health condition, prevention is easier than cure.

12 Causes of Osteoporosis

As the cases above illustrate, the causes of osteoporosis are wider ranging and more complicated than the simple estrogen deficiency or low calcium intake cited by conventional medicine as the culprits in the disease. If these were indeed the true culprits, then we could expect the rate of osteoporosis to be higher in countries where calcium intake is low and hormone replacement therapy is not the norm as it is in the United States.

Such is not the case. In Hong Kong, for example, the annual hip

Risk Factors of Osteoporosis

The following factors are linked to a higher risk of osteoporosis:[17]

- Small bone structure, thin build, and short in height
- High-protein diet
- Caucasian or Asian heritage (living in the U.S.)
- Fair skin, freckles, blonde or reddish hair
- Cigarette smoking
- Lack of exercise
- Lack of sunlight (less than 30 minutes three times weekly)
- High caffeine consumption (more than two cups of coffee daily)
- Early menopause (before age 43), either naturally or through surgery such as removal of the ovaries
- Absent or irregular menstrual periods
- Thyroid problems
- Premature gray hair (half gray by age 40)
- Use of certain conventional drugs, including glucocorticoids (e.g., Prednisone), anticonvulsants (e.g., Dilantin), tranquilizers, mood-altering drugs, Depo Provera, aluminimum-containing antacids (e.g., Maalox, Rolaids, Mylanta)
- Frequent indigestion, bloating, and gas
- Family history of osteoporosis
- Never having children
- Low calcium intake (less than 1,200 mg daily)
- High-salt diet
- High alcohol intake (more than two drinks daily)
- Celiac disease (intestinal malabsorption), kidney disease, or liver disease

Early Warning Signs of Osteoporosis

If you have several of the following symptoms, you could be suffering from osteoporosis. Bone screening for the condition may be advisable, especially if a number of the risk factors above are also present in your life.

- Height loss
- Brittle fingernails
- Leg cramps at night
- Transparent skin
- Tooth loss and periodontal disease
- Insomnia and restless behavior
- Joint pain

"The highest osteoporosis rates are found in the most prosperous and technologically advanced societies. Conversely, the lowest rates are typically found in poorer, less technologically advanced societies," says Susan Brown, Ph.D.

fracture rate per 100,000 people, age 35 and over, is 87.1 for women and 73 for men, compared to 319.7 women and 177 men in Rochester, Minnesota (in the U.S. dairy belt) over the same time period.[18]

Further evidence against the estrogen and calcium theories is found in history. A recent restoration of a London church opened a crypt which contained skeletons of women, ages 15 to 89, from the 18th and 19th centuries. In pre-industrial England, people's diets were not as calcium rich as ours today and women did not take estrogen. However, analysis of the women's bones revealed no significant premenopausal loss of bone density, and postmenopausal bone loss was less than our current figures. The findings were in striking contrast to the degree of bone loss in modern-day women.[19]

"The highest osteoporosis rates are found in the most prosperous and technologically advanced societies. Conversely, the lowest rates are typically found in poorer, less technologically advanced societies," says Dr. Susan Brown.[20] As discussed earlier, many aspects of modern life contribute to the development of osteoporosis. To ignore these factors in favor of taking estrogen and calcium supplements leaves the root causes untreated. The result is obvious.

While calcium is indeed essential to bone health, loading the body with more calcium does not address the deeper problems, namely, the body's inability to absorb the calcium and the factors that are robbing the body of calcium or preventing bones from repairing themselves. "Osteoporosis is a disease of excessive calcium loss caused by many factors," says Dr. John Lee. "In osteoporosis, calcium is being lost from the bones faster than it is being added, regardless of how much calcium a woman consumes."[21]

Another myth regarding calcium is widely accepted as fact: that taking certain antacid tablets will provide the body the calcium it needs for bone health, and thus prevent osteoporosis. This myth is advantageous for the manufacturers of these antacids, but not so for the unwitting consumer. There is no evidence that the calcium in the antacids accomplishes anything in the body. On the contrary, research has demonstrated that it is one of the "least absorbable" forms of calcium.[22]

Having laid the conventional myths of osteoporosis to rest, let's look at what really causes the disease, from the factors behind calcium loss and poor calcium absorption to hormonal imbalance, diet, hyperthyroidism, low body fat, lack of exercise, cigarette smoking, fluoride in your drinking water, conventional drugs, and environmental toxins and heavy metals.

1) Calcium Loss

Loss of calcium from bones leads to the thin, porous bones of osteoporosis. Excess consumption of caffeine and a variety of dietary factors can also contribute, as explained below. The body may also malabsorb dietary calcium, leading to a calcium deficiency (see pp. 131-132). Calcium malabsorption can be due to the excessive use of medications, anticonvulsant drugs, or anticancer drugs that interfere with calcium absorption. If your stomach has a low output of hydrochloric acid (that organ's basic digestive "juice") or if you take anti-ulcer drugs, such as cimetidine, which inhibits the secretion of stomach acid, your calcium stores may be low.[23]

High Caffeine Intake—Research has found that individuals who drink more than three cups of coffee a day increase their risk of osteoporosis by 82%.[24] Caffeine may produce this effect because it increases calcium excretion in the urine and allows more calcium to be secreted into the gastrointestinal tract.[25]

Other research clearly establishes the link between caffeine, calcium, and osteoporosis. In a study of women who consumed an average of two to three cups of coffee a day, among those who took 600 mg daily of a calcium supplement (which is slightly below the U.S. recommended daily allowance of 800 mg), caffeine consumption led to increased bone loss. By comparison, among women who took 900 mg of calcium daily, caffeine consumption had no negative effects on bone density. Since the majority of American women fall into the study's low-calcium group, caffeine intake in the popular forms of coffee and soda is an important risk factor in osteoporosis, the researchers concluded.[26]

Dietary Factors—The standard American diet of processed foods, carbonated soft drinks, and high protein, sugar, and salt consumption not only does not supply needed bone nutrients, but actually robs the bones of calcium. "Processed foods lead directly to calcium loss because these foods are nutrient deficient," says Dr. John Lee. "This in turn stimulates a need for protein, which, eaten in high amounts, can cause the

Nutrients and Drugs That Affect Calcium Levels

Based on an extensive review of clinical studies, Melvyn Werbach, M.D., has compiled a list of nutrients and other substances which aid or hinder calcium absorption and influence calcium levels. They are as follows:[28]

Nutrients that aid calcium absorption:

- Iron
- Lactose (milk protein)
- Lysine (an amino acid) in amounts up to 800 mg, if taken at the same time as a calcium source
- Potassium
- Sodium bicarbonate
- Vitamins D, B6, and A
- Glucose (simple sugar) can increase calcium absorption by 20% if taken at the same time as a calcium source

Nutrients that hinder calcium absorption:

- Fatty acids, fiber, phytates (found in the bran layer of cereal grains), and uronic acid (found in the fiber content of fruits and vegetables) decrease intestinal absorption of calcium
- Oxalates, concentrated in certain leafy green vegetables such as spinach, can block the absorption of

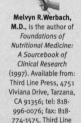

Melvyn R. Werbach, M.D., is the author of *Foundations of Nutritional Medicine: A Sourcebook of Clinical Research* (1997). Available from: Third Line Press, 4751 Viviana Drive, Tarzana, CA 91356; tel: 818-996-0076; fax: 818-774-1575. Third Line Press can also provide information on Dr. Werbach's series of health books, including *Nutritional Influences on Illness* (1996), and a CD-Rom of his collected works.

calcium if these foods are consumed alone, but not if they are eaten with other calcium-containing foods

- High daily zinc supplementation (140 mg) can reduce calcium absorption if at the same time a person has an especially low level (200 mg or less) of dietary calcium intake

Conventional drugs that affect calcium levels:

- Glucocorticoids (cortisol and cortisone) can reduce the amount of calcium in the blood
- Tetracyclines (a class of antibiotics), with prolonged use, can deplete calcium stores in the body
- Digoxin (a heart drug) and ethacrynic acid (used to induce urination) increase the amount of calcium excreted in the urine
- Isoniazid (an antibiotic for tuberculosis) curtails the production of vitamin D which is necessary for absorbing calcium
- Methotrexate (a chemotherapy agent), phenytoin (an anticonvulsant for epilepsy), and phenobarbital (a sedative), with prolonged use, can block calcium absorption and lead to calcium depletion

body to lose calcium."

This relationship between protein intake and calcium loss has been known to researchers since 1920, but a high protein intake continues to be considered synonymous with being well fed.[27] The body cannot store protein, and the excess is metabolized and excreted in urine. The breakdown of excess protein creates an excess of waste products, including ammonia and acids. Ammonia prevents calcium from being reabsorbed by the kidneys, and acids, which need to be buffered by calcium, deplete bones of this mineral.

The protein connection is supported by research which has found that vegetarians, who traditionally get less protein in their diets, experience less bone loss than those who eat meat. In one study of 1,600 women, lacto-ovo vegetarians (vegetarians who eat milk and eggs) who had been following this dietary regimen for 20 years had only 18% bone loss compared to omnivores (people who eat all types of food) who had lost 35% over the same time period.[29]

Nancy Appleton, Ph.D., a nutritional consultant in Santa Monica, California, states that a diet of excess protein, dairy products, sugar, soft drinks, alcohol, caffeine, and fried foods has an acidifying effect on the body, causing calcium to be drawn from the bones to buffer this condition.

A high salt intake, also common in the standard American diet, is another source of calcium loss. Women ingesting 3,900 mg of sodium daily excreted 30% more calcium than those getting 1,600 mg daily.[30] A diet high in sugar is similarly linked to loss of calcium and can cause metabolic problems which eventually lead to further mineral imbalances.[31]

By increasing the amount of calcium excreted in the urine, thereby decreasing overall calcium levels in the body, a high intake of protein, sugar, refined carbohydrates, sodium, and foods high in phosphorus (meat, grains, soft drinks) contributes to calcium loss, according to nutrition expert Melvyn R. Werbach, M.D., of Tarzana, California.

Consuming large amounts of soft drinks, which are high in phosphoric acid, can also raise the levels of phosphorus in the blood. The normal ratio of calcium to phosphorus in bones is about two to one, although a one-to-one ratio is adequate to maintain skeletal growth.[32] However, in the average American diet, this ratio is extremely skewed, with two, three, or even four parts phosphorus to calcium, according to Dr. Susan Brown. This causes the parathyroid glands (endocrine glands close to the thyroid), which help regulate calcium and phosphorus metabolism, to pull calcium from the bones to supplement blood calcium levels.[33]

2) Poor Calcium Absorption

The mere fact that you take calcium supplements or eat a calcium-rich diet doesn't ensure that your body is absorbing this essential nutrient. Specific interactions among nutrients affect calcium absorption and supplementation therefore should not be conducted at random.

For example, loading the body with calcium can actually interfere with bone health. "When large amounts of calcium are administered, your body turns off its production of the important vitamin D hormone, stopping the bone-remodeling process. This results in an unhealthy skeleton," states prominent vitamin D researcher Dr. Hector DeLuca.[34] People with even moderate osteoporosis often are deficient in vitamin D3, the hormonal form of the vitamin, which the body needs in order to utilize calcium in bone formation.[35]

Calcium is ingested in the form of relatively insoluble salts, whether the source is food or dietary supplements. For calcium to be absorbed, it requires vitamin D and adequate hydrochloric acid (HCl) in the stomach, says Dr. John Lee. Without adequate sunlight (a minimum of 30 minutes, three times per week), the body cannot manufacture vitamin D and calcium absorption will be compromised. In that case, it is advisable to add to the diet more natural sources of vitamin D, such as cod liver oil, oily fish such as salmon, herring and sardines, liver, egg yolks, and butter.[36] The vitamin is also added to milk, but long-term high intake of vitamin D in fortified foods has been linked to atherosclerosis and heart disease.[37]

With age, the amount of HCl secreted in the stomach decreases. Since 50% of those 70 or older produce less HCl than is needed for calcium absorption, Dr. Lee typically recommends taking a supplement of HCl or calcium citrate (a soluble form of calcium that is better absorbed than other calcium compounds when stomach acid is reduced) with meals.

3) Other Nutritional Deficiencies

In addition to calcium, essential fatty acids, and protein, there are 14 other nutrients vital for bone health, according to Dr. Susan Brown. They are: magnesium, boron, silica, copper, zinc, manganese, phosphorus, folic acid, vitamin A, vitamin B6, vitamin B12, vitamin C, vitamin D, and vitamin K.[38] Alan R. Gaby, M.D., of Seattle, Washington, cites 12 vital nutrients: magnesium, boron, silicon, copper, zinc, manganese, strontium, folic acid, vitamin B6, vitamin C, vitamin D, and vitamin K.[39]

To prevent osteoporosis, you must get sufficient levels and the proper ratio of these bone nutrients. Unfortunately, they are often deficient in the modern diet, which may be one of the reasons why osteoporosis is a disease of Western civilization. Dr. Gaby notes that our diets have a far lower vitamin and mineral content than those of our ancestors. "Studies indicate that modern farming practices deplete the soil of essential minerals, resulting in lower levels of these minerals in our foods," says Dr. Gaby. Added to this, overconsumption of nutrient-empty foods, such as sugar and white flour, further deprives us of vitamins and minerals.[40]

4) Hormonal Imbalance

Conventional medicine views osteoporosis primarily as an estrogen deficiency occurring at menopause. "While estrogen plays an important and complex role in bone health maintenance, osteoporosis cannot simply be attributed to lower estrogen levels," states Dr. Brown. If this were so, then all women around the world would get osteoporosis at menopause, she points out. As discussed earlier, this is not the case.[41]

Further, vegetarian women, who have lower estrogen levels than their meat-eating counterparts, still tend to have more bone mass.[42] Women also lose bone before menopause, when estrogen is still high, says women's health specialist Christiane Northrup, M.D., of Yarmouth, Maine. "Up to 50% of the bone that women lose over their lifespan is lost before menopause even begins," she says.[43]

Conventional medicine's standard use of estrogen replacement therapy (ERT) on women at menopause is problematic for a number of reasons (see "Read This Before You Agree to HRT," pp. 134-135), not the least of which is that it overlooks the role of progesterone in maintaining bone health. While estrogen can help prevent bone loss, progesterone is needed to build bone.

As cited earlier in the case of Elsie, Dr. Lee has discovered in his clinical practice that progesterone deficiency is actually more often the underlying cause of osteoporosis than low levels of estrogen. Progesterone deficiency begins as early as age 35; premenopausal and perimenopausal (on the verge of menopause) women often have

---

Graying Hair—An Early Sign of Osteoporosis?

Premature graying is associated with lower bone mineral density (BMD). A study of 293 postmenopausal women revealed that those whose hair had begun to turn gray when they were in their twenties had lower BMD throughout the skeleton than did women whose hair started graying later. Women whose hair was mostly gray by the age of 40 also had lower BMD.[44]

Read This Before You Agree to HRT

Despite research linking it to cancer, hormone replacement therapy (HRT)—also known as estrogen replacement therapy (ERT) since the hormone most often given is synthetic estrogen—has become conventional medicine's standard prescription for perimenopausal and menopausal women. The conclusion of a U.S. government–sponsored study analyzing the effectiveness and cost of hormone replacement therapy reflects the conventional position: "It would be reasonably cost effective to offer ERT at age 50 (the time of menopause) to all women who commit to a lifelong course of ERT."[45]

There are numerous flaws, not to mention health hazards, in this approach. First, it doesn't work. While estrogen may slow bone loss, it does nothing to promote new bone formation and its effects are temporary. Even a research review (of 31 studies) in the *American Journal of Medicine* concluded that estrogen did not have "significant benefit" in slowing osteoporosis onset.[46]

Since bone loss appears to resume at a pre-treatment rate once the ERT is stopped,[47] conceivably the therapy should be continued uninterrupted for twenty-plus years until bone loss abates around age 70. This is the reasoning behind the study's recommendation of a lifetime commitment. However, long-term use is not effective, according to Dr. John Lee. "Taking estrogen (as in hormone replacement therapy) can slow bone loss for those few (menopausal) years, but its effect wears off within a few years after menopause. Estrogen cannot rebuild new bone," he says.[48]

Second, research has clearly demonstrated that HRT increases the risk of breast and endometrial (uterine) cancers and that the risk goes up the longer a woman takes it.[49] Long-term use also increases the likelihood of side effects such as salt and water retention and increased fat synthesis, and serious secondary diseases such as uterine fibroids, gallbladder and liver disease, heart disease, and stroke, states Dr. Lee. To offset the risk of endometrial cancer, a synthetic progesterone (progestin) is now added to prescriptions to help balance the estrogen. While this seems to slightly improve osteoporotic bones, progestin may produce undesirable side effects of its own.[50]

Third, the causes of a woman's osteoporosis that have nothing to do with estrogen are entirely ignored in the ERT focus. Unchecked, these factors—such as diet, lack of exercise, toxic exposure, low progesterone levels, and the many other causes discussed in this chapter—continue to produce bone loss.

Fourth, the hormones prescribed in HRT are themselves suspect. "Replacement" therapy is a misnomer, as the synthetic hormones used have little resemblance to the hormones found in a woman's body. Premarin, the main synthetic estrogen prescribed by conventional physicians, is derived from pregnant (Pre) mare's (mar) urine (in). "Of the approximately 12 estrogens in horse urine, only two exactly match a woman's. In the 40 years we've been prescribing Premarin, there has not been adequate testing to discover what these ten other horse estrogens do to a woman," says Jesse Hanley, M.D., of Malibu, California.

If progesterone is considered in the HRT package at all, it is usually in the form of the synthetic Provera (medroxyprogesterone, a progestin) which, according to Jonathan Wright, M.D., is even less appropriate than Premarin for women. "It's never been found in people or anywhere else in nature, but was synthesized by a drug-company chemist so it could be patented and sold exclusively at a high price," states Dr. Wright.[51] In addition to producing water retention and depression, Provera increases your risk of blood clots, according to Dr. Hanley.

Dr. Lee also points to profit as the motive behind HRT. His research into natural progesterone revealed that its use had been studied as far back as the 1930s, but conventional medicine stopped using it in the 1950s. "It's money and control," says Dr. Lee. "The pharmaceutical companies discovered they couldn't patent natural progesterone. So, they created foreign chemical substitutes."[52] Like Dr. Wright and other alternative medicine physicians, he advises avoiding these drugs, as they block the action of real progesterone and have toxic side effects.

Dr. Susan Love concurs that the prevalence of HRT has to do with profit rather than medical necessity. "Until menopause became big business, American women were always told their symptoms were in their heads," she says. Dr. Love believes that drug companies have promoted the HRT myth by playing on the fear of aging which is integral to American culture. "One of the most powerful marketing techniques used to influence both doctors and patients is the manipulation of fears of aging and death," states Dr. Love.[53]

Perimenopausal and menopausal women are scared into taking the synthetic hormones, led to believe that if they don't, they will turn into dried-up old women.

With all of the evidence amassed against HRT, there is no logical reason for women to subject themselves to these toxic synthetic hormones; especially when there are safe, effective, natural methods to prevent and reverse osteoporosis. As none of these claims apply to HRT, the choice is obvious.

For more about **natural progesterone**, see this chapter, pp. 147-149, and Chapter 1: Fibrocystic Breast Disease, pp. 39-42. For a list of **progesterone products**, see Chapter 1: Fibrocystic Breast Disease, pp. 40-41.

excess estrogen and low progesterone up until the time of menopause, when estrogen drops, Dr. Lee explains.[54] "Progesterone and not estrogen is the missing factor…in reversing osteoporosis," he says.[55]

Research supports Dr. Lee's findings. One study of 66 pre-menopausal women, 21 to 41 years old, all of whom were marathon runners, measured hormone levels and bone loss over a year. The researchers found that "while there was no correlation between the rate of bone losses and serum levels of estrogen, there was a close relationship between indicators of progesterone and bone loss."[56]

5) Hyperthyroidism

In this book, hypothyroidism (an underactive thyroid gland) appears repeatedly as a causal factor behind a wide range of health conditions. In the case of osteoporosis, an overactive thyroid gland, hyperthyroidism, is more likely to be the problem. Thyroxin, a hormone secreted by the thyroid gland (SEE QUICK DEFINITION), stimulates minerals to be drawn out of the bones as part of the natural and ongoing process of bone remodeling. In hyperthyroidism, elevated levels of thyroxin result in too much mineral strength being drawn from the bones, causing depletion of bone mass.

The **thyroid gland**, one of the body's seven endocrine glands, is located just below the larynx in the throat, with interconnecting lobes on either side of the trachea. The thyroid is the body's metabolic thermostat, controlling body temperature, energy use, and, in children, the body's growth rate. The thyroid controls the rate at which organs function and the speed with which the body uses food; it affects the operation of all body processes and organs. Of the hormones synthesized in and released by the thyroid, T3 (triiodothyronine) represents 7%, and T4 (thyroxine) accounts for almost 93% of the thyroid's hormones active in all of the body's processes. Iodine is essential to forming normal amounts of thyroxine. The secretion of both these hormones is regulated by thyroid-stimulating hormone, or TSH, secreted by the pituitary gland in the brain. The thyroid also secretes calcitonin, a hormone required for calcium metabolism.

The thyroid issue becomes especially compelling later in life as thyroid hormone medication is prescribed for many postmenopausal women either to suppress an overactive thyroid gland or to stimulate an underactive thyroid. French researchers studied the results of 41 studies involving 1,250 women and found that taking a conventional synthetic thyroid hormone drug to suppress an overactive thyroid was associated with increased bone loss in women who had been through menopause. The drug did not have this effect on premenopausal women.

However, premenopausal women who took synthetic thyroid hormones to replenish deficient thyroid hormone levels experienced an increase in bone loss, especially in the spine and hip. The researchers warned that overuse of thyroid hormone therapy is widespread and that, in many instances, the use of this therapy is "overzealous or irrelevant."[57] Dr. Susan Brown advises: "If you use thyroid hormones, it would be wise to have your hormone levels carefully monitored and to take only the minimum necessary amount."[58]

6) Conventional Drugs

In addition to thyroid medication, a number of other conventional drugs can cause bone loss. Adrenal corticosteroid drugs such as Prednisone (commonly prescribed for arthritis and asthma) are particularly problematic. These drugs both impair calcium absorption and inhibit bone formation. Research has found that taking more than 7.5 mg of Prednisone daily for six months or longer significantly increases your risk of osteoporosis.[59]

For more about **drugs and osteoporosis**, see "Nutrients and Drugs That Affect Calcium Levels," p. 130.

Birth control pills also increase your risk by their tendency to create folic acid deficiency. Insufficient levels of folic acid allow homocysteine (a by-product of metabolism of the amino acid methionine, found in red meat, milk, and milk products) levels to rise. Research has linked homocysteine to osteoporosis development.[60]

According to Dr. Gaby, other conventional medications which increase your risk of osteoporosis include antibiotics such as tetracycline, anticonvulsants such as Dilantin (for seizures), anticoagulants (blood thinners), aluminum-containing antacids, certain chemotherapy drugs, and lithium, among others.[61] However, natural progesterone used concurrently with conventional medications can help protect against the dangerous side effect of bone loss, says Dr. John Lee.

7) Low Body Fat

Being excessively lean, whether from extreme dieting or exercise (such as marathon training), impairs hormone synthesis which in turn compromises bone health. Low body fat causes reduced progesterone and, if menstruation is irregular or ceases altogether (18% body fat is needed to maintain a normal menstrual period[62]), both progesterone and estrogen are lowered. Under these circumstances, the consequences for bone mass are the same as with menopause. In fact, studies show that bones bearing the weight of a large body are healthier than the bones of a small, thin person.[63] After menopause, estrogen levels are also higher in heavier women because the hormone is synthesized in adipose (fat) tissue.[64]

8) Lack of Exercise

The old saying "use it or lose it" applies directly to bones. Unless bones are stimulated by weight-bearing exercise, they become sluggish and lazy and stop building bone mass. The key is weight-bearing exercise, as in running, dancing, or brisk walking versus swimming. The force of impact such exercise delivers to bones is a stimulant to bone-building.[65] Lifting weights can also provide bone-building stimulation by exerting weight and pull on bones.[66]

In addition to stimulating bone growth, exercise also improves

In addition to stimulating bone growth, exercise also improves blood circulation to the bones, an important aid in preventing osteoporosis. Bones have a limited blood vessel network to begin with, so improving blood circulation optimizes the effects of that system in the bones.

blood circulation to the bones, an important aid in preventing osteoporosis. Bones have a limited blood vessel network to begin with, so improving blood circulation optimizes the effects of that system in the bones. Similarly, anything that impedes circulation, such as cigarette smoking, will gradually diminish the blood supply to the bones and cut off important nutrients.

Many studies have demonstrated that women who get regular weight-bearing exercise lower their risk for osteoporosis. A four-year study at the University of Vienna showed that regular running significantly reduced bone loss in middle-aged women.[67]

Another study found that athletic women (defined as engaging in a sporting activity for at least 20 years) who engaged in impact sports had denser bones than women with a sedentary or less active lifestyle. The study documented 80 women over the age of 40: 20 were active in high-impact sports such as basketball; 20 played middle-impact sports such as field hockey or tennis; 20 engaged in a non-impact sport such as swimming; and 20 women played no sport at all. Upon comparison, researchers found that all 60 athletes had more lean body mass than their sedentary counterparts. However, the middle- and high-impact athletes demonstrated a much higher bone mineral density than both the swimmers and the sedentary controls.[68]

Despite this evidence as well as many other positive health benefits, one in four adult Americans still spends their leisure time doing little or nothing, according to the American Medical Association (AMA). The AMA surveyed nearly 10,000 adults in the U.S. and found that 22% engaged in no physical activity during leisure time and 46% stated that they don't exercise regularly. A related study of 2,783 men and 5,018 women, 65 and older, indicated that only 37% of men and 24% of women in this age group exercise at least three times weekly, and when they do, the preferred activities are walking and gardening.[69]

While walking may help prevent bone loss, gardening, unless strenuous, will do little. The results of this survey may explain, in part, why osteoporosis is so prevalent in the United States. Between bad diet and no exercise, bones are not getting what they need to prevent the disease. When one remedy is as simple as taking a brisk walk for half an hour three times a week, it is unfortunate that more people don't make the effort on behalf of their bones.

9) Cigarette Smoking

Cigarette smoking appears to promote osteoporosis by lowering estrogen concentration in the bloodstream and reducing estrogen's inhibiting effect on osteoclast cells.[70] If you recall, the osteoclasts are the cells responsible for bone breakdown. In addition, with smoking, less carbon dioxide than normal leaves the body on an exhaled breath, and this too can exert a detrimental effect on bones. According to Dr. John Lee, carbon dioxide retention leads to higher blood levels of carbonic acid which the body attempts to neutralize with calcium taken from bones.

10) High Alcohol Intake

Research has linked alcohol consumption and bone loss; specifically, drinking more than a few ounces of alcohol a day inhibits calcium absorption, contributes to calcium loss, and disturbs mineral balance in the body. One study found that 31% of the male subjects under the age of 40 who drank beyond moderation had osteoporosis. That percentage is very high both for men and for that age group, which indicates the powerful impact of alcohol on bone health.[71] A second study at the Veteran's Affairs Medical Center in Portland, Oregon, found that even alcohol consumption of one to two drinks daily "is clearly linked with reduced bone mass."[72]

Impaired bone formation is one of the mechanisms by which alcohol causes bone loss; specifically, ethanol inhibits the activity of osteoblasts, the bone-building cells. Any substance that interferes with osteoblast function has a negative impact on bone density.[73]

11) Fluoride

Fluoride, which has routinely been added to public drinking water and toothpaste since the 1950s, is actually a poison second in toxicity only to arsenic. The fluoride compounds most commonly added to water are unrefined toxic waste products of phosphate fertilizer production. As early as 1953, scientists proved that fluoridated water did not reduce cavities in children, which was the rationale for adding it to water and consumer products.

"Fluoride, once touted as an osteoporosis treatment, is, in fact,

"Fluoride, once touted as an osteoporosis treatment, is, in fact, toxic to bone cells," says Dr. Lee. "When given in treatment doses, fluoride causes an apparent increase in bone mass, but the resulting bone is abnormal and lacks strength."

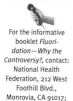

For the informative booklet *Fluoridation—Why the Controversy?*, contact: National Health Federation, 212 West Foothill Blvd., Monrovia, CA 91017; tel: 626-357-2181; fax: 626-303-0642.

toxic to bone cells," says Dr. Lee. "When given in treatment doses, fluoride causes an apparent increase in bone mass, but the resulting bone is abnormal and lacks strength." Recent studies in the United States and England have shown that even smaller amounts of fluoride in common drinking water increase the risk of hip fracture.[74]

Other research findings include:

■ Women who have had extensive exposure to fluoridated water fracture their hips from osteoporosis 2.6 times more than the norm.

■ A study of 500,000 cases proved a definite correlation between consumption of fluoridated water and the incidence of hip fractures; specifically, 41% more among men, 27% more among women.

■ Prolonged fluoride intake of more than 3 ppm (parts per million) can produce osteosclerosis, a spinal column disease.

■ A study of dog fetuses showed that fluoride consumed by the mother gets deposited in the bones of the fetus, making them brittle.

■ Fluoride contributes to the breakdown of collagen in bones, muscle, skin, cartilage, and lungs.

■ Fluoride blocks blood antibody formation, causes premature aging, depletes the energy reserves of white blood cells, and promotes bone cancer development.

Despite the weight of scientific evidence, the American Dental Association will not endorse any dental product unless it contains fluoride. Meanwhile, even though fluoridated water has been outlawed in 14 European countries plus Egypt and India as being too toxic for public health, the U.S. still regards up to 4 ppm as a "safe" level. California, often a trendsetter for the nation, has made fluoridation of public water supplies in that state mandatory, an ill-advised move opposed by many.[75]

12) Environmental Toxins and Heavy Metals

Dr. Alan Gaby points to the polluted world as another factor in the widespread incidence of osteoporosis in the United States and other industrialized countries. Heavy metals such as lead, cadmium, tin from tin cans, and aluminum are particularly at fault, he says. For example, excessive exposure to lead can cause a negative calcium balance, and high cadmium levels in the body can result in a decrease in the mineral content of bone.

These heavy metals are found in products to which we are exposed daily. They are also delivered to us by acid rain. "Acid rain leaches heavy metals out of the bedrock, moving them into our rivers and lakes, and eventually into the water we drink," says Dr. Gaby. "Acid rain has also caused our drinking water to become more acidic, which in turn challenges our body's buffering capacity, drawing calcium out of bones to provide alkalinity for balance. All this can lead to osteoporosis."

Aluminum which is especially pervasive in products used daily damages bone by interfering with the mineralization process, says Dr. Susan Brown. "Even small quantities of aluminum such as from aluminum-containing antacids can lead to negative calcium balance," she says. Other sources of aluminum include aluminum cookware, foil, and antiperspirants.[76]

Testing for Osteoporosis

If in reviewing the causes of osteoporosis discussed above, you conclude that you are at risk of developing the disease, you may want to be tested. Certain testing is also useful in establishing a baseline bone density before beginning a treatment program. In this way, the effectiveness of treatment can be monitored and adjustments made accordingly.

Currently, there are three methods of testing for osteoporosis: the first simply measures for height loss; the second uses X rays or light-beam scanning to determine bone density and assess bone loss; and the third option is a urinalysis to measure bone loss.

Height Loss—The initial test for osteoporosis, according to Katherine O'Hanlan, M.D., of Stanford University, is measuring for a loss in height, which is one of the earliest symptoms of the disease. "With osteoporosis, vertebrae shrink and this leads to height loss which can be observed," explains Dr. O'Hanlan. Height should be measured routinely at regular doctor visits. "A loss of one-half inch from what you've been all your life is significant," says Dr. O'Hanlan. If a loss of height is confirmed, bone density should then be measured.

Bone Density: DEXA Versus X Ray or DPA—Conventional bone X rays can only detect osteoporosis after 25% of the bone mass has been lost, according to Dr. O'Hanlan. Mary James, N.D., of Great Smokies Diagnostic Laboratory, in Asheville, North Carolina, places the number much higher—after 60% is lost. Another common technique, DPA or dual photon absorptiometry, uses photons (light beams) to determine bone density and is able to detect bone loss at much lower percentages than standard X rays.

However, the most accurate bone density testing method is DEXA or dual X-ray absorptiometry, says Dr. O'Hanlan. DEXA uses a lower radiation dose than conventional X rays, has a 98% to 99% accuracy rate,[77] and can detect even a bone mass change of 3% to 5%.[78]

In bone density testing, it is more effective to monitor the spongy (trabecular) areas rather the denser (cortical) parts of bone, says Dr. Lee. The turnover rate of the spongy bone is more rapid and changes will show much earlier. He recommends targeting vertebrae, particularly in the lumbar spine as four vertebrae can be measured, reducing the chance of an erroneous reading when only a single bone is tested. Lumbar bone mineral density can then be monitored at regular intervals as a progress check in treatment.

Bone Loss: Osteoporosis Risk Evaluation Test—This urinalysis assesses your risk for osteoporosis based on biochemical markers in your urine which signify bone loss. When it comes to osteoporosis, prevention is "everything," says Dr. James. The Osteoporosis Risk Evaluation Test, developed at the Great Smokies Diagnostic Lab, can also demonstrate whether a calcium supplementation program (or any prevention or treatment approach) is getting useful results in slowing bone loss.

As mentioned earlier, our bones are continually being remodeled. During the bone loss stage, the components of bone, including collagen, are broken down and collagen-binding fibers are released into the urine. These "collagen crosslinks" include two protein substances called pyridinium (Pyd) and deoxypyridinium (D-Pyd).

For information about the **Osteoporosis Risk Evaluation Test**, contact: Great Smokies Diagnostic Laboratory, 63 Zillicoa Street, Asheville, NC 28801; tel: 800-522-4762 or 704-253-0621; fax: 704-252-9303.

With dietary imbalances, nutritional deficiencies, hormonal fluctuations, or menopause, the cycle of bone loss and bone rebuilding is disturbed and more bone is lost than rebuilt, explains Dr. James. It turns out that Pyd and D-Pyd are excellent biochemical markers that show, through a simple urine analysis, how much bone loss is happening. Higher than average concentrations of either substance in the urine indicates progressive bone loss.

For the test, urine is collected from the second morning urination and sent by a licensed health practitioner to the Great Smokies lab for analysis, usually at a cost of $65 to $100.

Alternative Medicine Therapies for Osteoporosis

Once you have determined that you are at risk of osteoporosis or that bone loss is already under way, there are numerous steps you can take to prevent the development of the disease or to halt and reverse its progress. Many of these steps can be accomplished relatively easily by making dietary and lifestyle modifications and eliminating as many other of the known risk factors present in your life as possible.

For example, quitting smoking, keeping alcohol consumption to a moderate level, eliminating your use of aluminum products such as cookware and aluminum-containing antiperspirants, making sure to get enough exercise and sunshine, and cutting down on excessive protein consumption are all important preventive measures.

Quitting smoking, moderating alcohol consumption, eliminating your use of aluminum products, getting enough exercise and sunshine, and cutting down on protein consumption are all important preventive measures.

"A treatment plan for osteoporosis should recreate the conditions under which normal bone building occurs, including proper diet, nutritional supplements, hormone balance, exercise, and avoidance of known toxic factors such as fluoride and cigarette smoking," states Dr. John Lee. In addition to the therapies addressing these issues in the previous case studies, more information on dietary recommendations, the importance of exercise, natural progesterone therapy, nutritional supplements, and herbal medicine can be found in the following sections.

Dietary Recommendations

For osteoporosis prevention and reversal, Dr. Susan Brown typically recommends a nutrient-rich diet that avoids the high sugar, high

Simple Steps for Preventing and Treating Osteoporosis

Evidence suggests that osteoporosis is less a consequence of aging and more a result of our modern diet and lifestyle. In fact, exercising regularly and addressing certain dietary and lifestyle concerns may be sufficient to prevent this debilitating disease. Based on the findings of osteoporosis research, the following will help build stronger, healthier bones.[79]

■ Exercise regularly. Brisk walking, running, aerobics, tennis, and other weight-bearing exercise strengthens bones and lowers the risk of fracture.

■ Eat a whole-foods diet with plenty of fruits and vegetables. Avoid eating too much meat and other protein foods. Limit intake of caffeine and salt.

■ Use supplements wisely. Don't load up on calcium or take calcium only. Other nutrients, such as the B vitamins, vitamins C and D, phosphorus, magnesium, and zinc, are as important for bone health. Consult a qualified practitioner to determine what your individual nutritional needs are.

■ Make sure you are getting enough essential fatty acids (EFAs). Research has shown that two essential fatty acids, in particular, contribute to calcium balance and bone calcium content: EPA (eicosapentaenoic acid), an omega-3 EFA found in fish such as salmon, cod, and mackerel; and GLA (gamma-linolenic acid), an omega-6 EFA found in evening primrose, black currant, and borage oils.

■ Make sure you are getting enough boron, a mineral which helps prevent calcium loss and bone demineralization. Good dietary sources of boron include soybeans, almonds, peanuts, prunes, raisins, and dates. A beneficial supplemental dosage is 3 mg daily.

■ Quit smoking. Numerous studies have reported that quitting cigarette smoking reduces the risk of bone fractures due to osteoporosis. According to one study, stopping smoking lowered the risk of hip fracture by as much as 25%.

■ If you drink alcohol, do so only in moderation. Drinking to excess can interfere with bone formation, thus increasing the risk of osteoporosis.

CAUTION!
Before beginning any exercise program, consult your physician.

■ Avoid cooking with aluminum (pans, foil, and other kitchen items). Aluminum can suppress the parathyroid gland (involved in calcium metabolism), which can, in turn, result in osteoporosis.

■ Avoid taking steroids on a long-term basis. Research has linked this to a greater incidence of osteoporosis.

fat, high protein, and excess processed foods of the standard American diet. She also endorses adding a nutritional supplement program, noting that it is difficult to get enough bone nutrients on 1,500 calories or less daily, the limit observed by many women trying to control their weight.[80]

Dr. Brown's anti-osteoporosis diet includes the following: whole grains (1-3 servings per meal); vegetables (three to four cups of low-starch variety daily; 1-2 servings of starchy variety daily); dried beans or other legumes (one or more servings daily); fish, lean meat, or poultry (one 4- or 5-ounce serving daily); dairy (up to three servings daily, if tolerated); fruits (one to three daily); fats (2-3 tsp daily of cold-pressed or expeller-pressed oils); nuts and seeds (2-3 tbsp daily); and eight glasses of water daily.[81]

Research has found that a diet high in soy foods appears to help prevent osteoporosis. "Soy protein does not cause calcium excretion like animal protein," says fitness and nutrition consultant Linda Ojeda, C.N.C., Ph.D.[82] In addition, tofu, tempeh, and other soy foods contain calcium and plant estrogens, or phytoestrogens. "Recent work suggests that the isoflavones [phytoestrogens] in soybeans also have a direct benefit on bone health, possibly by inhibiting bone resorption," Dr. Ojeda says.[83] Phytoestrogens are so named because they can act like hormonal estrogen in the body, attaching to estrogen receptor sites and serving to restrain bone loss.

Phytoestrogens also are beneficial because they are predominantly estriol, which is the type of estrogen that is least carcinogenic, says Phyllis Bronson, a nutritional biochemist in Aspen, Colorado. By contrast, xenoestrogens, environmental toxins that "mimic" estrogen inside the body and attach to estrogen receptor sites, are mostly estradiol, the estrogen targeted as responsible for breast and uterine cancer, Bronson says.

Another myth of osteoporosis is that the best dietary preventives of the disease are milk and other dairy products. You will note that these food items are not among the main dietary recommendations included here. The promotion of a high dairy intake is, again, part of the calcium myth. As has already been established, loading up on calcium is not the solution for osteoporosis. In fact, a high dairy intake is linked to a high risk of osteoporosis.[84]

Further, dairy products are problematic foods; they are not easily digested, many people are lactose intolerant (without even knowing it), and the body cannot utilize the calcium in pasteurized dairy products. Pasteurization changes the calcium into an unusable form, according to Dr. M.T. Morter, Jr.[85] In addition, unless it is organic and raw, milk contains numerous toxins, from traces of the hor-

145

In a study of 20 postmenopausal women (between the ages of 58 and 83) conducted at California State University at Fullerton, ten months of aerobic exercise resulted in a 1.33% increase in bone mineral content and bone density compared to a 2.58% decrease in these measurements in the control group.

mones and other drugs given to the cattle and pesticides in their food supply to processing additives and residues.

There are many other foods that are high in calcium and which contain beneficial nutrients that help the body absorb calcium as well. Kale, for example, gives you far more assimilable calcium than milk.[86] Other leafy greens are also excellent sources, as are turnips, almonds, asparagus, and parsley.[87] For dietary calcium, many alternative medicine physicians emphasize these foods over milk for the reasons cited above.

Exercise Program

With a growing body of research demonstrating the link between exercise and osteoporosis prevention, there is every reason to make regular exercise part of your lifestyle. As mentioned earlier in the causes section, the key in anti-osteoporosis exercise is that it be weight-bearing, as in running, dancing, or brisk walking. Weight-lifting also has a stimulating effect on bones, but the higher-impact activities produce greater benefit.

If you are not an athlete or have not exercised much in your life, that doesn't mean you should resign yourself to osteoporosis. Research shows that beginning exercise even *after* menopause can help build bone strength. In other words, it's not too late to begin an exercise program and start reaping the benefits.

In a study of 20 postmenopausal women (between the ages of 58 and 83) conducted at California State University at Fullerton, ten months of aerobic exercise resulted in a 1.33% increase in bone mineral content and bone density compared to a 2.58% decrease in these measurements in the control group. There was no significant difference in bone mineral content and density between women who participated in aerobics alone and those who did aerobics plus upper-body weight training.[88]

Along with a healthy diet and appropriate nutritional supplements, integrating regular exercise into your life may be the best thing you can do for your bones. Exercise has so many other proven

A Comprehensive Osteoporosis Treatment Plan

Preventing or reversing osteoporosis requires a complete lifestyle and dietary program. Here is an example of a basic treatment plan, as recommended by John Lee, M.D. Variations on the dosages and suggestions may be indicated; check with your practitioner before beginning any treatment program.

Daily nutritional supplements:

- Vitamin D: 350-400 IU
- Vitamin C: 2,000 mg in divided doses
- Beta carotene: 15 mg (equivalent to 25,000 IU vitamin A)
- Calcium: 800 mg through diet and/or supplements
- Vitamins B6 and K, magnesium, zinc, manganese, strontium, boron, silicon, and copper (dosages depending on individual)
- Hydrochloric acid, if protein digestion is a problem (a certain type of urinalysis can determine if you are digesting proteins adequately)

Exercise:

- At least 20 minutes daily or half an hour of exercise three times a week

Dietary recommendations:

- Emphasize leafy green vegetables and whole grains
- Avoid excessive protein; limit red meat to three times per week or less
- Avoid all soft drinks and limit alcohol consumption
- Restrict intake of fat, caffeine, and salt
- As dietary sources of calcium, fish and beans are preferable to dairy products; if eating dairy, yogurt is best, especially for lactose-intolerant people

health benefits that it will be a major investment in your overall health as well.

Natural Progesterone Therapy

As illustrated in the case of Elsie at the beginning of the chapter, natural progesterone cream, applied topically and absorbed through the skin (transdermally), can add bone mass and prevent osteoporosis. Progesterone, as mentioned previously, actually builds bone while estrogen, the hormone which tends to be emphasized in conventional prescriptions for women, only slows bone loss but does not create new bone.

Transdermal use of natural progesterone is considered the best application because the hormone is absorbed directly into the bloodstream, bypassing any breakdown in the liver and in the digestive system. The transdermal cream also delivers progesterone in a more gradual manner, as needed by the body, while oral progesterone (either infused in oil or capsulized in powder form) is delivered all at once and

Testing Your Hormone Levels

A simple saliva test can give you an approximate idea of what your hormone levels are, so you can determine if natural progesterone cream is appropriate for you. The salivary hormone test can also be used to monitor your levels during treatment, enabling you to adjust your dosage as needed. For the test, all you have to do is collect samples of your saliva in the morning and send them to a laboratory for analysis of their hormonal content.

For **laboratories that perform the salivary hormone test** for non-medical individuals, contact: Aeron LifeCycles, 1933 Davis Street, Suite 310, San Leandro, CA 9577; tel: 800-631-7900 or 510-729-0375; fax: 510-729-0383. Diagnos-Techs, Inc., 6620 South 192nd Place, J-104, Kent, WA 98032; tel: 800-878-3787 or 425-251-0596; fax: 425-251-0637.

can therefore result in irregular effects on mood and energy.

Natural progesterone in any form does not produce the mood changes and more serious side effects associated with synthetic progesterone (such as Provera and other progestins) which is prescribed in conventional medicine for osteoporosis prevention and sometimes in hormone replacement therapy to offset the cancer-causing effects of synthetic estrogen.

Derived from sterols (a group of substances related to fats) found in wild yams, natural progesterone does not have the side effects because "it is virtually the same molecule as the progesterone the body makes," states Dr. John Lee. By contrast, the synthetic progestin has additional chemical groups that change its shape. The danger is that cells that bind progesterone accept the false progesterone, but it cannot function properly, Dr. Lee explains.

For example, with natural progesterone, sodium stays outside cells where it belongs. With progestin, sodium moves into the cells and brings water along with it; the result can be water retention and high blood pressure. This is only one of many dysfunctions associated with synthetic progesterone.[89]

The safety of natural progesterone has been confirmed by extensive testing at Vanderbilt University under Joel Hargrove, M.D., Department of Obstetrics and Gynecology.[90] Dr. Hargrove and his colleagues prescribe natural progesterone for premenstrual syndrome and as hormone replacement therapy for menopausal and postmenopausal women.

Dr. Lee has used natural progesterone in his medical practice with positive results since 1982. In a clinical trial of 100 of his patients, 38-83 years old, a treatment program of diet, nutritional supplementation, and natural progesterone cream was virtually 100% successful in building bone mass, reports Dr. Lee. "The average increase in bone mass was 15%. The bone status of women with relatively good initial BMD remained stable while the BMD of women with the lowest scores gained over 40%," he states. "Women with postmenopausal osteoporosis routinely showed true reversal of their disease, with significant improvement in bone mass and the virtual elimination of osteoporotic fractures."

The study also refuted the view that osteoporosis cannot be reversed in older women. Even women who went through menopause 25 years before the study measured a 10% to 15% increase in bone mineral density (BMD) after using natural progesterone cream, says Dr. Lee.[91]

Natural progesterone has the added benefit of helping to prevent breast cancer, says Dr. Lee. In studies of several thousand women followed over 18 years, "those who had a good, high-normal progesterone level had only one-tenth the amount of cancer as those who had low progesterone levels during their years of having normal periods," he observes. "They also had 5.4 times less breast cancer. So over 80% of the breast cancers were prevented if the progesterone levels were at a good, normal level."[92]

Dr. Lee's typical recommended dose for natural progesterone is one ounce of 3% cream per month. At bedtime, apply about ¼ teaspoon to soft tissue skin such as on the thighs, stomach, breasts, and inside the upper arms, alternating the sites of application; do this nightly for two to three weeks of your monthly cycle (the two weeks before your period if still menstruating; three weeks if postmenopausal).

To ensure that treatment is resulting in proper hormone levels, you might want to get a simple hormone test (see "Testing Your Hormone Levels," p. 148).

Natural progesterone cream is available at health food stores. For one brand, ProGest, contact: Transitions for Health, 621 S.W. Alder Street, Suite 900, Portland, OR 97205; tel: 800-888-6814 or 503-226-1010; fax: 800-044-2495. For the name of **a physician in your area who is knowledgeable about natural hormones**, contact: American College for Advancement in Medicine, 23121 Verdugo Drive, Suite 204, Laguna Hills, CA 92653; tel: 800-532-3688 or 949-583-7666; fax: 949-455-9769.

For more about **synthetic hormones**, see "Read This Before You Agree to HRT," pp. 134-135. For more about **progesterone**, see this chapter, pp. 133-136, and Chapter 1: Fibrocystic Breast Disease, pp. 39-42. For a **list of natural progesterone products**, see Chapter 1: Fibrocystic Breast Disease, pp. 40-41.

Nutritional Supplements

When most people think of nutritional supplements for bone health, they think of calcium. However, as discussed earlier, numerous other nutrients are essential to keep your bones healthy, particularly magnesium, boron, phosphorus, silica, zinc, manganese, copper, folic acid, and vitamins D, C, B6, and K. Dr. Alan Gaby notes that the recommended daily allowance (RDA) for most of these nutrients is too low. "Because of genetic factors, combined with the effects of stress and environmental pollution, some individuals may need more than the RDA for particular nutrients to achieve optimal bone health," he says.[93]

Keep in mind as you read this section that nutritional supplementation is most effective when it is tailored to the individual. In addition, the complex interaction of nutrients makes taking supplements a delicate balancing act to ensure optimal absorption and to avoid creating further imbalances. For these reasons and especially in the case of a serious disease such as osteoporosis, it is best to consult a qualified health-care practitioner to determine your exact nutritional status. The dosages presented here are merely rough guidelines and may not be applicable to everyone.

Calcium—For the reasons cited throughout this chapter, even if your diet has enough calcium, you could be calcium deficient and supplementation may be advisable. There are several types of calcium supplements, the most common being calcium carbonate. Michael T. Murray, N.D., of Bellevue, Washington, a prominent natural health author and teacher, prefers the more soluble forms—calcium citrate, calcium lactate, and calcium aspartate.

Honora Lee Wolfe, Dipl. Ac., of Boulder, Colorado, usually recommends taking a supplement of natural microcrystalline calcium hydroxyapatite complex (MCHC), which is a compound of calcium, phosphorus, magnesium, and fluoride in amounts equal to the normal physiological proportions found in bone. MCHC, available through health-care practitioners, has been found to not only halt bone loss but also to restore bone mass in cases of osteoporosis.[94]

Ralph Golan, M.D., of Seattle, Washington, concurs in the compound supplement approach. He generally recommends balanced bone nutrient supplements (i.e., not just calcium alone) such as Osteoprime Forte (two capsules twice a day) or Osteoporosis Formula (three capsules, three times daily).[95] However, the daily dosage of calcium he advises is 800 mg.[96] The National Institutes of Health places the dosage higher: at 1,000 mg daily for premenopaual women (ages 25 to 50); 1,500 mg daily for postmenopausal women not on estrogen drugs and for women over 65; and 1,000 mg daily for postmenopausal women taking estrogen.[97] Dr. Susan Brown often recommends a daily dosage of 1,000-1,500 mg.

Dr. Nancy Appleton cautions about possible side effects associated with calcium supplementation. "Excess calcium can be redistributed in the body, and is often deposited in soft tissues, possibly causing arthritis, arteriosclerosis, glaucoma, kidney stones, and other problems," she says. "Excess calcium can also imbalance stores of other minerals in the body."[98]

Dr. Werbach agrees that calcium supplementation should be done with care and offers the following guidelines and cautionary notes:[99]

■ **Bioavailability.** This term indicates the body's ability to process, absorb, retain, and use a nutrient from a dietary or supplemental source. If you are taking a calcium supplement, the most efficient absorption typically occurs in individual doses of 500 mg or less; late evening is the most effective absorption time. Taking a calcium supplement with foods increases your absorption by 10%. You are also likely to absorb more calcium if you take vitamin D concurrently. Calcium in a whole-bone extract tends to be better absorbed than simple calcium salts. Of calcium salts, calcium citrate appears to be among the most bioavailable, but caution is advised, because calcium citrate can increase your absorption of dietary aluminum.

■ **General cautions.** Keep your calcium-to-phosphorus intake at a ratio of less than 2:1 to avoid an excess of calcium which can cause reduced bone strength. Consuming calcium in excess of 2 g daily can make your parathyroid gland (located in the throat and concerned with calcium metabolism) overactive. Calcium also needs to be maintained in ratio to magnesium.

> ## Vitamin C is Bone-Friendly
>
> Long-term vitamin C supplementation can increase bone mineral density. A study of 1,892 women found that those between the ages of 55 and 64 who had not been on estrogen replacement therapy and who took vitamin C supplements for ten years or longer had a higher bone mineral density (BMD) than women in the same age group who took no supplements. The researchers observed that dietary intake of vitamin C seemed to have no effect on BMD.[100]

If you are a woman taking estrogen and have a low magnesium intake, calcium supplementation may increase your risk of thrombosis (blood clotting that can lead to a heart attack). Calcium carbonate, such as from ground oyster shells, can produce constipation. Calcium supplements, especially from natural materials (such as limestone rock) may contain toxic metals such as lead. In one study of 70 different brands, 25% exceeded lead safety levels, while a second study of one brand of dolomite (a calcium-magnesium compound found in limestone) revealed higher than desirable levels of aluminum, arsenic, cadmium, and lead.

Dr. Susan Brown's
Anti-Osteoporosis Supplement Program

Susan Brown, M.D., generally recommends the following bone nutrients to help prevent and reverse osteoporosis:[102]

- Calcium: builds healthy bones (1,000-1,500 mg daily)
- Magnesium: helps regulate calcium metabolism (450 mg daily)
- Boron: helps regulate calcium, magnesium, and phosphorus metabolism (no more than 3 mg daily)
- Copper: aids in bone formation (1.5-3 mg daily)
- Manganese: needed for bone cartilage and collagen (3.5-7 mg daily)
- Phosphorus: combines with calcium to form essential bone mineral salt (1-to-1 ratio with calcium)
- Silica: needed for bone collagen (no established rate, possibly 20-30 mg daily)
- Zinc: necessary for osteoblast and osteoclast formation and helps manufacture collagen matrix that holds bones together (12 mg daily)
- Vitamin A: helps increase osteoblasts, the bone-building cells (4,000-5,000 IU daily)
- Vitamin B6: necessary for hydrochloric acid production, which is required for calcium absorption (2 mg daily)
- Vitamin B12: required by bone-building cells to maintain optimum functioning (2-3 mcg daily)
- Folic acid: detoxifies homocysteine, a substance that can cause osteoporosis (400 mcg daily)
- Vitamin C: helps form bone collagen (250-2,000 mg daily)
- Vitamin D: essential for calcium absorption (200 IU daily)
- Vitamin K: required to manufacture the bone protein matrix (70-140 mcg daily)
- Protein: builds bones and needed to absorb calcium (44 g daily)
- Essential fatty acids: help bone structure and development (omega-3s and omega-6s, dosages vary per individual)

Magnesium—Women with osteoporosis have lower than average dietary intake and bone levels of magnesium. Magnesium deficiency can compromise calcium metabolism and hinder the body's production of vitamin D, further weakening bones. According to one study, postmenopausal women with osteoporosis were able to halt further bone loss by taking 250-750 mg of magnesium daily for two years; of these women, 8% experienced a net increase in bone density. Another study showed that by taking magnesium lactate (1,500-3,000 mg daily for two years), 65% of the women were completely free of pain and had no further degeneration of spinal vertebrae.[101]

Dr. Gaby usually recommends 200-600 mg daily and Dr. Brown 450 mg daily.

Boron—This trace mineral helps to regulate calcium, magnesium, and phosphorus metabolism. "Boron helps in the conversion of vitamin D to its active form, which is necessary for the absorption of calcium," says Dr. Murray. He notes that although 5 mg of boron daily is the optimum intake, the average American is only consuming 1 mg to 3 mg. Whole plant foods (whole grains, nuts, seeds, fruits, and vegetables) are good sources of boron. Dr. Brown recommends no more than 3 mg daily.

Additional Supplements—Zinc and copper have a particular relationship to hormones. This makes maintaining the proper levels and ratios of these two minerals important during perimenopause and menopause when hormone levels change and osteoporosis becomes of special concern. A healthy ratio is 8 (zinc) to 1 (copper), according to nutrition specialist Ann Louise Gittleman, M.S., C.N.S.

However, in estrogen-dominant women (meaning an excess of estrogen in relation to progesterone), the ratio can be as high as 25 (copper) to 1 (zinc), she says. Zinc levels tend to rise and fall with progesterone while copper goes up and down with estrogen. In general, explains Gittleman, women in perimenopause tend to be copper-heavy and zinc-deficient.

This supports the view of Dr. John Lee and others that progesterone deficiency rather than estrogen deficiency is the imbalance in perimenopause and menopause, and the hormonal factor in osteoporosis. Given that copper and zinc are important bone minerals, a skewed ratio has obvious implications for osteoporosis. Dr. Lee points out that zinc, like magnesium, is lost in grain refining, so the standard American diet is deficient in this important mineral.[103]

Dr. Brown often recommends 1.5 mg to 3 mg daily of copper and 12 mg daily of zinc. Again, to ensure that you are addressing your specific deficiencies and imbalances, it is best to base your supplementation on the results of a nutritional status test.

In addition to calcium, magnesium, boron, copper, zinc, manganese, silicon, folic acid, vitamin B6, vitamin C, vitamin D, and vitamin K, Dr. Gaby recommends strontium as an aid to bone strength and suggests a dosage of 0.5 mg to 3 mg daily.[104]

Herbal Medicine

Master herbalist Susun Weed of Woodstock, New York, has found

To contact **Susan Brown, Ph.D.**: Nutrition Education and Consulting Services, 605 Franklin Park Drive, East Syracuse, NY 13057; tel: 315-432-9231; fax: 315-463-7706. For information on **Osteoporosis Formula**: Enzymatic Therapy, 825 Challenger Drive, Green Bay, WI 54311-8328; tel: 800-783-2286 or 920-469-1313; fax: 920-469-4444.

Anti-Osteoporosis Formula From Brazil

A special algae found off the coast of Chile contains not only a highly absorbable form of calcium (oxide organic calcium, which is 90% absorbable compared to the 7%-8% of calcium carbonate and the 30%-40% of chelated calcium), but the minerals the body needs in order to utilize calcium as well.

"If we had spoken with God, and special ordered the algae, we could not have gotten a more perfect natural balance of bone-building nutrients and micronutrients," states Milton L. Brazzach, Ph.D., the researcher at the University of Sao Paulo, in Brazil, who headed the team that developed Osteoporex™, an anti-osteoporosis supplement containing the algae.

The Osteoporex formula also includes vitamin D from shark oil and the herbs zedoary and *Panax ginseng.* The vitamin D aids calcium's solidification into new bone mass. Zedoary (*Curcuma zedoaria*) is a plant long known to Asian medicine for its powerful anti-inflammatory properties; painful inflammation often accompanies osteoporosis. The saponin compounds in ginseng resemble hormones in structure and may therefore aid in calcium absorption and utilization, according to the researchers.

The result of this combination is a supplement that can help stop osteoporosis, increase bone mass, and relieve inflammation. In 300 treatment studies, taking Osteoporex resulted in significant bone mass increases in 95% of the patients. In the remaining 5%, their osteoporosis involved complications of cancer or other serious disease.

Bone mass increases occur much more quickly with Osteoporex than with conventional drugs—and without the side effects. Dr. Brazzach and his team of researchers reported increases as much as 3% in as little as three to six months. Osteoporex also has the advantage over conventional drugs in that it doesn't need to be taken every day for the rest of your life. The researchers recommend that in the first year, you take Osteoporex for about six months; after that, you may only need to take it for two to three months out of a year.[106]

For **Osteoporex**, contact: PI New Era Natural Products, 1491 South Miami Avenue, Miami, FL 33130; tel: 800-516-9796 or 305-379-5900; fax: 305-379-5611.

---

that herbal medicine (SEE QUICK DEFINITION) can enhance an osteoporosis prevention and treatment program. Here are some of the more helpful herbs she typically uses, which are particularly effective when combined with bone-promoting dietary and lifestyle changes, as discussed elsewhere in this chapter.[105]

■ Horsetail (*Equisetum arvense*): restores bone density; take as a daily tea made from dried herb or use the Bone Brew infusion below.

■ Dandelion root tincture: improves absorption of minerals by hydrochloric acid, ten to 15 drops before meals.

■ Bone Brew—calcium-rich infusion of three dried herbs: nettle (*Urtica dioica*), 1 tbsp; horsetail (*Equisetum arvense*), 1 tbsp; and sage (*Salvia officinalis*), 1 tbsp. Put the first two herbs in a quart container, crush, and then add the sage. Fill container with boiled water and close cap tightly. Let sit for a minimum of four hours. When ready, remove herbs and drink tea hot or cold. One cup of tea has as much calcium as a cup of milk, according to Weed.

Dr. Linda Ojeda generally suggests that certain herbs be incorporated into an osteoporosis prevention program because they have hormone-stimulating properties. As mentioned previously, progesterone builds bone and estrogen inhibits bone loss, so these herbs can contribute to bone health. Unlike synthetic hormone replacement therapy, they do so safely and gently. The herbs can be taken as supplements or teas. Dr. Ojeda cites the following herbs as estrogen-stimulating: black cohosh, alfalfa, hops, sweetbriar, horsetail, buckwheat, sage, rose, and shepherd's purse. Among the herbs she recommends to support progesterone are: wild yam, chastetree berry, sarsaparilla, and yarrow.[107]

The word "herb" as used in **herbal medicine** means a plant or plant part that is employed in medicine, food flavors (spices), or aromatic oils for soaps and fragrances. An herb can be a leaf, a flower, a stem, a seed, a root, a fruit, a bark or any other plant part used for its medicinal, food-flavoring, or fragrant property.

For **herbs used in the treatment of osteoporosis:** Gaia Garden Herbal Dispensary, 2672 West Broadway, Vancouver, BC, V6K 2G3 Canada; tel: 604-734-4372; fax: 604-734-4376.

For more information on **hormonal imbalances and the menstrual cycle**, see *Alternative Medicine Guide to Women's Health 1* (Future Medicine Publishing, 1998; ISBN 1-887299-12-2); to order, call 800-333-HEAL.

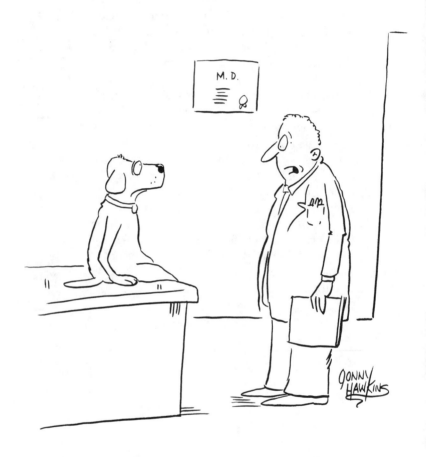

"*That's not the kind of bone loss we talk about.*"

More than 3 million people
in the U.S. and 90 million worldwide suffer
from chronic fatigue syndrome. However,
CFS and its close relatives—fibromyalgia and
environmental illness—can be successfully
turned around by treating the multiple
underlying causes which are often overlooked.

Chronic Fatigue Syndrome,

FIBROMYALGIA, AND ENVIRONMENTAL ILLNESS

WHEN THE FIRST CASES of chronic fatigue syndrome (CFS) were identified in the 1980s among patients in a small Nevada town, the strange disease—marked principally by deep fatigue and muscle aches—was dubbed "Yuppie flu." It seemed to be concentrated among young, affluent white professionals. Due to this and to the subjective nature of the symptoms, CFS was the butt of jokes and its sufferers were often not taken seriously, even by many physicians.

A decade later, CFS has become an epidemic and crossed all ethnic and demographic barriers. It is now recognized as a severe, debilitating illness, although the previously dismissive attitude persists in some doctors. Yet despite recognition of the disorder, conventional medicine still does not know what causes chronic fatigue syndrome—blaming it variously on the Epstein-Barr virus, candidiasis, and the herpes virus—and has no answers for treating it.

The Multiple Factors That Contribute to CFS

- Multiple infections (viruses, bacteria, candidiasis, parasites)
- Immune dysfunction
- Thyroid and hormonal problems
- Mercury toxicity
- Enzyme deficiencies
- Allergies
- Nutritional deficiencies
- Lifestyle issues (stress, psychological/emotional factors)

The CDC reports that 80% of diagnosed cases are women, the majority of whom are white and between the ages of 25 and 45. However, these figures reflect underreporting among nonwhite populations.[1] Meanwhile, the number of chronic fatigue cases continues to rise. The U.S. Centers for Disease Control (CDC) offers a typically conservative estimate of four to ten cases per 100,000 adults (or 10,440 to 26,100 Americans),[2] but other sources place the numbers much higher.

According to Murray R. Susser, M.D., of Santa Monica, California, chronic fatigue syndrome (also known as chronic fatigue and immune dysfunction syndrome, CFIDS) afflicts an estimated 3 million Americans and 90 million people worldwide. Jesse A. Stoff, M.D., co-author of *Chronic Fatigue Syndrome: The Hidden Epidemic* and director of Integrative Medicine for Integramed, in Tucson, Arizona, believes it is even more widespread, estimating that the number of people with CFS in North America alone exceeds by 4 million the number of people with AIDS.[3]

Alternative Medicine Therapies for CFS
■ Acupressure
■ Acupuncture
■ Anti-*Candida* treatment
■ Anti-parasite therapy
■ Applied kinesiology
■ Chelation therapy
■ Detoxification
■ Dietary recommendations
■ Enzyme therapy
■ Glandular extracts
■ Herbal medicine
■ Homeopathy
■ Immunomodulators
■ Magnet therapy
■ Massage therapy
■ Nutritional supplements
■ Nambudripad Allergy Elimination Technique (NAET)
■ Stress management

Closely Related Severe Chronic Fatigue States

Two close relatives of chronic fatigue syndrome—fibromyalgia and environmental illness—are also becoming more prevalent. Fibromyalgia (from "fibro," connective tissue, and "myalgia," muscle pain) is a painful muscle disorder in which the thin film or tissue (myofascia) holding muscle together becomes tightened or thickened, causing pain. Fibromyalgia, also called fibrositis, shares many of the same symptoms as CFS, including debilitating fatigue, muscle and joint pain, sleep disorders, depression, anxiety, mental confusion, and digestive problems.

Understanding the Basic Terms

CHRONIC FATIGUE SYNDROME (CFS) is an umbrella term for a multiple symptom disorder characterized most commonly by the sudden onset of extreme, debilitating fatigue, pain in the muscles and joints, headaches, and poor concentration. The fatigue is not alleviated by rest and results in a substantial reduction in previous levels of daily activity. CFS is often cyclical, with periods of relative health followed by debilitation. Other symptoms include depression, anxiety, digestive disorders, memory loss, allergies, recurring infections, and low-grade fever. According to the U.S. Centers for Disease Control, CFS predominantly affects white women, 25-45 years old.

FIBROMYALGIA is a multiple-symptom syndrome primarily involving widespread muscle pain (myalgia) which can be debilitating in its severity. The pain seems to be caused by the tightening and thickening of the myofascia, the thin film of tissue which holds the muscle together. Typical tender sites include the neck, upper back, rib cage, hips, and knees. Other symptoms include general fatigue and stiffness, insomnia and sleeping disorders, anxiety, depression, mood swings, allergies, carpal tunnel syndrome, headaches, the sense of "hurting all over," tender skin, numbness, irritable bowel symptoms, dizziness, and exercise intolerance. Post-traumatic fibromyalgia is believed to develop after a fall, whiplash, or back strain, whereas primary fibromyalgia has an uncertain origin. The majority of fibromyalgia sufferers are women between the ages of 34 and 56.

ENVIRONMENTAL ILLNESS is a multiple-symptom, debilitating, chronic disorder involving prolonged, heightened, and often incapacitating allergies or sensitivities to numerous common substances found in one's environment. Symptoms may include headaches, fatigue, muscle pain and/or weakness, coughing or wheezing, asthma, weight loss, infections, and emotional fluctuations, depression, and irritability. The illness is sometimes referred to as "20th century disease" because patients become allergic to and functionally incompatible with many products and substances found in the modern world, such as car exhaust, synthetic carpets, plywood and other building materials, cleaning agents, office machines, and plastics, among others.

Jacob Teitelbaum, M.D., a specialist in the two syndromes, calls CFS the "drop-dead" flu and fibromyalgia the "aching-all-over" disease. Given the similarity that these descriptive names embody, Dr. Teitelbaum prefers to put CFS and fibromyalgia in a single category he calls severe chronic fatigue states.[4] An estimated 3 million to 6 million Americans, 86% of whom are women, suffer from fibromyalgia. The level of disability caused by fibromyalgia is severe enough that 25.3% of women and 27% of men affected are unable to work, according to a recent study.[5]

The symptoms of environmental illness similarly overlap with those of CFS and fibromyalgia. Also known as multiple chemical sensitivity, the syndrome involves numerous and extensive allergies, often to nearly everything in one's environment and to such a degree that many sufferers must isolate themselves in their homes and avoid exposure to such commonplace items as chemically treated building materials, plastics, synthetic carpets, newsprint, perfume, soap, and car exhaust, to name a few. Since the sensitivities seem to be focused on (although not limited to) manufactured products, many people view environmental illness as a response to the increasing level of toxins in our environment.

Some practitioners believe that environmental illness is an extreme extension or outcome of prolonged chronic fatigue syndrome. Shari Lieberman, Ph.D., C.N.S., a nutritional specialist based in New York City, is among them. She has treated several hundred people with chronic fatigue syndrome to date and reports: "I see patients with environmental sensitivities who have come to me after three to five years of chronic fatigue. If they've only had CFS for six months, they don't tend to have environmental sensitivities."

Multiple Causes Require Layers of Treatment

Symptoms of CFS

allergies
anxiety
brain fog and confusion
cough
decreased appetite
depression
digestive disorders
dizziness
dry eyes and mouth
general stiffness
headaches
increased thirst
irritability
joint and muscle pain
low body temperature
low-grade fever
memory loss
muscle weakness
nausea
night sweats
PMS (women)
poor concentration
prolonged fatigue after exertion
rashes
recurring infections
severe fatigue
sleep problems
sore throat
swollen lymph nodes
visual blurring

The alternative medicine view is that CFS, fibromyalgia, and environmental illness share the same cluster of underlying causes. Therefore, the information about chronic fatigue syndrome in this

Symptoms of Fibromyalgia

allergies

anxiety

carpal tunnel syndrome

depression

dizziness

dry eyes alternating with watery eyes

dysmenorrhea (women)

exercise intolerance

fingernail ridges

general fatigue

general stiffness

headaches

heightened sensitivity to light, sound, smell, touch ("irritable everything syndrome")

"hurting all over"

irritability

irritable bowel symptoms

mood swings

numbness or tingling sensations

sensitivity to cold

sleeping disorders

tender skin

widespread muscle and joint pain

chapter is equally useful if you are suffering from one of the other disorders. The first point to understand in order to effectively treat any of the three syndromes is that, as with breast cancer discussed in Chapter 2, there is no *one* underlying cause. Multiple causes combine to overload the body and produce the breakdown known as CFS or one of its relatives.

Alternative medicine physicians regard the conventional medicine approach of seeking a single CFS cause, such as a virus, as misguided. Dr. Leon Chaitow, N.D., D.O., of London, England, is one of these physicians, believing strongly that CFS is and must be treated as a multi-causal condition. He describes it as "similar to an onion in which each peeled layer reveals another layer, or symptomatic factor, underneath. Focus on immune function would be more beneficial than focus on the virus, which is simply taking advantage of the situation," Dr. Chaitow observes. The multiple causes of the three syndromes and, therefore, the necessity for a combination of treatment methods make these disorders ideal candidates for alternative medicine's multimodal approach to healing.

Treating the Individual

The second important point to understand about CFS is that no two people with the disorder have exactly the same causal factors. Treatment must therefore be tailored to each patient. Misdiagnosis and failure to address individual factors are common and create additional pain and frustration, which could likely have been avoided by an individualized approach to the patient. Treating each person as unique is a hallmark of alternative medicine.

The following case illustrates both the multi-causal nature of CFS (and environmental illness) and how vital the individualized approach is in unraveling the complexities of the syndrome and designing an effective treatment program. It also features a number of the underlying causes which are discussed in more detail later in this chapter.

Success Story: Reversing CFS and Environmental Illness

Millicent, 33, poses an all too common case of a person with entrenched, debilitating symptoms who consulted many doctors and ended up trusting none—that is, until she met Constantine A. Kotsanis, M.D., medical director of the MindBody Health Center International, in Grapevine, Texas. Millicent had a long history of chronic conditions, including fatigue, sinusitis, multiple infections, bronchitis, and pain, none of which were improved by repeated rounds of antibiotics or any other drugs or therapies offered.

At one point in her two years of "bouncing around" among physicians, Millicent went to a clinic specializing in environmental medicine. They tested her for allergies to multiple substances and determined that she was reactive to certain chemicals. Millicent received allergy desensitization injections, nutritional supplements, saunas, and dietary advice, but rather than experiencing improvement, her condition continued to deteriorate. She fit the classification of both CFS and environmental illness.

When Millicent first consulted Dr. Kotsanis, she was debilitated to the point that she could no longer maintain her former high-stress, demanding job and felt more ill when she left her house. She couldn't sleep at night, but often fell asleep during the daylight hours. She was highly frustrated and a bit despondent about the seeming intractability of her condition, says Dr. Kotsanis. "The core of her problem was a breakdown of her immune system," he says. "It had become hyperactive trying to deal with the multiple infections

Symptoms of Environmental Illness

allergies (multiple)
anxiety
asthma
coughing or wheezing
depression
digestive problems
fatigue
headaches
infections
irritability
mood swings
multiple chemical sensitivities
muscle pain and/or weakness
weight loss

What is CFS, According to the U.S. Centers for Disease Control?

In March of 1988, the U.S. Centers for Disease Control (CDC) released criteria for a diagnosis of CFS, which it revised in 1994 to encompass the broader symptom spectrum of those afflicted. In order to be diagnosed with CFS, a person has to be suffering from:

1) New, unexplained, persistent or relapsing chronic fatigue which is not a consequence of exertion, not resolved by bed rest, and severe enough to significantly reduce previous daily activity

2) Four or more of the symptoms below for at least six months:

- unexplained or new headaches
- short-term memory or concentration impairment
- muscle pain
- pain in multiple joints unaccompanied by redness or swelling
- unrefreshing sleep
- post-exertion malaise which lasts for longer than 24 hours
- sore throat
- tender lymph nodes in the neck or armpits

and allergies; then the antibiotics injured her digestive system and this contributed to her fatigue." A newlywed, Millicent had lost all interest in sex as a consequence of her illness and her marriage was at risk. "She was in a state of hopelessness—a young woman with no hope, no desire to do anything."

Detoxifying the Body

Initially, Millicent "tested" Dr. Kotsanis by agreeing to some acupuncture treatment. Millicent soon moved away, however, and did not return to the area for a year. Feeling only marginally better than when she left, Millicent again sought Dr. Kotsanis' help. Calling on the services of a consulting acupuncturist, Dr. Kotsanis had Millicent tested for heavy metal toxicity; he was concerned about the potential mercury leakage from her eight amalgam dental fillings. The acupuncturist, using electrodermal screening (see p. 169), determined that Millicent did have significant toxicity in her body owing to mercury leakage. An analysis of Millicent's urine confirmed the mercury diagnosis.

Over the next six months, Millicent had her mercury fillings (SEE QUICK DEFINITION) carefully removed. To assure the elimination of mercury residues from her body once the fillings were out, Millicent underwent chelation therapy which involved infusions of a special nontoxic chemical called DMPS (SEE QUICK DEFINITION) to chelate, or bind up, the heavy metal and prepare it for excretion from the body. After six DMPS infusions over a space of three months, Dr. Kotsanis assessed that the mercury had been removed from her body. Prior to the DMPS infusions, Millicent had worn a surgical mask all the time to filter out allergens and toxic materials from the air she breathed. She no longer required this mask once the mercury toxicity was eliminated, Dr. Kotsanis notes.

Concurrent with administering the DMPS, Dr. Kotsanis made nutritional and dietary recommendations for Millicent. These included flaxseed oil (two tablespoons daily); extra virgin olive oil (for cooking and in salads) to help the liver; raw flaxseeds (two teaspoons daily); organic foods; lean meats, such as organically raised chicken, venison, or lamb; and less common grains such as quinoa, amaranth, and teff.

The more common grains, such as wheat and corn as well as soybeans, have been far too genetically manipulated and, in Dr. Kotsanis' view, are best avoided by the chronically ill. Millicent was also instructed to avoid dairy products, red meats (due to antibiotic-hormonal residues), and fish (due to potential mercury contamination). Organic brown rice and oats were acceptable; the consumption of $^3/_4$-1 gallon of pure water every day was advised to help her system flush out toxins.

As a further aid in detoxifying, Dr. Kotsanis prescribed three products from Metagenics, taken in sequence: UltraClear-Plus, UltraClear, and UltraClear-Sustain. These were taken in powder form, at the rate of two scoops daily, mixed with juice or water. To complement this daily regimen, Millicent took Metagenic's multivitamin (without iron) in a dosage of one tablet, two times daily. "Nutritional problems account for perhaps 50% of the problem in patients with chronic disease," says Dr. Kotsanis.

Emotional Detoxification

But Millicent still had discomfort and fatigue, and was subject to bouts of crying and serious depression. "Millicent was steadily getting better, but still dragging herself around. She was going through a lot of emotional distress," says Dr. Kotsanis. "I decided she should do some emotional detoxification because everyone who has a chronic disease needs this." To Dr. Kotsanis, it is not only important to detoxify the internal organs, such as

QUICK DEFINITION

Mercury fillings, or amalgams, have been used in dentistry since the 1820s, but not until 1988 did the routine use of mercury raise serious enough questions for the Environmental Protection Agency (EPA) to declare scrap dental amalgam a *hazardous waste*. Evidence now shows that mercury amalgams are the *major* source of mercury exposure for the general public, at rates six times higher than those found in fish and seafood. Studies by the World Health Organization show that eight amalgams in a single mouth can release 3-17 mcg of mercury per day, making dental amalgam a major source of mercury exposure. A Danish study of a random sample of 100 men and 100 women showed that increased blood mercury levels were related to the presence of more than four amalgam fillings in the teeth. Mercury toxicity has been shown to have destructive contributory effects on kidney function and in cardiovascular disease, neuropsychological dysfunction, reproductive disorders, and birth defects, to name a few. Symptoms of mercury toxicity make a very long list: anorexia, depression, fatigue, insomnia, arthritis, multiple sclerosis, moodiness, irritability, memory loss, nausea, diarrhea, gum disease, swollen glands, headaches, and many more.

DMPS (2,3-dimercapto-propane-1-sulfonate) is the chelating (binding-up) agent of choice for the removal of elemental mercury from the human body. It can be given orally, intravenously, or intramuscularly, and is useful for people who have been exposed to mercury amalgam through their dental fillings, or for those who show evidence or suspicion of heavy metal toxicity from other sources.

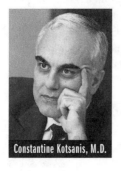

Constantine Kotsanis, M.D.

To Dr. Kotsanis, it is not only important to detoxify the internal organs, such as the liver, pancreas, and intestines, of toxic materials, but also to purge the emotions of buried pain, grief, and unresolved trauma to achieve a lasting cure.

To contact
Constantine A. Kotsanis, M.D.:
MindBody Health Center International, Baylor Medical Plaza, 1600 West College Street, Suite 260, Grapevine, TX 76051; tel: 817-481-3131; fax: 817-488-8903. For **UltraClear-Plus, UltraClear, Sustain,** and **UltraFlora Plus,** contact: Metagenics West, Inc., 12445 East 39th Avenue, Suite 402, Denver, CO 80239; tel: 800-321-6382 or 303-371-6848; fax: 303-371-9303. For the **Adrenal Stress Index saliva test,** contact: Diagnos-Tech, Inc., 6620 South 192nd Place, J-104, Kent, WA 98032; tel: 800-878-3787 or 425-251-0596; fax: 425-251-0637. For **phosphatidylserine Phos-serine,** contact: Thorne Research, P.O. Box 3200, Sandpoint, ID 83864; tel: 800-228-1966 or 208-263-1337; fax: 208-265-2488.

the liver, pancreas, and intestines, of toxic materials, but also to purge the emotions of buried pain, grief, and unresolved trauma to achieve a lasting cure.

Dr. Kotsanis worked with psychologist Stephen Vasquez, Ph.D., of Bedford, Texas, who employs a combination of skillful psychological questioning and a form of strobic light therapy to elicit buried emotions. Up to 12 different colored lights are emitted from a device and, after being registered by the eyes, can provoke emotional reactions from a patient. As the lights provoke emotional memories, the patient regressing slowly backwards in time, the psychologist asks them questions about their condition.

In Millicent's case, says Dr. Kotsanis, it was revealed that, as a child, she was treated like a soldier by her father, a military man, and she felt abandoned by her mother who suffered from a terrible illness. Millicent said also that she had been sexually abused by relatives. As an adult, she married a man much like her authoritative father.

"These difficult emotional memories can contribute to an already debilitating condition and need to be acknowledged by the patient," says Dr. Kotsanis. "The light therapy approach allows your brain to regress to the point where the affliction formed," he adds. "Once you re-live the original problem, you completely cleanse yourself of it." Typically, there are 15 color treatments, lasting one hour daily, five days per week. "What psychotherapy takes three years to achieve, this approach can produce in three weeks," Dr. Kotsanis says. The light therapy moved Millicent a couple of steps closer to recovery, he adds.

Correcting Hormonal Imbalance

After these treatments—mercury amalgam removal, DMPS chelation, dietary changes, nutritional supplements, detoxification, and light therapy—Millicent was about 60% improved. To complete the recovery, Dr. Kotsanis analyzed Millicent's hormone levels. Using a saliva test called Adrenal Stress Index (ASI), Dr. Kotsanis was able to examine the rhythm and secretory activity of Millicent's adrenal glands. He learned that Millicent's cortisol levels (an adrenal gland secretion indicative of stress) were exceptionally high, which is often the case in CFS. This meant her adrenal glands were virtually exhausted; hence, her chronic fatigue. In addition, Dr. Kotsanis determined that Millicent's thyroid was mildly underactive, a condition called hypothyroidism (SEE QUICK DEFINITION) characterized by many of Millicent's symptoms.

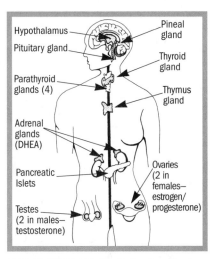

THE ENDOCRINE SYSTEM. Endocrine glands, including the testicles, ovaries, pancreas, adrenals, thyroid, parathyroid, and pituitary, are central to the regulation and normalization of all the body's complex, interconnected systems, from metabolism and heat production to spermatogenesis and uterine preparations for pregnancy.

Instead of supplementing the adrenal glands or thyroid, Dr. Kotsanis prescribed a formula that would correct the balance of brain chemicals (neurotransmitters) that directly affect the adrenal glands. He had Millicent take a formula (three times daily) containing brain nutrients, such as phosphatidylserine and phosphatidylcholine (both derived from lecithin). Dr. Kotsanis says that had he attempted to correct the brain chemical axis controlling the adrenal glands before removing Millicent's mercury fillings and flushing out residual mercury with DMPS, it would have failed. "The adrenal glands and most of the endocrine system would have been shut down by the mercury," he explains.

After ten days on this supplement, the brain chemicals in effect realigned themselves and "her whole life turned around—Millicent's energy level skyrocketed," reports Dr. Kotsanis. "She was happy and began telling everyone how wonderful she felt." Millicent's self-esteem soared, her vitality returned to normal, and for the first time in many months, she was glad that she was alive again. Her sex drive, absent for years, returned. Typically this is the last to return when you are chronically ill, according to Dr. Kotsanis. Millicent's husband was delighted. "I have my wife back," he told people. About one month later, Millicent became pregnant and felt herself to be "the happiest woman in town."

This case illustrates Dr. Kotsanis' principle of illness causation and health restoration. "Many factors in Millicent's life led to a gradual breakdown of her immune system. To reverse this, you must clean out the system starting with the basics: clean the colon, liver, and spleen; remove the heavy metals and toxins; resolve the emotional issues; and put the good nutrition back."

It is "extremely essential," says Dr. Kotsanis, to know how the body's detoxification system works. You also must understand that if the immune system is perpetually occupied with inflammation, allergies, and detoxification, it will not have the time or resources to do anything else, such as promote a lasting recovery. Dr. Kotsanis cautions that it's prudent to expect lasting recovery from a complex case of chronic fatigue syndrome to take at least nine to 12 months.

Diagnosing CFS and Its Causes

Millicent's case clearly demonstrates the complexity that characterizes CFS, making diagnosis and treatment complex as well. Getting a clear picture of an individual's CFS is often difficult due to the tendency of symptoms to fluctuate in degree and severity, not only over a period of weeks or months, but even from day to day. A cyclical pattern of illness and reasonable health is the result.

Frequently, after a severe bout of CFS, a patient resumes normal activity and exercise, only to relapse into extreme fatigue after a period of time. But if a number of CFS symptoms persist for six months (see "What is CFS, According to the U.S. Centers for Disease Control," p. 164) and other causes have been eliminated, it is considered likely that the person has CFS.[6]

However, alternative medicine physicians are less focused on getting a definitive diagnosis of CFS than they are in gathering as much information as possible on the underlying causes that are producing the patient's symptoms. Without determining precisely what is happening in the patient's body, treatment is guesswork. A careful medical history, a physical examination, and selected laboratory tests can pinpoint the imbalances, deficiencies, infectious agents, and specific immune system weaknesses which are contributing to your CFS and provide the physician with an inventory of the pattern of symptoms.

Most of the testing involves simple blood, urine, and stool analyses, but your conventional doctor may not be aware of the specific parameters to investigate. The following section on the causes of CFS can serve as a guideline for testing; these factors are often present in the syndrome and should be investigated in the individual case as symptoms warrant.

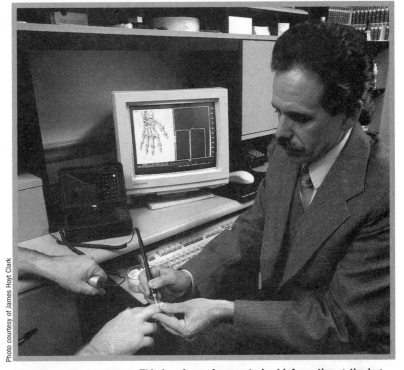

Photo courtesy of James Hoyt Clark

ELECTRODERMAL SCREENING. This is a form of computerized information gathering which is based on physics, not chemistry. A blunt, noninvasive electric probe is placed at specific points on the patient's hands, face, or feet, corresponding to acupuncture points at the beginning or end of energy meridians. Minute electrical discharges from these points serve as information signals about the condition of the body's organs and systems, useful for the physician in evaluation and developing a treatment plan.

In addition to blood, urine, and stool analyses, electrodermal screening is a quick method to identify most of these factors, especially those involving toxic (as illustrated in the case of Millicent) or allergic substances. The normal waiting period of laboratory analysis is avoided through the immediate feedback provided by this computerized testing of the body's organs and systems via acupuncture points. As a cross-reference, specific blood, urine, and stool analyses can then be ordered to serve as confirmation of electrodermal results.

By quickly pinpointing problems, EDS can prevent unnecessary, guesswork testing. For example, if EDS indicates that a person has a specific type of parasite, running a stool analysis for that parasite eliminates the trial and error of the often long process of testing to see if parasites, in general, are a problem. EDS can also be helpful in determining the body's tolerance to medications or remedies which may be prescribed.

Eight Causes of CFS and How to Treat Them

For more about **electrodermal screening**, contact: James Hoyt Clark, Biosource Inc., 1388 West Center Street, Orem, UT 84057; tel: 801-226-1117.

Candida albicans is a yeast-like fungus found widely in nature, in the soil, on vegetables and fruits, and in the human body. It is frequently present in small quantities in the intestines and in a woman's vagina. When its numbers are few, *Candida* is generally not harmful to the human body. A *Candida* overgrowth, a condition called **candidiasis**, can become pathogenic and cause allergic reations throughout the body. These reactions can lead to a wide range of symptoms, including depression, fatigue, weight gain, anxiety, rashes, headaches, and muscle cramping.

As a syndrome, CFS is an array of symptoms which may appear unrelated, but which, according to alternative medicine, are all products of an underlying imbalance in the body produced by multiple simultaneous infections and accompanying physical, mental, and environmental factors.

The eight underlying causes (multiple infections, immune dysfunction, thyroid and hormonal problems, mercury toxicity, enzyme deficiencies, allergies, nutritional deficiencies, and lifestyle issues) covered in this chapter are those most often present—in various combinations and to varying degrees—in CFS patients. As discussed earlier and evidenced in the case of Millicent, it is usually a combination of these factors that produce CFS. Included in the discussion of each cause is information on testing and alternative medicine treatment methods.

1) Multiple Infections

Viruses, candidiasis (SEE QUICK DEFINITION), bacterial infections, and/or intestinal parasites (SEE QUICK DEFINITION) are often factors in chronic fatigue syndrome. Whether these infections in combination are the cause of CFS or opportunistic invaders of an already weakened immune system has not been conclusively determined. In either case, compromised immunity is a central feature of the syndrome and the infections involved perpetuate and deepen immune dysfunction by further taxing an already overloaded system. "One infection puts demand on the immune system which can't kick it, and another infection may join in, leading from one to another in a domino effect," Dr. Murray Susser explains.

"The most common infections we find are yeast [*Candida albicans*] and parasites," reports Dr. Susser. "We also find hidden bacterial infections such as Lyme disease [*Borrelia burgdorferi*] and abscesses in the teeth and sometimes chronic sinusitis and chronic gastritis." Elevated levels of antibodies (SEE QUICK DEFINITION) to certain viruses are frequently found in the blood of CFS patients. These include Epstein-Barr, cytomegalovirus, human herpes virus–6, herpes simplex, rubella, and Coxsackie.

The damage caused by parasites in particular can be quite extensive. Parasites can destroy cells faster than they can be regenerated; they can release toxins that damage tissues, resulting in pain and inflammation; and, over time, they can depress, even exhaust, the immune system.

Testing for Multiple Infections

In addition to electrodermal screening (see pp. 169-170), the following tests are useful in determining if you have a viral or bacterial infection, candidiasis, and/or intestinal parasites.

The Anti-Candida Antibodies Panel—Candidiasis can be determined by stool or blood analysis. One blood test, called the Anti-Candida Antibodies Panel, measures the levels of the IgG and IgM antibodies against *Candida*; the IgG levels indicate both past and ongoing infection, while the IgM may be a truer reflection of present infection.

The Comprehensive Digestive Stool Analysis—Conducted by Great Smokies Diagnostic Laboratory, in Asheville, North Carolina, this test provides useful indications of general parasitic activity. In addition to parasites, this stool analysis can identify many other intestinal factors that may be play-

QUICK DEFINITION

A **parasite** is any organism that lives off another organism (called a host), and draws nourishment from it. Specifically, parasites are the protozoa (single-cell organisms), arthropods (insects), and worms that infect the body and cause serious damage to tissues and organs. Common forms of the protozoan parasites are *Giardia lamblia*, which causes giardiasis; *Entamoeba histolytica*, which causes dysentery; and *Cryptosporidium*, which causes diarrhea, particularly in people with immunologic diseases such as AIDS. The most common arthropod parasites are lice, mites, ticks, and fleas. Worm parasites include pinworms, roundworms, tapeworms, *Trichinella spiralis* (worms usually acquired from eating tainted pork), hookworms, Guinea worms, and filaria (threadlike worms that inhabit the blood and tissues).

An **antibody** is a protein molecule containing about 20,000 atoms, made from amino acids by B-lymphocyte cells in the lymph tissue and set in motion by the immune system against a specific foreign protein, or antigen. An antibody is also referred to as an immunoglobulin and may be found in the blood, lymph, colostrum, saliva, and the gastrointestinal and urinary tracts, usually within three days after the first encounter with an antigen. The antibody binds tightly with the antigen as a preliminary for removing it from the system or destroying it.

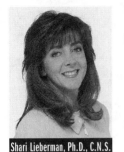

Shari Lieberman, Ph.D., C.N.S.

Dr. Lieberman developed a multivitamin/ mineral formula which she uses as the basis of an antiviral, antibacterial nutritional supplement program for CFS patients. To date, she has treated several hundred people with CFS using this program.

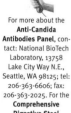

For more about the **Anti-Candida Antibodies Panel,** contact: National BioTech Laboratory, 13758 Lake City Way N.E., Seattle, WA 98125; tel: 206-363-6606; fax: 206-363-2025. For the **Comprehensive Digestive Stool Analysis,** contact: Great Smokies Diagnostic Laboratory, 63 Zillicoa Street, Asheville, NC 28801; tel: 800-522-4762 or 704-253-0621; fax: 704-252-9303.

ing a role in your illness. Problems that begin in the intestines have far-reaching effects on the body and can contribute to the development of serious illnesses. Digestive problems, such as diarrhea, constipation, irritable bowel syndrome, bloating, gas, or indigestion, are usually part of the symptom picture in CFS, fibromyalgia, and environmental illness.

Treating Multiple Infections

Alternative medicine physicians usually employ a two-pronged approach to treating the infections associated with chronic fatigue syndrome. One, they strengthen the immune system (see pp. 178-180) and thus bolster the body's own defense mechanisms against disease-producing microorganisms; and two, they address the infection directly, via parasite and candidiasis elimination programs and antimicrobial agents to reduce the viral and bacterial load on the body.

Useful antimicrobial herbs include echinacea, goldenseal, citrus seed extract, aloe vera, tea tree oil, and pau d'arco bark (from a Brazilian tree). Lita Lee, Ph.D., an enzyme therapist in Lowell, Oregon, cites coconut oil as well. In addition to its antiviral properties, it also promotes thyroid function, regulates blood sugar, and protects mitochondria (the cells' energy "factories") against stress injuries, says Dr. Lee.

An extract of shiitake mushroom called LEM (*Lentinus edodes mycelium*) is another potent agent, having been shown to inhibit viruses and stimulate the immune system.[7] *HealthWatch*, the newsletter of the CFIDS (chronic fatigue and immune dysfunction syndrome) Buyers Club, reports that LEM is the "all-time best-selling nutritional supplement used by CFIDS sufferers."[8]

An Antimicrobial Nutritional Program—Shari Lieberman, Ph.D.,

C.N.S., developed a multivitamin/mineral formula called Optimum Protection which she uses (at a dosage of four tablets daily) as the basis of an antiviral, antibacterial nutritional supplement program for CFS patients. Along with that formula, here are the other components of her program, with typical dosages (the components and dosages will vary, depending upon the individual):

■ Kyolic Premium EPA: a combination of garlic and fish oil (EPA or eicosapentaenoic acid, an omega-3 essential fatty acid); four capsules a day

■ Quercetin: a bioflavonoid (vitamin C helper) with antihistamine, anti-inflammatory, and antiviral properties; 1,000-1,500 mg per day

■ N-acetyl cysteine (NAC): an antiviral and amino acid precursor for the production of glutathione which reduces free radical (SEE QUICK DEFINITION) damage and prevents antioxidant (SEE QUICK DEFINITION) depletion; 500 mg twice a day

■ Glycyrrhizinate: an antiviral derived from licorice; two to three capsules daily or $1/2$ teaspoon of the gel form twice a day

■ Echinacea: an antimicrobial and immune stimulant; 30-50 drops of Echinaguard tincture (available in health food stores) once a day, in an ongoing cycle of four days on, four days off

■ Coenzyme Q10: an antioxidant; 100 mg once or twice daily

■ Maitake D-Fraction: an immune-enhancing extract of the maitake mushroom, used for viruses; mix tincture with Echinaguard at the same dosage, 30-50 drops once a day, four days on, four days off

■ *Acidophilus*: a beneficial bacteria to help restore intestinal balance; $1/2$ teaspoon of the powdered, refrigerated variety once or twice a day, mixed with water or juice or sprinkled on food

■ Aloe Vera: for gastrointestinal complaints; $1/4$ cup, twice daily (may need to start at low dosages and gradually build to the full amount)

■ Diet: avoid dairy, gluten (a vegetable protein found in wheat, rye, oats, and barley), fat, and sugar

A **free radical** is an unstable, toxic molecule of oxygen with an unpaired electron that steals an electron from another molecule and produces harmful effects. Free radicals are formed when molecules within cells react with oxygen (oxidize) as part of normal metabolic processes. Free radicals then begin to break down cells, especially the cell membranes, often in a matter of minutes to a hours. A single free radical can destroy a cell. Their work is enhanced if there are not enough free-radical quenching nutrients, such as vitamins C and E, in the cell. While free radicals are normal products of metabolism, uncontrolled free-radical production plays a major role in the development of degenerative disease, including cancer and heart disease. Free radicals harmfully alter important molecules, such as proteins, enzymes, fats, even DNA. Other sources of free radicals include pesticides, industrial pollutants, smoking, alcohol, viruses, most infections, allergies, stress, even certain foods and excessive exercise.

An **antioxidant** (meaning "against oxidation") is a natural biochemical substance that protects living cells against damage from harmful free radicals. Antioxidants work against the process of oxidation—the robbing of electrons from substances. If unblocked or left uncontrolled, oxidation can lead to cellular aging, degeneration, arthritis, heart disease, cancer, and other illnesses. Antioxidants in the body react readily with oxygen breakdown products and free radicals, and neutralize them before they can damage the body. Antioxidant nutrients include vitamins A, C, and E, beta carotene, selenium, coenzyme Q10, pycnogenol (grape seed extract), L-glutathione, superoxide dismutase, and bioflavonoids. Plant antioxidants include *Ginkgo biloba* and garlic. When antioxidants are taken in combination, the effect is stronger than when they are used individually.

Parasites can be fought with high-dosage probiotic substances such as *Lactobacillus acidophilus, Bifidobacterium bifidum,* and *Lactobacillus bulgaricus.*

Eliminating Candidiasis

Avoiding certain foods is important in a candidiasis treatment protocol. Yeast feeds on sugar, refined carbohydrates such as white flour, and fermented products such as vinegar and pickles. These foods should therefore be eliminated from your diet. Yeast-containing products, alcohol, coffee, and caffeinated tea are also to be avoided.

In addition to dietary changes, nutritional supplements can be effective in the treatment of candidiasis. James Braly, M.D., of Fort Lauderdale, Florida, offers the following regimen:

- Vitamin C (8-10 g daily)
- Vitamin E (one 400 IU capsule daily)
- Evening primrose oil (six to eight capsules daily)
- Essential fatty acids (omega-3 oil, 920 mg, and omega-6 oil, 460 mg, three times daily)
- Pantothenic acid (250 mg daily)
- Taurine (500-1,000 mg daily)
- Zinc chelate (25-50 mg daily)
- Goldenseal root extract with 5% hydrastine (250 mg twice a day)
- *Lactobacillus acidophilus* (one dry teaspoon, three times daily; if allergic to milk, use nonlactose *acidophilus*)

Dr. Braly recommends supplementation of hydrochloric acid (HCl). He notes that the aging process, alcohol abuse, food allergies, and nutrient deficiencies deplete HCl in the stomach, which prevents food from being digested and permits *Candida* overgrowth. HCl supplementation, he says, helps restore the proper balance of intestinal flora. Dr. Braly typically recommends one capsule of HCl and pepsin (a digestive acid in the stomach) at the start of meals, increasing cautiously to 2-4 capsules with each meal, if needed.

A general nutritional support program is frequently needed to correct nutritional deficiencies, build up depleted immune function, and reverse digestive inefficiency—all results of months or years of chronic candidiasis, according to Dr. Leon Chaitow. He usually recommends the following supplements (dosages will vary according to the individual):

- Individual B vitamins: increase antibody response and are used in nearly every body activity

■ Vitamin C: stimulates adrenaline and is essential to immune processes

■ Vitamin E: a lack depresses immune response

■ Vitamin A: builds resistance to infection and increases immune response

■ Beta carotene: a vitamin A precursor which increases T cells

■ Antioxidants such as selenium, calcium, and zinc: immune-boosters useful in combating candidiasis

■ Chromium, magnesium, and adrenal glandular extracts: stimulate adrenal function

■ Probiotic supplements: repopulate the intestines with "friendly" bacteria and correct the imbalance of flora created by *Candida* overgrowth

■ Essential fatty acids such as evening primrose oil: for healthy metabolism

Eliminating Parasites

If you know or suspect that you have intestinal parasites, certain dietary practices are recommended. It is advisable to eliminate all uncooked foods from your diet and cook all meats until well done; soak both organic and inorganic vegetables in salted water (one tablespoon per five cups) for a minimum of 30 minutes before cooking. It is also suggested that you avoid coffee, all sugars including fruits and honey, and all milk and dairy products, with the possible exception of raw goat's milk. Raw goat's milk contains secretory IgA and IgG (immunoglobulins), which help protect the intestinal lining from infectious agents. According to Steven Bailey, N.D., of Portland, Oregon, IgA and IgG have been found to be helpful in the treatment of parasites.

To treat parasitic infection, Dr. Chaitow advises pursuing a comprehensive supplement approach rather than medication. "In many cases, anti-parasitic prescriptive drugs have not proved to be lastingly effective," he points out. "They may diminish symptoms for one or two months, but the symptoms later return with full force." Parasites can be fought with high-dosage probiotic substances such as *Lactobacillus acidophilus, Bifidobacterium bifidum, and Lactobacillus bulgaricus.* Treatment may last from eight to 12 weeks. Dr. Chaitow reports an 80% success rate in cases of seriously ill people afflicted with parasites and yeast overgrowth using this method.

In addition, herbal remedies have been reported to be safe and effective for the treatment of parasitic infections. These remedies can

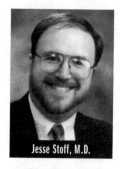

Jesse Stoff, M.D.

"It is essential to address both the structure *and* function of the immune system because a person's immune system can be structurally intact yet not functioning well," says Dr. Stoff. Dr. Stoff and other alternative physicians use tests to identify what immune areas are malfunctioning or weak and then to track treatment progress so necessary adjustments can be made.

also be used as a preventive measure against parasitic infection when water or food conditions are questionable:

■ Citrus seed extract: highly active against viruses, bacteria, yeast, and parasites; can be administered for up to several months, which may be required to eliminate *Giardia* and the candidiasis that often accompanies it

■ *Artemisia annua*: especially effective against *Giardia*; some caution is advisable because it can initially worsen symptoms or cause allergic reactions and some intestinal irritation; often prescribed with citrus seed extract

■ *Artemisia absinthium*: wormwood, used to expel worms; should be used in combination with other herbs to nullify its toxicity

According to Dr. Leo Galland, it is advisable to continue any treatment regimen until at least two parasitological tests, performed one month apart on "purged stool" specimens, are negative.

2) Immune Dysfunction

While infecting organisms, as described above, are frequent sources of chronic fatigue, a depleted immune system (SEE QUICK DEFINITION) is also a central feature in CFS. The immune system is the body's basic defensive system by which it resists infection and disease formation—it keeps the body immune from illness. In someone with CFS, the immune system has been operating at a constant, heightened level of activity for a prolonged period. Ironically, this heightened level of activity is marked by diminished competency; it seems to work harder, but it is actually incapacitated.

Testing for Immune Dysfunction

Even if you recognize that your immune system is deficient, it is necessary to identify the specifics of that deficiency before an effective treatment program can be designed and implemented. "It is essential to address both structure *and* function of the immune system because a person's immune system can be structurally intact yet not functioning well," says Jesse Stoff, M.D.

"By analogy, this is like having an expensive, perfectly crafted Swiss clock that you forgot to wind; it could keep excellent time, but it isn't even functioning." Dr. Stoff and other alternative physicians use tests to identify what immune areas are malfunctioning or weak and then to track treatment progress so necessary adjustments can be made. The following are useful tests for both purposes:

T and B Cell Panel and NK Cell Function—Both the T and B Cell Panel, which gives information about 25 immune system components, and the blood test for NK cell (natural killer cell, SEE QUICK DEFINITION) function are relatively inexpensive standard laboratory tests that any physician can order. Through these tests, the clinician can see where the hole exists in the person's immune defense and whether the deficiency is in T, B, or NK cells. Then he or she can determine which immunomodulators (substances that can regulate, or modulate, the activities of the immune system) will work best to plug the hole.

Biological Terrain Assessment—Biological terrain is a phrase used to describe the conditions, general health, and activity level of cells. This includes the status of both beneficial and harmful microorganisms at the cellular level. Components of the blood, urine, and saliva reveal this cellular information. By monitoring biochemical changes in these fluids and by making appropriate changes in diet, lifestyle, and medical treatment, health can be reestablished.

Biological Terrain Assessment, or BTA, is a test designed to provide this monitoring. Specifically, it measures the parameters of cellular health: 1) optimal pH (acid-base balance); 2) optimal oxidation-reduction potential (the degree of "oxidative stress" or free radical damage); and 3) resistivity (the opposite of electrical conductivity). In

Natural killer (NK) cells are a type of non-specific, free-ranging immune cell produced in the bone marrow and matured in the thymus gland. NK cells can recognize and quickly destroy virus and cancer cells on first contact. "Armed" with an estimated 100 different biochemical poisons for killing foreign proteins, they can kill target cells without having encountered them previously. As with antibodies, their role is surveillance, to rid the body of aberrant or foreign cells before they can grow and produce cancer or infection.

In addition to multiple infections, the accumulation of toxins in the body is often a feature of CFS and creates a further burden on the immune system. Whether from stress, poor diet, or chemicals in food and the environment, these toxins need to be removed from the body if the immune system is to be restored to health. For more about detoxification, see Chapter 1: Fibrocystic Breast Disease, pp. 35-39.

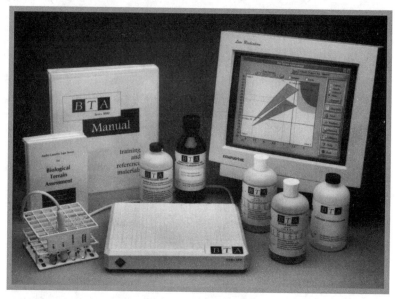

BIOLOGICAL TERRAIN ASSESSMENT. This unit analyzes blood, urine, and saliva samples and displays information about an individual's cellular health on its monitor.

only ten minutes, a computerized device called a BTA S-1000, which uses a pen-shaped microelectrode, can determine these values from blood, saliva, and urine samples obtained following a 12-14 hour fast.

Treating Immune Dysfunction

Two powerful tools in restoring compromised immune function are immunomodulators (which can include nutritional supplements and herbs) and acupuncture.

Immunomodulators—An immunomodulator is a substance that can tune, adjust, regulate, or focus—modulate—the activities of the immune system to reverse illnesses. Homeopathic remedies, herbs, hormones, amino acids and other nutritional supplements, and specif-

To contact **Jesse Stoff, M.D.**: Integramed, 3402 East Broadway, Tucson, AZ 85716; tel: 520-319-9074; fax: 520-319-9073. For **NK Daily** and **NK Support**, contact: Solstice Vitamin Company, 982 Stuyvesant Avenue, Union, NJ 07083; tel: 800-765-7842 or 908-810-0909; fax: 908-810-9207. For *Stibium* and *Carduus Marianus*: Weleda Pharmacy, P.O. Box 49, Congers, NY 10920; tel: 800-289-1969 or 914-268-8572; fax: 800-280-4899 or 914-268-8574. For **DHEA**: Mountain View Pharmacy, 10565 N. Tatum Blvd., Paradise Valley, AZ; tel: 800-942-7065 or 602-948-7065; fax: 602-948-9489. For **L-glutamine** (Doctors Brand): Genesist, 1321 S. Grant Street, Longmont, CO 80501; tel: 303-651-2522; fax: 303-772-4566. For **METBAL**®: Southwest Nutraceuticals, 1955 W. Grant, Suite 125U, Tuscon, AZ 85745, tel: 520-740-1993; fax: 520-624-4028. For more about the **BTA-S 1000**, contact: Biological Technologies International, P.O. Box 560, Payson, AZ 85547; tel: 520-474-4181; fax: 520-474-1501.

ic dietary changes can all operate as immunomodulators. The following are immunomodulators Jesse Stoff, M.D., generally uses to rebuild a depleted immune system:

- **NK Daily**: from purified colostrum (first mother's milk after birth) from cows; stimulates NK cells

- **NK Support**: a natural immune-building compound containing Larix (derived from the Western larch tree, *Larix occidentalis*); stimulates NK cells and macrophages (immune cells that "eat" germs); take with vitamin C and iodine to help dissolve cell membranes of bacteria and other foreign proteins

- **Amino acids arginine and lysine**: support NK cell function

- **Homeopathic *Stibium***: aids T cells and helps reorganize immune system

- **DHEA**: hormone that activates T4 cells

- **Amino acid L-glutamine**: helps maintain white blood cell population and T-cell production; supports intestinal health

- **Milk thistle (*Carduus marianus*)**: aids liver detoxification which assists the immune system by reducing the toxic load in the body

- **METBAL®**: super vitamin to trigger the immune system, supply nutrients for tissue repair and rebuilding, and increase cell nutrient absorption

For information about **Dr. Stoff's approach to cancer**, see *Alternative Medicine Definitive Guide to Cancer* (Future Medicine Publishing, 1997; ISBN 1-887299-01-7); to order, call 800-333-HEAL.

Acupuncture—William M. Cargile, B.S., D.C., F.I.A.C.A., former chairman of research for the American Association of Oriental Medicine, has successfully treated CFS patients with acupuncture, concentrating on the points which relate to the immune system. Dr. Cargile notes that the immune system uses 60% of the body's energy-storage compound called ATP (SEE QUICK DEFINITION), which manufactures proteins to make immune antibodies. "You don't have enough energy because your immune system is using all the ATP for the production of antibodies," explains Dr. Cargile.

By using acupuncture to stimulate both the immune system and the production of ATP, Dr. Cargile has achieved striking results with his CFS patients. One such patient, a 54-year-old woman named Emily, was diagnosed with idiopathic chronic fatigue, meaning her condition did not have a known cause such as cancer or thyroid or

ATP stands for adenosine triphosphate, a substance found in all cells, particularly muscle, and responsible for energy. When enzymes split ATP, energy is released (12,000 calories/mole of ATP) from the high-energy phosphate bonds. This bond can be instantly split on demand whenever energy is required to run cellular functions. Then ATP becomes ADP. When energy is returned, it becomes ATP again. ATP is often called the cell's energy currency because it can be continually spent and remade again in a matter of minutes.

The good news is that once hypothyroidism and hormonal imbalances are identified, they are relatively easy to treat through supplementation with thyroid glandular extracts.

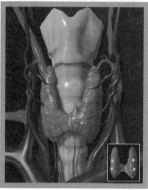

The **thyroid gland**, one of the body's seven endocrine glands, is located just below the larynx in the throat, with interconnecting lobes on either side of the trachea. The thyroid is the body's metabolic thermostat, controlling body temperature, energy use, and, in children, the body's growth rate. The thyroid controls the rate at which organs function and the speed with which the body uses food; it affects the operation of all body processes and organs. Of the hormones synthesized in and released by the thyroid, T3 (tri-iodothyronine) represents 7%, and T4 (thyroxine) accounts for almost 93% of the thyroid's hormones active in all of the body's processes. Iodine is essential to forming normal amounts of thyroxine. The secretion of both these hormones is regulated by thyroid-stimulating hormone, or TSH, secreted by the pituitary gland in the brain. The thyroid also secretes calcitonin, a hormone required for calcium metabolism.

For more about **hypothyroidism**, see Chapter 1: Fibrocystic Breast Disease, p. 31, and Chapter 5: Depression, pp. 217-223.

endocrine abnormalities. She often lacked the motivation to leave her bedroom, spending up to 20 hours a day in bed. Within five acupuncture treatments with Dr. Cargile, Emily was walking three miles daily, her energy level completely restored.

3) Thyroid and Hormonal Problems

Thyroid problems, particularly an underactive thyroid gland (hypothyroidism), are often implicated in chronic fatigue syndrome. While hypothyroidism is technically considered a separate illness and not a cause of CFS, many CFS patients have not been properly tested for thyroid problems and distinct categorization of the two illnesses is not necessarily of benefit to the patient. Eliminating or confirming the thyroid as a factor should be a first step in the investigation of what is causing your CFS.

Hormonal (SEE QUICK DEFINITION) imbalances are also common in CFS; specifically, imbalances or deficiencies in the adrenal hormones DHEA (SEE QUICK DEFINITION) and cortisol and the hormone ACTH (adreno-cortico-tropic hormone, secreted by the pituitary gland and essential for adrenal health). Since the adrenal glands play a central role in maintaining the body's energy levels, when these glands are functioning poorly, the result is fatigue. Low amounts of melatonin, the pineal gland hormone which regulates the body's sleep cycle, may also be contributing to the overall symptom picture of CFS.

The good news is that once hypothyroidism and hormonal imbalances are identified, they are relatively easy to treat through supplementation with thyroid glandular extracts (SEE QUICK DEFINITION) or the appropriate hormones. The bad news is that these conditions are frequently overlooked or misdiagnosed and the patient fails to receive the proper treatment. With the correct tests, you can circumvent this medical myopia.

Testing for Thyroid and Hormonal Problems

TRH Test—To assess thyroid function, doctors will often measure blood levels of the two thyroid hormones, thyroxine (T4) and tri-iodothyronine (T3), and thyroid stimulating hormone (TSH) secreted by the pituitary gland. However, a person's thyroid hormone levels may test normal while their thyroid is underfunctioning. The TRH (thyrotrophin-releasing hormone) test is a far more sensitive laboratory measure than routine thyroid blood tests and can show conclusively that a patient is suffering from an underactive thyroid, explains Raphael Kellman, M.D., a New York City physician who specializes in thyroid-related cases and uses the test regularly in his clinical practice.

For the TRH test, the physician measures the patient's level of TSH through a simple blood test, then gives an injection of TRH (a completely harmless synthetic hormone modeled after the TRH secreted by the hypothalamus gland in the brain), and finally draws blood 25 minutes later to remeasure the TSH. The TRH injection stimulates the pituitary gland which produces TSH; if the thyroid is underfunctioning, the pituitary gland will secrete excess TSH upon stimulation. If the second TSH blood test measures are high (above 10), it tells us the patient's thyroid is underactive. A TSH reading of 15 is suspicious, while 20 strongly points to hypothyroidism.

In checking for hormonal imbalances, the following tests can provide useful information:

Aeron LifeCycles Saliva Assay Report—Most of our key hormones—estrogen, testosterone, DHEA—decline as we age, leaving us vulnerable to reduced physiolog-

QUICK DEFINITION

Hormones are the chemical messengers of the endocrine system that impose order through an intricate communication system among the body's estimated 50 trillion cells. Examples include the "male" sex hormone (testosterone), the "female" sex hormones (estrogen and progesterone), melatonin (pineal), growth hormone (pituitary), and DHEA (adrenal).

DHEA (dehydroepiandrosterone) is naturally produced by the human adrenal glands and gonads with optimal levels occurring around age 20 for women and age 25 for men. After those ages, DHEA levels gradually decline so that a person 80 years old produces only a fraction of the DHEA they did when they were 20. As an antioxidant, hormone regulator, and the building block from which estrogen and testosterone are produced, DHEA is vital to health. Low DHEA levels have been associated with cancer, diabetes, multiple sclerosis, hypertension, obesity, AIDS, heart disease, Alzheimer's, and immune dysfunction illnesses. Test subjects using supplemental DHEA reported improved sleeping patterns, better memory, an improved ability to cope with stress, decreased joint pain, increases in lean muscle, and decreases in body fat. No serious side effects have been reported to date, although acne, oily skin, facial hair growth on women, deepening of the voice, irritability, insomnia, and fatigue have been reported with high DHEA doses.

A **glandular extract** is a purified nutritional and therapeutic product derived from one of several animal glands including the adrenal, thymus, thyroid, ovaries, testes, pancreas, pineal, and pituitary. It is prescribed by a physician for a person whose corresponding gland is underfunctioning and not producing enough of its own hormone. The various glands are part of the endocrine system which, along with the nervous system, coordinates the functioning of all of the body's systems.

Self-Test for Thyroid Function

A simple temperature test can tell you if your thyroid is underactive. While it may not detect all thyroid dysfunction, if your temperature falls within a certain range, it would be advisable to get laboratory testing. Called the Barnes basal temperature test, it was developed by Broda O. Barnes, M.D., Ph.D., a pioneer in hypothyroidism. You can use a standard oral thermometer, but it's easier and faster with a digital thermometer which gives an electronic readout in about five seconds versus the ten minutes of its oral counterpart. Also, a built-in memory saves the last temperature reading, so you can record it for later reference.

Take the reading under your armpit while still lying in bed in the morning, before getting up or doing anything else. Wait until the thermometer beeps, signaling the temperature has registered. (If you're using an oral thermometer, wait ten minutes. Make sure you shake it down before using). Keep a record of the temperatures. If you are still menstruating, start testing on the first day of your period, when temperatures are lowest. Take the temperature for three or four days. Temperatures averaging below 97.8° F may reflect hypothyroidism.

For more about **thyroid health**, contact: Broda O. Barnes Research Foundation, P.O. Box 98, Trumbull, CT 06611; tel: 203-261-2101. The Broda O. Barnes Research Foundation is a nonprofit information and education organization that disseminates the work of Dr. Barnes and other experts in the field of endocrine function. They offer information packets, audios and videos, physician referrals, a 24-hour urine test, and consultation services for doctors.

For more about the **Aeron LifeCycles Saliva Assay Report**, see Chapter 1: Fibrocystic Breast Disease, p. 26.

ical functioning and possibly disease, states John Kells, president of Aeron LifeCycles in San Leandro, California, a laboratory that offers a saliva-based test for measuring levels of eight different hormones. The Aeron LifeCycles Saliva Assay Report, which can be ordered by both laypeople and physicians, provides graphs of individual hormone levels.

DHEA Challenge Test—The hormone DHEA is often deficient in people with CFS, and taking a DHEA supplement to raise the levels is relatively easy. However, while many people taking DHEA report significant improvement in sleeping patterns, energy level, and ability to cope with stress, some people actually experience the opposite effect.

Depending upon a person's genetic makeup, a certain amount of DHEA from a supplement may be converted by the body into the hormones testosterone and estradiol (a type of estrogen). If you are genetically predisposed to convert DHEA, you may experience unwanted side effects with supplementation as a result of increased amounts of these two hormones. These side effects can include fatigue, insomnia, irritability, acne, oily skin, deepening of the voice, and an increase in body hair.

Through a simple saliva sample, the DHEA Challenge Test determines whether, in your particular case, DHEA supplements will improve or worsen your health. The test works by measuring levels of the two hormones (testosterone and estradiol) in the saliva both before and after a five- to seven-day treatment with the DHEA hormone (15 mg daily for women, 25 mg for men). If your testosterone and estradiol levels are too high following the "challenge" to the system, continuing to take DHEA supplements is probably not advisable.

Adrenal Stress Index—The Adrenal Stress Index (ASI) can pinpoint whether an imbalance in the adrenal glands might be contributing to CFS. This test evaluates how well one's adrenal glands are functioning by tracking hormone levels over a 24-hour cycle (circadian rhythm). Four saliva samples taken at intervals throughout the day are used to reconstruct the adrenal rhythm in the laboratory and determine whether the three main stress hormones are being secreted in proper proportion to each other, and at the right times. Based on the results, a physician can prescribe the appropriate treatment to restore the balance of hormones and correct the circadian rhythm.

4) Mercury Toxicity

The accumulation of the heavy metal mercury in body tissues can lead to chronic fatigue, immune breakdown, hypothyroidism, and many other health disorders. The major source of mercury exposure for the U.S. population is mercury dental fillings. Euphemistically called "silver" fillings, mercury amalgam dental fillings are actually only 35% silver. Mercury makes up 50% of the mix, with tin, copper, and zinc comprising the rest. Every year, more than 100 million mercury amalgam fillings are put into the mouths of U.S. dental patients, despite the negative health effects and the fact that, in 1988, the Environmental Protection Agency (EPA) declared scrap dental amalgam a *hazardous waste.*

Other symptoms and conditions linked to mercury tox-

For more about the **TRH test,** contact: Raphael Kellman, M.D., The Center for Progressive Medicine, 140 West 69th Street, New York, NY 10023; tel: 212-721-6633; fax: 212-721-6714. For the **Aeron LifeCycles Saliva Assay Report,** contact: Aeron LifeCycles, 1933 Davis Street, Suite 310, San Leandro, CA 94577, tel: 510-729-0375 or 800-631-7900; fax: 510-719-0383. For the **Adrenal Stress Index test** and the **DHEA Challenge test,** contact: Diagnos-Tech, Inc., 6620 South 192nd Place, J-2204, Kent, WA 96032; tel: 800-878-3787 or 425-251-0596; fax: 425-251-0637.

For more about **mercury toxicity,** see Chapter 2: Breast Cancer, pp. 73-74.

Extreme care must be taken to protect the body from mercury poisoning during mercury amalgam removal. For this reason, you should only have the procedure done by a dentist who specializes in amalgam removal. Further, mercury residues throughout the body must be carefully removed through the use of some form of chelating agent, such as garlic, seaweeds, vitamin C, etc., which will bind with the mercury and help to remove it safely from the body.

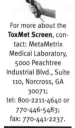

icity make a very long list, including anorexia, depression, fatigue, insomnia, arthritis, multiple sclerosis, moodiness, irritability, memory loss, nausea, diarrhea, gum disease, swollen glands, and headaches, among many others.

Testing for Mercury Toxicity

Electrodermal screening and hair analysis can reveal the levels of mercury in the body. Another test, the ToxMet Screen, provides an inexpensive but detailed analysis of the levels of mercury as well as other heavy metals in a patient's system. Based on a urine sample, ToxMet tests for four highly toxic heavy metals (mercury, arsenic, cadmium, and lead); it also reports on levels for ten potentially toxic elements, including aluminum, bismuth, boron, nickel, and strontium. Finally, information is gathered on a patient's status regarding 14 essential metals and minerals, such as copper, calcium, chromium, molybdenum, selenium, and vanadium. The test typically costs about $100 and is ordered by a physician.

Treating Mercury Toxicity

Mercury detoxification methods can only provide temporary relief of symptoms if the source of mercury exposure is not eliminated. Thus, if you have mercury dental fillings and testing reveals a high level of mercury in your body, you might want to consider having your fillings replaced with composite fillings which contain no mercury. Once the mercury has been removed from your mouth, you can proceed with detoxification protocols to remove the mercury stored in your tissues.

Chelation therapy (SEE QUICK DEFINITION) is an effective method for accomplishing this. Here, DMPS, the chelating agent for mercury, is delivered intravenously. It binds with the mercury in your body and both are then eliminated through the urine and feces. Garlic and chlorella (blue-green algae) also aid in chelation and can be taken as oral supplements to support the intravenous program.

5) Enzyme Deficiencies

Enzymes (SEE QUICK DEFINITION), essential in the breakdown of nutrients and the clearing of toxins in the blood, come from two sources: they are manufactured in the pancreas and we get them from our food. If our food doesn't contain the necessary enzymes, which is

Conditions Associated With Enzyme Deficiency

Note how many of these symptoms or conditions also characterize chronic fatigue syndrome.

allergies

anxiety

bacterial and viral infections

bronchial and respiratory conditions

candidiasis

chronic fatigue syndrome

depressed immunity

depression

environmental illness

frequent sore throats

gastrointestinal problems

hypothyroidism

indigestion

insomnia

irritability

lack of concentration

lymphatic congestion with swollen glands

memory loss

mental sluggishness

mood swings

sinusitis and sinus infections

often the case in the highly processed standard American diet, then the pancreas must work overtime to produce more enzymes. This taxes the pancreas and also depletes the number of enzymes available to circulate in the blood and clear toxins. When this state of affairs is prolonged, you will be unable to absorb the nutrients from food and supplements properly and toxins will accumulate beyond your body's ability to eliminate them. Immune dysfunction results and chronic fatigue syndrome can follow.

Again, as with the viruses associated with CFS, it is unclear which comes first—the weakened immune system or the enzyme deficiencies. In either case, supplementing with plant enzymes can correct the enzyme imbalance and break the cycle of ill health, in which dysfunction in one system worsens dysfunction in another. Enzyme therapy, the precise supplementation with enzymes and other nutrients, can therefore be an important component in treating CFS. In addition, before implementing dietary changes and a regimen of nutritional supplements as part of a total CFS treatment program, it is advisable to determine if enzyme deficiencies are present. Without enough or the proper enzymes, the most careful diet and highest quality supplements will have little or no effect because the body will be unable to absorb the nutrients.

QUICK DEFINITION

Enzymes are specialized living proteins fundamental to all living processes in the body, necessary for every chemical reaction and the normal activity of our organs, tissues, fluids, and cells. Enzymes are essential for the production of energy required to run cellular functions. There are hundreds of thousands of these Nature's "workers." Enzymes enable the body to digest and assimilate food. There are special enzymes for digesting proteins, carbohydrates, fats, and plant fibers. Specifically, protease digests proteins, amylase digests carbohydrates, lipase digests fats, cellulase digests fiber, and disaccharidase digests sugars. Enzymes also assist in clearing the body of toxins and cellular debris.

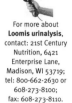
For more about
Loomis urinalysis,
contact: 21st Century
Nutrition, 6421
Enterprise Lane,
Madison, WI 53719;
tel: 800-662-2630 or
608-273-8100;
fax: 608-273-8110.

Testing for Enzyme Deficiencies

In her work as an an enzyme therapist, Lita Lee, Ph.D., of Lowell, Oregon, relies on the urinalysis developed by Charles Loomis, D.C., founder and president of 21st Century Nutrition, in Madison, Wisconsin. Dr. Lee emphasizes that a 24-hour urine sample is the only way to pinpoint enzyme deficiencies.

Specific parameters of the Loomis test reveal the status of digestive function in three food groups: protein, carbohydrates, and fats. Abnormal values in uric acid indicate a deficiency of protease, the enzyme which digests protein. If calcium phosphate values are abnormal, it means there is a deficiency of amylase, the enzyme which digests carbohydrates. Lastly, the calcium oxalate component is linked to lipase, the enzyme which digests fats.

In addition to enzyme deficiencies, the Loomis test isolates digestive disorders and nutrient deficiencies. For the test, the client collects urine over 24 hours and the sample is then analyzed by someone who specializes in Loomis urinalysis.

6) Allergies

Allergies are a common complaint of people who suffer from chronic fatigue syndrome and fibromyalgia and they are the defining feature of environmental illness. Characterized by multiple and extensive allergies, environmental illness could be called the "ultimate allergy." Allergies in all three syndromes further stress an already taxed immune system. Allergies and the immune response they generate can be a factor in up to 80% of patients with chronic fatigue.[9] As a contributor to immune overload, ongoing allergic reaction is an essential condition to address in the treatment of CFS.

Allergies, like immune dysfunction and enzyme deficiencies, are closely linked to intestinal disorders. For example, candidiasis (overgrowth of the intestinal fungus *Candida albicans)* and allergies are often paired. The intestinal dysfunction created by candidiasis can lead to "leaky gut" syndrome. Here, undigested food particles pass through the intestinal walls into the bloodstream where the body launches an allergic reaction against these foreign substances.

When the condition is chronic, the development of an allergy to that food may be the result. A delayed allergic reaction (hours to days after eating a food) is common and means you can have food allergies and not know it. Continued dysbiosis (SEE QUICK DEFINITION) leads to more allergies and serious health disorders such as chronic fatigue syndrome. "Dysbiosis and delayed food allergies are almost universally present in people with autoimmune disorders [such as CFS]," observes Serafina Corsello, M.D., director of the Corsello Centers for Nutritional Complementary Medicine, in New York City and Huntington, New York.

Testing for Allergies

Identifying and taking steps to eliminate allergies or avoiding exposure to the offending substances is a vital part of reducing the burden on the immune system. In the case of environmental illness, the extent of the allergies presents a daunting prospect, but the level of disability created by the constant allergic reaction makes the process of identification all the more necessary.

There are numerous tests to identify allergens, or allergy-causing substances, but two of the most effective are electrodermal screening, mentioned previously, and the Nambudripad Allergy Elimination Technique. In addition, the IgG ELISA blood test can pinpoint food allergies, including delayed food allergies which are the most difficult to identify.

Nambudripad Allergy Elimination Technique (NAET)— Developed by Devi Nambudripad, D.C., L.Ac., R.N., Ph.D., this highly effective method of both detecting and permanently eliminating allergies and sensitivities combines applied kinesiology's (SEE QUICK DEFINITION) muscle response testing with acupuncture and chiropractic.

To identify an allergen, the patient holds a vial containing the suspected allergy-causing substance in one hand while the practitioner tests the muscle strength of the patient's arm or leg. A weak muscle response indicates an allergy or sensitivity to that substance. Treatment involves the patient again holding the substance while the NAET practitioner uses acupuncture or acupressure to retrain the brain and nervous system to no longer respond to the substance allergically.

The IgG ELISA—Conventional allergy blood tests measure the presence of IgE (immunoglobulin E, SEE QUICK DEFINITION) antibodies, but most food allergies are dealt with in the body by the IgG (immunoglobulin G) antibodies. The IgG ELISA (enzyme-linked

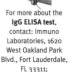

For more about the **IgG ELISA test,** contact: Immuno Laboratories, 1620 West Oakland Park Blvd., Fort Lauderdale, FL 33311; tel: 800-231-9197 or 954-486-4500; fax: 954-739-8583.

immunoabsorbent assay) offers new hope for food allergy sufferers. It is currently the only commercially available test of its kind for delayed food allergies. (NAET identifies this type of allergy as well.)

"We know that one of the fundamental causes behind food allergies is the penetration of undigested or partially digested food from the digestive tract into the bloodstream," explains James Braly, M.D., medical director of Immuno Laboratories, in Fort Lauderdale, Florida.

"With the IgG ELISA test, we can measure the actual presence of specific foods and their specific IgG antibodies in the blood to precisely determine which foods a person is allergic to." Convenient and automated, the IgG ELISA involves computer analysis of a blood sample for the presence of IgG antibodies against over 100 foods. The test can be done through the mail, as long as samples reach testing labs within 72 hours after the blood is drawn.

Treating Allergies

Often, avoiding allergenic foods while treating the underlying intestinal condition, such as candidiasis, which created the allergies in the first place is sufficient to eliminate the allergy. However, as discussed above under testing, the Nambudripad Allergy Elimination Technique is an excellent method for permanently ending allergies, not just to food, but to all substances.

For the last 15 years, Dr. Nambudripad has used her technique to eliminate the allergies of between 80% and 90% of her patients. Today, over 600 practitioners—including M.D.s, acupuncturists, and chiropractors—have joined her and are using NAET with equal success. They have seen numerous cases of CFS reversed by getting rid of the person's allergies; many of these patients had been going to CFS clinics for years with little result.

Such was the case with Marta, 35, who had been treated for CFS for three years. In spite of this and a healthy diet, she was getting progressively worse and had already been on disability for three years when she came to Dr. Nambudripad. A thorough evaluation determined that she was allergic to almost all foods and fabrics. However, Marta was relieved to learn that she was suffering from allergies rather than some incurable illness. Within a couple of

Success Story:
A Three-Point Program for Fibromyalgia

Ellen, 54, suffered from chronic low back pain, muscle soreness, general achiness, fatigue, and depression. She endured years of clinical testing and various drug treatments without getting a diagnosis or relief of her symptoms. Frustrated by her lack of progress with conventional doctors, Ellen sought help from Mary Olsen, D.C., a chiropractor based in Huntington, New York. Dr. Olsen identified Ellen's condition as fibromyalgia by testing the 18 trigger points associated with that disorder. Eleven of these points must be sore to the touch to qualify as fibromyalgia, according to the conventional medical definition. In Ellen's case, 16 of the sites were tender.

Dr. Olsen prescribed a three-part treatment program for Ellen. First, she used acupressure (based on acupuncture, but using gentle pressure of the fingers instead of needles) on Ellen's trigger points, applying pressure in eight-second intervals and repeating three times at each site. The trigger points in fibromyalgia are actually muscles in spasm and those near the spine often pull it out of alignment. Dr. Olsen administers acupressure to massage the trigger point, chiropractic to realign the spine, and applied kinesiology to prevent the trigger point from reinjuring the spine. Ellen saw Dr. Olsen three times a week until her spine began to respond to treatment, and monthly thereafter.

Second, Dr. Olsen prescribed vitamin supplements tailored to fibromyalgia. From her clinical experience, Dr. Olsen has found that fibromyalgia sufferers tend to have low levels of B vitamins and malic acid. The supplement formula she typically uses for this deficiency includes vitamin B1 (25 mg), vitamin B6 (75 mg), manganese (2.5 mg), and malic acid (300 mg). "In most cases, I notice a dramatic improvement within 48 hours of beginning the vitamin therapy," Dr. Olsen says. Ellen took this formula two to eight times daily, as needed.

Third, Ellen began a moderate exercise program, performing a ten- to 15-minute stretching routine five days a week and walking for 20 minutes three times weekly. The exercise would help raise her serotonin (a brain neurotransmitter which influences mood) levels which, in turn, would reduce her fatigue. Dr. Olsen emphasizes that her patients never exercise to the point of pain and this aspect of treatment needs to vary according to the individual. Dr. Olsen usually waits until the person's condition has improved through vitamin therapy before beginning the exercise program. In Ellen's case, she was able to start exercising relatively quickly.

After one year of treatment, Ellen reported that her low back pain was gone, her muscle aches had subsided, and her energy level had increased considerably. As her condition improved, Ellen began exercising more which further boosted her energy level. Her increased energy (and relief from pain) also elevated her mood and Ellen no longer suffers from depression.

To contact **Mary Olsen, D.C.:** 42 High Street, Huntington, NY 11743; tel: 516-421-1248; fax: 516-421-1249.

To design an effective program of nutritional supplementation, it is necessary to identify all deficiencies. Thorough testing can avoid prescribing the wrong supplement and save time and expense in the long term.

months of beginning NAET treatment, she started showing marked improvement. In all, it took six months (with three to four visits per week) to clear all of her allergies. At the end of that period, Marta felt almost normal and began to work at a regular job.

7) Nutritional Deficiencies

Nutritional deficiencies are often a feature of chronic fatigue syndrome. As with most of the factors involved in this disorder, it is difficult to tell which came first, the deficiencies or the immune breakdown. The immune and other physiological systems of the body need proper nutrients in order to maintain health. Without enough or the right kinds of nutrients, these systems cannot operate at an optimum level.

If the nutritional deficiency becomes chronic, breakdowns in function will occur. In addition, a body whose immune system is continually overactive, as it is in CFS, requires far more nutrients to keep it going than a healthy body does. Conversely, this overactive immune system with its accompanying nutritional drain can in itself lead to deficiencies in key nutrients.

As with an underactive thyroid, hormonal imbalances, and enzyme shortages, nutritional deficiencies are relatively simple to reverse, requiring precise supplementation of specific nutrients. As with the other deficits, testing is important to provide guidelines for this nutritional therapy.

Testing for Nutritional Deficiencies

Unfortunately, a person with CFS is likely to be receiving *fewer* nutrients than someone who is healthy. This is because the various viruses, parasites, fungal overgrowths, and other infections characteristic of CFS are draining nutrients from the person suffering from the disorder. In addition, with gastrointestinal disorders, such as candidiasis and the "leaky gut" syndrome which can result, many of the nutrients from food and even supplements are not being absorbed by the body.

As with other aspects of treatment, in order to design an effective program of nutritional supplementation, it is necessary to identify all deficiencies. Thorough testing can avoid prescribing the wrong supplement and save time and expense in the long term. Among the laboratory tests for nutrient status, the four discussed below are relatively inexpensive and provide detailed, practical information.

Individualized Optimal Nutrition (ION)—Using a blood and a urine sample, the ION (Individualized Optimal Nutrition) Panel measures 150 biochemical components. The test is highly useful for physicians who need detailed biochemical assessment of patients who have chronic fatigue or other immune disorders, multiple chemical sensitivities, cancer, heart disease, learning difficulties, or obesity. Specifically, ION checks for nutritional status in categories including vitamins, minerals, amino acids, fatty and organic acids, lipid peroxides, general blood chemistries (cholesterol, thyroid hormone, glucose), and antioxidants. In each category, a patient's levels are compared with predetermined limits.

FIA™ (Functional Intracellular Analysis)—These tests (as Comprehensive Profile 3000, B-Complex Profile 1100, Primary Profile 1500, Cardiovascular Profile 1600, or Antioxidants

Using Acupressure to Relieve an Allergy— A Self-Help Approach

Michael Reed Gach, Ph.D., director of the Acupressure Institute, in Berkeley, California, has found that allergic reactions can often be relieved through acupressure, the use of fingertips in place of needles to stimulate acupoints. Dr. Gach explains, "As soon as you begin experiencing an allergic reaction, apply pressure on the point in the center of the webbing of your hand, between your thumb and index finger." (See LI 4 on illustration below.)

"Gradually apply firm pressure onto the point, angling the pressure toward the bone that connects with the index finger," Dr. Gach instructs. He recommends keeping a constant pressure for at least two minutes while taking slow, deep breaths. Then repeat the process with the same point on your other hand. "This point works like an antihistamine," Dr. Gach further explains. "I have found that this simple technique can often quickly arrest an allergy attack, making it a useful self-help remedy that anyone can use."

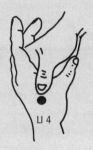

LI 4

All chronic fatigue patients do not have the same psychological or emotional makeup, but all chronic fatigue patients have a psychological and emotional component to their illness.

Profile 1400) measure the function of key vitamins, minerals, antioxidants, amino acids, fatty acids, and metabolites (choline, inositol) at the cellular level. They also assess the status of carbohydrate metabolism in terms of insulin function and fructose intolerance.

Pantox Antioxidant Profile™—Using a small blood sample, this diagnostic screen measures the status of more than 20 nutritional factors as a way of determining the body's antioxidant defense system. It then compares the results against a database of 7,000 normal and healthy profiles. Specifically, the screen reports on lipoproteins (cholesterol, triglycerides), fat-soluble antioxidants (vitamins A and E, carotenoids, coenzyme Q10), water-soluble antioxidants (vitamin C, uric acid, bilirubin), and iron balance. The Pantox Profile is displayed in bar graphs with accompanying explanatory medical text, telling you if your levels of a specific nutrient are low and pose a health risk. The test cost to patients is about $300 and is often covered by health insurance, including Medicare.

Oxidative Protection Screen—This test can provide your physician with an actual biochemical analysis of how well your body is handling free radicals. This information, in turn, is valuable to the physician in assessing your overall health, the degree of your antioxidant "protection," and the possible need for further nutrient supplementation. The test works by determining the amount of lipid peroxides in the plasma of a blood sample. When lipids (fatty acids and other oily organic compounds) are damaged by free radicals, they form lipid peroxides which circulate in the blood.

For more about **ION**, contact: MetaMetrix Medical Laboratory, 5000 Peachtree Industrial Blvd., Suite 110, Norcross, GA 30071; tel: 800-221-4640 or 770-446-5483; fax: 770-441-2237. For **Functional Intracellular Analysis**, contact: SpectraCell Laboratories, Inc., 515 Post Oak Blvd., Suite 830, Houston, TX 77027; tel: 800-227-5227 or 713-621-3101; fax: 713-621-3234; website: http://www.spectracell.com. The **Pantox Antioxidant Profile** must be ordered by a licensed health-care practitioner. Contact: Pantox Laboratories, 4622 Santa Fe Street, San Diego, CA 92109; tel: 888-726-8698, 800-726-8696, or 619-272-3885; fax: 619-272-1621. **Oxidative Protection Screen** must also be ordered by a licensed health-care practitioner. Contact: Antibody Assay Laboratories, 1715 East Wilshire, #715, Santa Ana, CA 92705; tel: 800-522-2611 or 714-972-9979; fax: 714-543-2034.

A Glossary of Herbs for CFS

The following are some of the many herbs that can help alleviate the symptoms of chronic fatigue, combat the multiple infections involved, and strengthen depleted body systems.

■ Astragalus (*Astragalus membranaceus*): immune stimulant, increases the production of white blood cells; antiviral and antibacterial; facilitates digestion

■ Dandelion (*Taraxacum officinale*): supports the liver and gastrointestinal system; blood cleanser and diuretic (urine-increasing agent); aids in detoxification of the body

■ Echinacea (*Echinacea angustifolia*): immune-enhancer, increases white blood cell numbers and function

■ Garlic (*Allium sativum*): antibiotic, antifungal, and antiviral; aids immune function

■ Ginkgo (*Ginkgo biloba*): antioxidant; sharpens memory and other cognitive functions by improving blood circulation to the brain

■ Ginseng (*Panax ginseng, P. quinquefolius, Eleuterococcus senticosus*): sharpens mental abilities, concentration, and alertness; improves stamina and delays the onset of fatigue after physical exercise; aids the body in coping with stress by supporting the adrenal glands; antioxidant; stimulates immune and endocrine systems

■ Goldenseal (*Hydrastis canadensis*): immune stimulant; antimicrobial

■ Hops (*Humulus lupulus*): calming and sleep-inducing for anxiety and sleep disorders

■ Kava-kava (*Piper methysticum*): natural tranquilizer for anxiety

■ Milk thistle (*Silybum marianum*): supports the liver; helps reverse toxic liver damage and protect liver from chemicals

■ Nettle (*Urtica dioica*): circulatory and immune stimulant; promotes lymphocyte production; assists the body in flushing toxins

■ St. John's wort (*Hypericum perforatum*): antidepressant

8) Lifestyle Issues

Lifestyle choices can contribute to chronic fatigue syndrome. For example, high stress and high-paced overachievement—some call it workaholism—characterize the lives of many CFS sufferers prior to their becoming sick. Getting laid out with unremitting fatigue is the only way some people will ever take the time to focus on their *internal* world and the emotional and psychological issues which are screaming for attention.

All chronic fatigue patients do not have the same psychological or emotional makeup, but all chronic fatigue patients have a psychological and emotional component to their illness. The elements of this component have a constant impact on the physiological factors involved and vice versa. (The body-mind link and the effect of emotions on healing has been well established in numerous studies.) As a result, unless stressful lifestyle practices and the mental and emotional factors contributing to your illness are thoroughly addressed, no cure will ever be complete and lasting.

Stress-management counseling and psychotherapy can be important tools in this process. In addition, homeopathic remedies can help you access and release stored emotions. Herbal medicines are also useful to provide palliative relief of difficult emotional states. For example, valerian and St. John's wort are known, respectively, for their anti-anxiety and antidepressant properties.

This discussion should not be interpreted as support of the view that CFS is all in the sufferer's head. It only highlights how essential it is to address all levels in the treatment of this complex disorder. For many people, the depression characteristic of CFS often disappears when the physical components of the illness are treated. However, the lifestyle and psychological and emotional factors referred to here are those deep, underlying patterns which, in combination with the physical elements, produced the condition and must be attended to if recovery is to be permanent.

Success Story: Reversing CFS and Its Multiple Causes

The following case history involves a number of the eight causes discussed above and shows the interrelationship of emotional, psychological, and physical factors. It also illustrates, once again, the complexity of chronic fatigue syndrome and exemplifies alternative medicine's multimodal approach.

When Elinor, 45, came to see Milton Hammerly, M.D., medical director of the American Whole Health Clinic, in Littleton, Colorado, she had been suffering from a long list of symptoms for 18 years. They included severe fatigue, depression, brain fog, concentration troubles, muscle spasms and aches, night sweats, premenstrual syndrome (PMS—SEE QUICK DEFINITION), frequent infections including bronchitis and sore throats, "migratory" rashes that sprang up on different areas of her body, and not feeling refreshed after sleeping.

Elinor also had digestive problems, including frequent

constipation and bloating. She had been taking Synthroid, a synthetic thyroid drug for an underactive thyroid for 12 years. She was also taking a battery of standard drugs to address her other symptoms, including prescription synthetic progesterone for her PMS, and had become dependent on many of them.

Elinor was generally unable to function; she couldn't hold a job or engage in normal social interactions. Elinor's husband had to drive her around and handle most of the domestic chores. Over the years, Elinor had seen many specialists and experimented with many drugs, but nothing had really helped. "Her symptoms were typical of CFS and fibromyalgia, both of which have come to be umbrella-like terms for this type of condition," observes Dr. Hammerly.

From Hormones to Magnets

A blood test revealed that Elinor was deficient in the hormone DHEA. While the range for DHEA is 130 to 980, Elinor's 136 was characteristic of a woman of 80, not 45, notes Dr. Hammerly. To start off her treatment, he put her on 25 mg once daily of DHEA. After a month of supplementation, a follow-up blood test showed her levels had climbed to a more acceptable 522. With the raising of her DHEA levels, Elinor observed that her sleeping was improved and she had fewer aches and pains, but she was still very tired.

At the same time as Dr. Hammerly had Elinor taking DHEA, he started her on digestive enzymes, taken with meals, to address her gastrointestinal disorders. He also gave her a product called Bioflora® (containing beneficial bacteria needed by her intestines for better digestion and absorption); and 500 mg twice daily of chelated magnesium citrate (to help reduce muscle spasms). To complete his nutritional recommendations, Dr. Hammerly suggested a variety of key antioxidants, including vitamin A (15,000-25,000 IU daily), vitamin C (2,000 mg daily), vitamin E (400-800 IU daily), and grapeseed extract (100 mg daily).

Dr. Hammerly taught Elinor a pain relief healing technique called electrostatic massage (SEE QUICK DEFINITION). He also suggested an energy therapy in the form of magnets (SEE QUICK DEFINITION) which he had Elinor apply to the pained muscles. A negative magnetic field has been

QUICK DEFINITION

Electrostatic massage (EM) is a therapeutic technique which uses static electricity to relieve pain by normalizing the malfunctioning nervous system, organs, and cells. A negatively charged PVC pipe is moved over the painful area of the body; this pushes electrons to the symptomatic area where they facilitate the normal healing process, stimulating the metabolism and increasing the amount of oxygen to the cells. EM can reduce swelling due to water retention (edema) by moving the water that accumulates in an area of inflammation. EM is used on patients suffering from general muscular pain, arthritis, fibromyalgia, headaches (tension and sinus), and tendinitis.

Magnet therapy works with the body's own electromagnetic fields to effect important metabolic changes in the body. Commonly, small, simple magnets are employed, providing a "calming" negative charge which helps to normalize pH, oxygenate the blood, reduce swelling, and cancel out free radicals, among other functions.

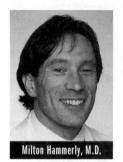
Milton Hammerly, M.D.

After the healing touch session, Elinor reported having a lot more energy and for the first time in 18 years she felt ready and able to start an exercise program. This change occurred two months into Dr. Hammerly's program.

To contact **Milton Hammerly, M.D.**: Centura Health, 2525 S. Downing #12-L, Denver, CO 80210; tel: 303-788-5893; fax: 303-788-7252. For **Bioflora®**, contact: PhysioLogics®, 6565 Odell Place, Boulder, CO 80301; tel: 800-765-6775 or 303-530-4554; fax: 303-516-5233 or 303-530-2592. Bioflora contains five principal beneficial or "friendly" bacteria in capsule form, including *Lactobacillus acidophilus, L. bulgaricus, Bifidobacterium bifidum, B. longium,* and *Streptococcus thermophilus.* For more information about the *Candida* **Antibodies Panel**, contact: National BioTech Laboratory, 13758 Lake City Way N.E., Seattle, WA 98125; tel: 206-363-6606; fax: 206-363-2025.

found to be therapeutic for a range of conditions, including chronic pain and sleep disorders. Dr. Hammerly also recommended that Elinor get a magnetic mattress pad so that the energy of the magnets could gently work on her physiology (organs, tissues, and cells) during sleep. After using this mattress for only a week, she reported sleeping better and decided to continue using it regularly.

Yet, Elinor was still very tired. At this point, two months into Dr. Hammerly's program, a registered nurse at the center treated Elinor with therapeutic touch, which is a way of delivering subtle healing energy through the hands. "Due to her degree of soreness, Elinor would not have responded well to massage, but needed a gentler 'hands off' approach, such as therapeutic touch which works with the body's energy fields rather than muscles." Dr. Hammerly notes that after the healing touch session, Elinor reported having a lot more energy and for the first time in 18 years she felt ready and able to start an exercise program.

Treating Her Allergies and Candidiasis

The healing benefits of therapeutic touch were, of course, working synergistically with the other components of the program. Elinor continued with this program, but three months later, her fatigue returned, accompanied by pressure in her head, sores in her nose and mouth, upper respiratory problems, and hair loss.

When he examined her, Dr. Hammerly found swollen lymph nodes and muscle tenderness. A food allergy test, called the IgG Antibody, which shows a patient's delayed reaction to allergenic substances and

For more about **DHEA**, see this chapter, pp. 180-183.

screens for reactions to 96 foods and 24 spices, indicated she was allergic to dairy products, eggs, gluten, and wheat.

The Anti-*Candida* Antibodies Panel (see p. 171) showed that there was a *Candida* yeast overgrowth in Elinor's mucosal cells lining the intestines, lungs, and mouth. As discussed previously, candidiasis can create leaky gut syndrome which can, in turn, lead to the development of allergies, as undigested food particles find their way from the intestines into the bloodstream where the immune system launches an allergic reaction against them. *Candida* infestation was also robbing Elinor's system of needed energy.

Dr. Hammerly prescribed Nystatin, an antifungal drug commonly given for *Candida* overgrowth. He also recommended dietary changes; Elinor needed to stop eating sugar and avoid the foods to which she was allergic. In addition, Dr. Hammerly wanted to build her nutrient status, as it is the foundation for energy and was depleted by the candidiasis and continual allergic reaction. He started Elinor on a series of Meyer's Cocktails (SEE QUICK DEFINITION), which involve a slow injection (lasting ten minutes) of mainly B-complex and C vitamins and magnesium. After four "cocktails" given over a four-week period, "her energy was significantly better." Elinor's *Candida* symptoms had also cleared up.

At this point, Elinor's psychiatrist started to reduce her antidepressants, telling Dr. Hammerly this was the first time in many years that Elinor had not seemed depressed to him. Her husband called Dr. Hammerly to exclaim, "I have my wife back for the first time in 18 years!" Two months later, Elinor had a slight relapse, feeling tired again, so Dr. Hammerly put her through a series of six Meyer's Cocktails, one per week; after this she was fine. "She is out in the world, doing things. She's exercising. Her aches and pains are gone and her energy is good. Her husband is having a hard time keeping up with her," says Dr. Hammerly.

The **Meyer's Cocktail** is an intravenous vitamin and mineral protocol developed in the 1970s by John Meyers, M.D., a physician at Johns Hopkins University, in Baltimore, Maryland. It contains magnesium chloride hexahydrate (5 cc given), calcium gluconate (2.5 cc), vitamin B2 (1,000 mcg/cc; 1 cc given), vitamin B5 (100 mg/cc; 1 cc given), vitamin B6 (250 mg/cc; 1 cc given), the entire vitamin B complex (100 mg/cc; 1 cc given), and vitamin C (222 mg/cc; 6 cc given). The solution is slowly injected over a 5-15 minute period. The "Cocktail" is indicated for patients with chronic fatigue, depression, muscle spasm, asthma, hives, allergic rhinitis, congestive heart failure, angina, ischemic vascular disease, acute infections, and senile dementia.

See *Alternative Medicine Guide to Chronic Fatigue, Fibromyalgia & Environmental Illness* (Future Medicine Publishing, 1998; ISBN 1-887299-11-4); to order, call 800-333-HEAL.

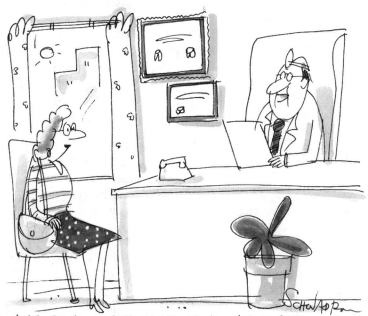

"I JUST STICK TO THE FACTS. IF YOU WANT CARING AND COMPASSION, I'LL REFER YOU TO OUR NURSE'S ASSISTANT."

Twice as many women as men suffer from serious depression, many to such a degree that they can't function without an antidepressant and have to endure the side effects. Using alternative medicine to identify and treat the underlying causes of your depression—from thyroid problems to biochemical imbalances—can permanently end the need for Prozac.

CHAPTER

5

Depression

AN ESTIMATED 17.6 MILLION Americans are affected by depression each year and the number of women afflicted is double that of men.[1] Christiane Northrup, M.D., of Yarmouth, Maine, a nationally recognized expert in women's health, estimates that 25% of women experience serious depression at some time in their lives. She cites the typical symptoms of women's depression as: sleep problems, poor concentration, memory problems, guilt, self-blame, and a sense of hopelessness. Susan Swedo, M.D., scientific director of the National Institute of Mental Health, defines true depression as when

Causes of Depression

- Hormonal imbalances
- Amino acid deficiencies
- Serotonin deficiency
- Underactive thyroid gland
- Diet and nutritional deficiencies
- Allergies and sensitivities
- Low blood sugar
- Stress and weakened immunity
- Toxic exposure
- Lack of exercise
- Lack of light

"the woman gives up hope of ever feeling better and feels helpless to improve her life." This kind of despair distinguishes depression from the occasional blues or grief after loss of a loved one which we all experience, says Dr. Swedo.[2]

Depression can be so debilitating that you don't have the energy, motivation, or will to seek help. However, recognizing the depression for what it is can begin the process of overcoming it. If you have not done so already, you need to determine if you are in fact clinically depressed. If you fit the criteria described here, it is strongly advised that you seek help from a qualified health-care practitioner, however difficult that may seem. According to the National Institute of Mental Health, the criteria for a diagnosis of clinical depression is five or more of the symptoms below, lasting for two weeks or longer:[3]

■ Persistent sad, anxious, or "empty mood"

■ Loss of interest or pleasure in activities, including sex

■ Restlessness, irritability, or excessive crying

■ Feelings of guilt, worthlessness, helplessness, hopelessness, pessimism

■ Sleeping too much or too little, early-morning awakening

■ Appetite and/or weight loss or overeating and weight gain

■ Decreased energy, fatigue, feeling "slowed down"

■ Thoughts of death or suicide, or suicide attempts

■ Difficulty concentrating, remembering, or making decisions

■ Persistent physical symptoms that do not respond to treatment, such as headaches, digestive disorders, and chronic pain

Alternative Medicine Therapies for Depression
■ Amino acid therapy
■ Biofeedback training
■ Chelation therapy
■ Detoxification
■ Dietary recommendations
■ Herbal medicine
■ Hormonal therapy
■ Light therapy
■ Nutritional supplements
■ Stress management
■ Glandular extracts

Along with these more recognizable symptoms, physicians have found that some seeming characteristics of personality—including lack of assertiveness, oversensitivity to rejection, or excessive shyness—can actually be hidden forms of depression. Physicians treating people for depression noticed that after their patients began taking the popular antidepressant drug Prozac, these traits diminished, leading to speculation that the seeming personality traits were actually manifestations of the depression, reports Steven Bratman, M.D., of Fort Collins, Colorado.[4]

Many people think that psychological counseling or antidepressants are their only choices when it comes to treatment of depression. In this chapter, you will learn that depression is frequently the result of biochemical imbalances and other physiological factors. As with any health condition, there may be emotional/psychological factors as well, but they are not necessarily the main cause of your depression. Even if your depression arises predominantly from such factors, there are usually physical components involved which, when addressed, can help restore mental balance.

With its approach of treating the individual and identifying *all*

Many people think that psychological counseling or antidepressants are their only choices when it comes to treatment of depression. But with its approach of treating the individual and identifying *all* sources of imbalance (emotional, physical, and psychological), alternative medicine can provide more comprehensive solutions for depression.

sources of imbalance (emotional, physical, and psychological), alternative medicine can provide more comprehensive solutions for depression. Once again, instead of only treating the symptoms, alternative medicine physicians look for the underlying causes in order to design treatment that will produce lasting results.

Before we turn to a discussion of factors which may be playing a role in creating your depression, along with case studies illustrating the range of therapies available to treat them, let's briefly consider the problems with conventional medicine's "solution" to depression.

A **neurotransmitter** is a brain chemical with the specific function of enabling communications to happen between brain cells. Chief among the 100 identified to date are acetylcholine, gamma-aminobutyric acid (GABA), serotonin, dopamine, and norepinephrine.

Acetylcholine is required for short-term memory and all muscle contractions. GABA works to stop excess nerve signals and thus keeps brain firings from getting out of control; serotonin does the same and helps produce sleep, regulate pain, and influence mood, although too much serotonin can produce depression. Norepinephrine is an excitatory neurotransmitter.

Quitting antidepressants should be overseen by a qualified physician. Do not attempt this on your own.

Why Antidepressant Drugs Might Not Be Your Best Option

The United States is in the midst of an antidepressant love affair, or epidemic, depending on your viewpoint, with Prozac, the latest drug of choice. Six million people in the U.S. and 12 million worldwide have prescriptions for Prozac and the pharmaceutical industry is expanding the antidepressant market to children. In 1996 alone, 600,000 children and adolescents in the U.S. were given Prozac or a similar antidepressant, such as Paxil or Zoloft—despite a lack of evidence showing benefits for children.[5] Even pets are targets of the pharmaceutical industry's desire for market expansion, with some conventional veterinarians enthusiastically prescribing Prozac for pets' emotional problems and compulsive behaviors such as excessive licking.

While it is true that antidepressants have saved lives and made many unbearable lives worth living, that is no justification for the massive overuse of these drugs and the lack of investigation of alternative methods for lifting depression. Antidepressants have a long list of side effects and fail to address the underlying factors causing depression. As a result, if patients wish to go off the drug, they are back where they started—or worse.

Antidepressant drugs work by altering the balance of chemical messengers in your brain called neurotransmitters (SEE QUICK DEFINITION). Prozac and Zoloft, for example, belong to a class of drugs called selective serotonin reuptake inhibitors (SSRIs). SSRIs prevent the movement of the neurotransmitter serotonin, a mood elevator, into nerve endings. This forces the serotonin to remain in the spaces around nerve endings, where it helps improve mood and mental alertness.[6] However, what is the price of these positive results?

Peter Breggin, M.D., a Harvard-trained psychiatrist, points out that drug therapy, while suppressing the symptoms of depression and other mental disorders, can also make a person chemically toxic, which will actually deepen the problem.[7] Sherry Rogers, M.D., of Syracuse, New York, also points to the worsening effects of long-term antidepressant use. "A lifetime of medications, by not uncovering the real causes, can not only lead to an escalation of

Side Effects of Conventional Antidepressants

According to the *Physicians' Desk Reference*, the following are reported as side effects of three commonly prescribed antidepressants. The first listing is of those symptoms shared by all three drugs. The individual listings are additional side effects of each.

All three (Prozac, Zoloft, Elavil): Headache, dry mouth, heart palpitations, nausea, vomiting, dizziness, blurred vision, insomnia, anxiety, tremor, excessive sweating, skin rash, weakness/fatigue, difficulty concentrating, urine retention, gastrointestinal problems (constipation, diarrhea, indigestion), sexual dysfunction (decreased libido, delayed ejaculation, impotence)

Prozac (fluoxetine): nervousness, somnolence, sinusitis, hot flashes, muscle and joint pain

Zoloft (sertraline): nervousness, somnolence, sinusitis, hot flashes

Elavil (amitryptiline): anemia, hypertension, numbness, tingling in extremities, nightmares, drowsiness, edema (fluid retention), breast enlargement (in women), testicular swelling (in men)

symptoms, but to the creation of new and seemingly unrelated symptoms," she cautions. In fact, over time, antidepressants generate "a slow, insidious, and escalating depression" by depleting the body of valuable nutrients, observes Dr. Rogers.[8]

Among the many reported antidepressant side effects are insom-

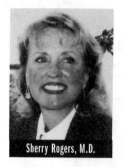

Sherry Rogers, M.D.

Over time, antidepressants generate "a slow, insidious, and escalating depression" by depleting the body of valuable nutrients, says Dr. Rogers. "It is only when the total body burden of mental and physical stressors has been sufficiently reduced that the body is able to reverse damages from years of overload and heal."

nia, anxiety, heart palpitations, headaches, dry mouth, nausea, and concentration problems (see "Side Effects of Conventional Antidepressants," p. 203). Another side effect, impairment of female sexual function, does not seem to get much public discussion. The *Physicians' Desk Reference* makes no mention of sexual dysfunction specific to women, although male dysfunction in this area is cited.

However, it is this side effect that causes many patients of Dr. Steven Bratman to give up on antidepressants, he reports.[9] Drugs such as Zoloft, he says, can rob women of the ability to achieve an orgasm, a condition called anorgasmia. Dr. Bratman, in discussing one of his female patients who went off antidepressants, describes her anorgasmic reaction to Zoloft: "She had no touble becoming aroused, but she 'felt like a train all revved up with nowhere to go.'"[10]

As you can see, antidepressants are not the "magic bullet" they are touted to be. Even for those who are lucky enough not to experience uncomfortable or disturbing side effects, the essential condition for which you are taking the medication remains untouched. Until the causes of this condition are treated, your Prozac or other prescription drug is only masking your depression.

11 Causes of Depression and How to Treat Them

For more about **testing**, see Chapter 4: Chronic Fatigue Syndrome, pp. 170-194.

In the majority of cases, depression's hidden causes are both identifiable and correctable, says Dr. Rogers. While no two people with depression have exactly the same causes, depression can result from multiple problems such as toxins accumulated in the body, allergies, high stress, chemical and hormonal imbalances, and nutrient deficiencies. "It is only when the total body burden of mental and physical stressors has been sufficiently reduced that the body is able to reverse damages from years of overload and heal," states Dr. Rogers.

To contact **Sherry Rogers, M.D.**: SK Publishing, P.O. Box 40101, Sarasota, FL 34242. Dr. Rogers is the author of *Depression, Cured at Last!* (Sarasota, FL: SK Publishing, 1997). For information about Dr. Rogers' other books, contact: Prestige Publishing, P.O. Box 3068, Syracuse, NY 13220; tel: 800-846-6687 or 315-455-7862; fax: 800-884-8119.

In order to identify the underlying causes, she recommends that patients have a complete biochemical workup including a urine analysis, thyroid test, and blood chemistry profiles that indicate nutrient status. A liver detoxification panel, urinary D-glucaric acid test, or mercapturic acid test will help indicate if the liver is overloaded through chemical exposure and is thereby unable to perform its detoxification functions. Dr. Rogers also advises a stool analysis to assess digestion, nutrient absorption, and intestinal microfloral composition.

The results of these tests then form the basis for a comprehensive healing program, involving dietary changes, detoxification, biochemical and nutrient replenishment, a change in the components of one's living environment, and a shift in attitude, as appropriate, says Dr. Rogers. Reversing chronic depression usually requires the guidance of a competent, holistically trained practitioner—and a patient who is aware of the medical realities of their reversible condition, she advises.

Through clinical experience with depression, alternative medicine physicians have determined that the 11 factors discussed below are common causes of depression. Often, more than one factor is involved and, when undetected and untreated, they together result in chronic depression. Case studies throughout illustrate how women have successfully reversed their depression by correcting these underlying causes.

1) Hormonal Imbalances

For women, imbalances in the reproductive hormones (see "A Glossary of Depression-Related Hormones," pp. 207-208), which are intimately linked to emotions and mood, can prove to be a major source of depression. Many factors can influence hormone levels, including diet, stress, exercise, toxic exposure, and the more obvious ones of childbirth and menopause. Postpartum (after childbirth) depression is a common occurrence and, for some women, the wild changes in hormones during this time create symptoms severe enough to warrant a diagnosis of clinical depression. Postpartum depression

A Depression by Any Other Name...

In addition to clinical depression (as defined by the National Institute of Mental Health, see pp. 200-201) and manic depression (a "bipolar" disorder in which the patient alternates between extreme highs and lows), two other diagnoses of depression are in common usage by medical and psychiatric practitioners. They are dysthymia and seasonal affective disorder.

Dysthymia refers to mild to moderate depression or chronic low-grade depression, similar to malaise or melancholy. Dysthymia doesn't incapacitate a person, but gnaws at quality of life on a day-to-day basis, draining joy, enthusiasm, and brightness. People suffering from dysthymia are good candidates for herbal antidepressants, such as St. John's wort, described later in this chapter.[11]

Acknowledged only recently as a distinct condition, seasonal affective disorder (SAD), or winter depression, affects some 10.8 million North Americans. Caused by sunlight deprivation, SAD strikes during the fall and winter months, when days grow shorter and natural light is in short supply. SAD victims typically experience chronic depression, along with hypersomnia (increased sleep), fatigue, lethargy, and carbohydrate cravings accompanied by significant weight gain. For women, a worsening of PMS (premenstrual) symptoms is also common. Light therapy is one method of reversing SAD.

For more about **St. John's wort**, see this chapter, p. 217. For information on **light therapy**, see this chapter, pp. 239-242.

has a history of being dismissed as a woman's maladjustment to motherhood, but there are clear physiological foundations for this plunge into despondency.

The same is true of the depression associated with perimenopause and menopause, which has likewise been attributed to a woman's psychological difficulties in making the transition to this new stage of life. Although there is certainly a psychological component, hormonal changes may play a larger role in the attendant depression.

Perimenopause is the time when hormone levels begin to shift in preparation for menopause (the cessation of menstruation). It is not so much the decrease in hormones that produces the uncomfortable symptoms associated with perimenopause, but rather the changing ratio between the two primary female hormones, estrogen and progesterone. Perimenopause can begin as long as ten to 15 years before a woman's periods finally stop, although a shorter duration is more typical. With the average American woman starting perimenopause after the age of 45 and entering menopause around age 52, that's still enough years for hormonal shifts to create emotional havoc. Chronic or episodic depression, severe mood swings, and anxiety are frequent manifestations of these

A Glossary of Depression-Related Hormones

Estrogen is a female sex hormones produced mainly in the ovaries (some in the fat cells) which regulates the menstrual cycle. Estrogen is important for adolescent sexual development, prepares the uterus for receiving the fertilized egg by stimulating the uterine lining to grow, affects all the body's cells, and declines after menopause. Estrogen slows down bone loss that leads to osteoporosis and can help reverse the incidence of heart attacks; it also improves skin tone, reduces vaginal dryness, and can act as an antiaging factor. For the first 10-14 days in a woman's cycle and peaking at ovulation, her uterus is mainly under the influence of the hormone estrogen. Estrogen levels begin to climb right after menstruation, from about day 7-14. There are three natural types of estrogen: estradiol (produced directly from the ovary); estrone (produced from estradiol); and estriol (formed in smaller amounts in the ovary). Estradiol is the most potent of the three, and prepares the uterus for the implanatation of a fertilized egg; it also helps mature and maintain the sex characteristics of the female organs.

Progesterone is a female sex hormone (produced in the *corpus luteum* of the ovaries) which prepares the uterus for a fertilized egg and stops the cell proliferation in the uterus begun under estrogen when a pregnancy does not occur. When estrogen is high during days 7-14 of the woman's cycle, the level of the hormone progesterone is at its lowest; climbs to a peak from around day 14 to 24 then dramatically drops off again just before the start of menstruation. When the cells stop producing progesterone, it's a signal to the uterus to let go of all the new cells each month and to start afresh. In a sense, menstruation is progesterone withdrawal. Starting at age 35, a woman's progesterone production begins to decline.

DHEA (dehydroepiandrosterone) is naturally produced by the adrenal glands and gonads with optimal levels occurring around age 20 for women and age 25 for men. After those ages, DHEA levels gradually decline so that 80-year-olds produce only a fraction of the DHEA they did when they were 20. As an antioxidant, hormone regulator, and the building block from which estrogen and testosterone are produced, DHEA is vital to health.

Low DHEA levels have been associated with cancer, diabetes, multiple sclerosis, hypertension, obesity, AIDS, heart disease, Alzheimer's, and immune dysfunction illnesses. Test subjects using supplemental DHEA reported improved sleeping patterns, better memory, an improved ability to cope with stress, decreased joint pain, increases in lean muscle, and decreases in body fat. No serious side effects have been reported to date, although acne, oily skin, facial hair growth on women, deepening of the voice, irritability, insomnia, and fatigue have been reported with high DHEA doses.

A Glossary of Depression-Related Hormones (cont.)

Testosterone is the primary male sex hormone, made in the testes, and important for the development of male sexual characteristics. It declines after "male menopause" at midlife. Testosterone can help reverse male impotence, heighten virility, and increase muscle mass. Women have testosterone, too. As testosterone levels decline, one of the safest ways to make it available to your system is through a skin-absorbed (percutaneous) gel. The gel is apply topically to the skin and absorbed slowly into the blood stream. Restoring testosterone levels increases sperm count in men and, in both sexes, raises lowered libido.

Pregnenolone is a hormone produced in the brain and adrenal cortex from cholesterol; in turn, pregnenolone is the "parent" hormone for DHEA and other key hormones. Usually, starting at age 45, pregnenolone production slows down, and by the time one turns 75, the body produces 60% less pregnenolone than in one's youth. As a brain power hormone, pregnenolone enhances memory, improves concentration, reduces mental fatigue, and generally keeps the brain functioning at peak capacity. A typical recommended dose for brain-power enhancement is 50 mg daily, best taken in the morning. Generally, one can expect a "modest improvement" in brain power within hours after taking pregnenolone, but as this hormone's effect is cumulative, the full beneficial effects will emerge over time.

Melatonin, a hormone produced by the pea-sized, light-sensitive pineal (pronounced pie-NEEL) gland in the center of the brain, regulates the body's internal clock, or circadian rhythm, which determines the 24-hour sleep-wake cycle. With aging, the peak in melatonin secretion is about one hour later than normal (normal peak secretion time is about 2 a.m.), and the maximum peak of melatonin is only one-half the level of young adults. Low melatonin levels have been associated with sleeping disturbances and light-related conditions such as seasonal affective disorder (SAD). Eating vitamin- and mineral-rich foods and increasing your exposure to bright light can improve the body's natural melatonin production.

midlife hormonal fluctuations.

Phyllis Bronson, a Ph.D. candidate in biochemistry, and Harold Whitcomb, M.D., directors of the Aspen Clinic for Preventive and Environmental Medicine, in Aspen, Colorado, report that almost all of the perimenopausal women they see are suffering from either depression or anxiety caused by hormonal imbalance. "Only a very small percentage feel great naturally," says Bronson. Anxiety is the result in those who have too much estrogen in relationship to other hormones (estrogen dominance), says Bronson, and depression occurs when the woman has too little estrogen in the hormonal equation (estrogen deficiency).

The following case from **Phyllis Bronson** and **Dr. Whitcomb** illustrates the powerful influence hormones have on mood and how even chronic depression can be reversed with the proper balance of supplements and natural hormone therapy:

Success Story: Hormonal Deficiency Caused Her Ten-Year Depression

Margaret was 50 when she came to see us. At that age, she was nearing menopause and had irregular periods. She suffered from chronic depression, for which she had been prescribed numerous antidepressants over the last ten years. She also had sleeping difficulties and a lack of clarity in her thinking, a condition referred to as brain fog. Our blood tests revealed that Margaret was low in estrogen, progesterone, DHEA, and testosterone (see "A Glossary of Depression-Related

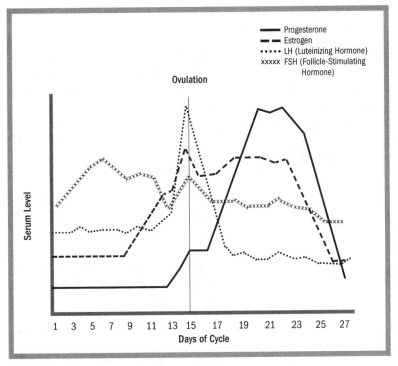

HORMONE LEVELS DURING THE MENSTRUAL CYCLE.

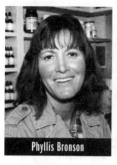

Phyllis Bronson

Anxiety is the result in those who have too much estrogen in relationship to other hormones (estrogen dominance), says biochemist Phyllis Bronson, and depression occurs when the woman has too little estrogen in the hormonal equation (estrogen deficiency).

Hormones," pp. 207-208).

Margaret told us she was lethargic and lacked motivation even to get to a therapist to help relieve her depression. She experienced persistent sadness, cried frequently, continually gained weight, and retained water (a symptom associated with progesterone deficiency). Other symptoms associated with estrogen deficiency can include hot flashes, sex drive loss, mood swings, and weight gain. (These are also typical of perimenopause.) An estrogen-deficient woman may run a higher risk of cardiovascular disease and osteoporosis as well.

Margaret's depression was consistent with low levels of estradiol, which is how we measure estrogen status. Her estrogen level was 54.3, whereas a woman her age should have a level between 90 and 130. Margaret's progesterone level was 0.2, whereas a normal reading for her would have been 25. Her testosterone was around 14; the acceptable reference range for women is 14 to 76, but for menopausal women we like to see it around 40 to 60. With a low level of 14, Margaret had no sex drive.

We also checked her DHEA level, which was 90. For a woman of this age to be optimally healthy with a low risk of degenerative disease, the DHEA count should be above 400 and preferably 500 to 600. Low DHEA levels such as Margaret's are often correlated with extreme exhaustion and flu-like symptoms (which she had) without apparent medical basis.

Estrogen-deficient women often are low in pregnenolone (see "A Glossary of Depression-Related Hormones," pp. 207-208), an essential hormone which is a precursor to progesterone. Pregnenolone may be a significant factor in depression for the following reason: it is abundant in the brain where it improves the transmission of nerve impulses and facilitates communication between brain cells. In a sense, people who are depressed may have poor communication, neuronally speaking, between the different parts of their brain because they are deficient in pregnenolone. This hormone appears to have a great calming effect because it activates receptor sites in brain cells for GABA (itself a calming agent), enabling more GABA to be absorbed by the cells.

Using electrodermal screening (SEE QUICK DEFINITION), we discovered that Margaret had many food sensitivities, specifically to grains such as wheat, rice, rye, kamut, and spelt. A further blood test showed us that Margaret was deficient in histidine, an amino acid (SEE QUICK DEFINITION) associated with allergies; histidine deficiencies are often correlated with a hormonal imbalance such as Margaret's. To address the food allergies and depression, we prescribed histidine (200 mg, once daily) and another amino acid, tyrosine (500 mg, before meals), vitamin B5 (pantothenic acid; 500 mg, with meals), and a supplement called Doctor's Brand 007, containing amino acids needed to produce serotonin, a key brain chemical involved in mood regulation.

Many estrogen-deficient women come to us already taking Prozac or another prescription antidepressant; such women, typically, are low in the amino acid tryptophan, which is a precursor to serotonin. While depression is multifaceted in origin, the role of amino acids is central to any discussion on the biochemistry of depression (see pp. 213-215). These women usually respond well to amino acid supplementation.

Amino acids and natural hormones are the basis of our natural antidepressant program which has enabled many women, with their doctor's supervision, to be weaned off their prescription drugs. When people take Prozac for depression, they're actually trying to biochemically elevate their serotonin levels. What we do is substitute the natural neurotransmitters or their amino acid precursors for the psychotropic drugs. The result is a more thorough healing with no side effects.

We also gave Margaret a natural estrogen called E1, E2, E3 Tri-estrogen (E123), which contains 100 mg of progesterone in cream form and a transdermal DHEA gel. Margaret applied the E123 cream twice daily and the DHEA gel once daily, rubbing them into the skin at soft tissue sites such as the stomach and thighs; applying each in a different place and spacing the applications

QUICK DEFINITION

Electrodermal screening is a form of computerized information gathering, based on physics, not chemistry. A blunt, noninvasive electric probe is placed at specific points on the patient's hands, face, or feet, corresponding to acupuncture points at the beginning or end of energy meridians. Minute electrical discharges from these points serve as information signals about the condition of the body's organs and systems, useful for the physician in evaluation and developing a treatment plan.

Amino acids are the basic building blocks of the 40,000 different proteins in the body, including enzymes, hormones, and the key brain chemical messenger molecules called neurotransmitters. Eight amino acids cannot be made by the body and must be obtained through the diet; others are produced in the body but not always in sufficient amounts. The body's main "amino acid pool" consists of: alanine, arginine, aspargine, aspartic acid, carnitine, citrulline, cysteine, cystine, GABA, glutamic acid, glutamine, glycine, histidine, isoleucine, leucine, lysine, methionine, ornithine, phenylalanine, proline, serine, taurine, threonine, tryptophan, tyrosine, and valine.

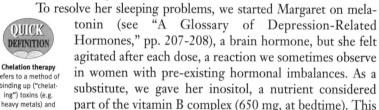

Depression can be caused by amino acid deficiencies accompanied by hormonal imbalances and shortages of the neurotransmitter serotonin. As you can see by Margaret's transformation, symptoms can improve dramatically by taking the proper supplements, says Dr. Whitcomb.

at least an hour apart.

To resolve her sleeping problems, we started Margaret on melatonin (see "A Glossary of Depression-Related Hormones," pp. 207-208), a brain hormone, but she felt agitated after each dose, a reaction we sometimes observe in women with pre-existing hormonal imbalances. As a substitute, we gave her inositol, a nutrient considered part of the vitamin B complex (650 mg, at bedtime). This quickly ended her sleeping difficulties.

A hair analysis for heavy metals revealed that Margaret had unacceptable levels of arsenic, lead, and cadmium. These created a toxic load, particularly on her nervous system, which contributed to her chronic depression. We gave her a product called OC Packs, a multinutrient package that would bind up (chelate, SEE QUICK DEFINITION) the heavy metals and remove them from her system. She also started taking vitamin C buffered with calcium and magnesium (2,000 mg, four times daily). High doses of vitamin C, with calcium and magnesium, bind with toxic metals to form a new compound called ascorbogen which can be safely excreted from the body, thereby removing some of the metals. A hair analysis some months later confirmed that Margaret's heavy metal load was much lower.

After the first six weeks, Margaret's energy picked up, and she started sleeping deeply and woke feeling refreshed. She reported a marked clarity in her thinking, as one of her most significant symptoms, brain fog, had lifted. Her libido returned and, with it, the interest for a romantic relationship. Four months into the program, Margaret's progesterone level had climbed to 5.6. Her estrogen levels came up more slowly, which is often the case with natural estrogens.

Chelation therapy refers to a method of binding up ("chelating") toxins (e.g. heavy metals) and metabolic wastes and removing them from the body while at the same time increasing blood flow and removing arterial plaque. One type of chelation therapy involves the chelating agent disodium EDTA given as an intravenous infusion over a 3½ hour period. Usually 20 to 30 treatments are administered at the rate of one to three sessions per week. Chelation therapy is especially beneficial for all forms of atherosclerotic cardiovascular disease including angina pectoris and coronary artery disease.

For more information on **hormonal imbalances and menstruation,** see *Alternative Medicine Guide to Women's Health 1* (Future Medicine Publishing, 1998; ISBN 1-887299-12-2); to order, call 800-333-HEAL.

Now, more than a year after beginning with us, Margaret's estrogen is at 95, progesterone at 8, DHEA at 350, and testosterone at 42. Margaret says she "feels great" and has plenty of energy. Her hormones have been rebalanced naturally. As you can see by Margaret's transformation, depression caused by a deficiency of estrogen and related amino acids can be improved dramatically by taking the proper supplements. ∎

2) Amino Acid Deficiencies

As Margaret's case demonstrated, amino acid deficiencies can accompany hormonal imbalances and deficiencies of serotonin, both of which contribute to depression. Since amino acids are the building blocks for hormones and neurotransmitters (such as serotonin and norepinephrine), a shortage in amino acids is frequently behind deficiencies in these other vital substances.

Numerous alternative practitioners have found that supplementing with amino acids and supporting vitamins and minerals relieves depression by restoring the balance of the neurotransmitters. Priscilla Slagle, M.D., of Encino, California, calls this process "precursor loading," because the amino acids are the precursors of the amines or neurotransmitters.[12]

Amino acid deficiency is a perfect example of what is left untreated when conventional antidepressants are applied as the solution to depression. They may raise serotonin levels, but the original deficiency (for example, of tryptophan) that created the lack of serotonin in the first place is not amended and, therefore, true healing has not occurred. The clinical use of amino acids, on the other hand, produces no side effects or health risks while generating lasting healing results. Tryptophan, because of its contribution in making serotonin, has been used effectively for many years for depression and sleep disorders. Found in turkey, milk, and bananas, tryptophan is what's behind the

Phyllis Bronson is a nutritional biochemist and a Ph.D. candidate in biochemistry with 20 years of clinical experience in the nutrient effects of depression and anxiety. **Harold Whitcomb, M.D.,** is a board-certified internist with an emphasis in environmental and preventive medicine. They may be contacted at: Aspen Clinic for Preventive and Environmental Medicine at Internal Medicine Associates, 100 East Main Street, Aspen, CO 81611; tel: 970-920-2523 or 970-925-5440; fax: 970-920-2282. For information about **Doctor's Brand 007**, contact: Livingston Health Foods, Inc., 1324 South Sherman Street, Longmont, CO 80501; tel: 303-651-2522 or 800-672-4566; fax: 303-772-4566. For **E1, E2, E3 Tri-estrogen** (by prescription only), contact: Women's International Pharmacy, 13925 Meeker Blvd., Suite 13, Sun City West, AZ 85375; tel: 800-699-8143 or 602-214-7700; fax: 602-214-7708. For **DHEA Transdermal Gel** (by prescription only), contact: College Pharmacy, 833 N. Tejone Street, Colorado Springs, CO, 80903; tel: 800-888-9358 or 719-634-4861; fax: 800-556-5893 or 719-634-4513. For **OC Packs**, contact: Advanced Medical Nutrition, Inc., 2247 National Avenue, P.O. Box 5012, Hayward, CA 94540; tel: 800-437-8888 or 510-783-6969; fax: 510-783-8196. For **Buffered Vitamin C**, contact: Allergy Research Group, 400 Preda Street, San Leandro, CA 94577; tel: 800-545-9960 or 510-639-4572; fax: 510-635-6730.

Numerous alternative practitioners have found that supplementing with amino acids and supporting vitamins and minerals relieves depression by restoring the balance of the neurotransmitters.

For more about **tryptophan**, see this chapter, p. 216. For information on **testing your nutritional status**, see Chapter 4: Chronic Fatigue Syndrome, pp. 190-192.

folk remedy of warm milk for insomnia.

The following case demonstrates how amino acid supplementation, combined with the appropriate hormones, vitamins, and minerals, can solve even intransigent chronic depression.

Success Story: Seven Years of Bedbound Depression Reversed

When Jackie, 55, first met Eric R. Braverman, M.D., a physician practicing in Penndel, Pennsylvania, and New York City, she had been so deeply depressed for the past seven years that she spent most of her days in bed, sleeping. "She was treatment resistant, therapy resistant, and bedbound, and she had failed to respond to multiple antidepressant drug trials," recalls Dr. Braverman. In retrospect, he accords her the dubious honor of having "the worst case of depression for which I have seen a recovery."

Jackie's problems had begun at the age of 48 when she showed signs of perimenopause, or menopause onset, says Dr. Braverman. Her hair started to thin, she developed chronic fatigue, she became increasingly dysfunctional, and soon she took to her bed. Before Jackie consulted Dr. Braverman, her physicians tried most of the standard conventional antidepressants on her, but they produced little benefit.

After running a series of blood tests to determine Jackie's hormonal status, Dr. Braverman settled on a natural hormonal supplementation program to include estrogen, progesterone, testosterone, and DHEA. "When women reach age 40, they often start losing progesterone and some estrogen," comments Dr. Braverman. "But you never know which hormone will run out first. Then around age 47 to 52, a woman may become deficient in testosterone and psychiatric symptoms may develop. Any number of symptoms, such as depression, anxiety, memory loss, or diminished sexual drive, can occur as a result of missing key nutrients and hormones."

Specifically, his daily prescription for Jackie included testosterone (2.5 mg at bedtime), estradiol (one of the estrogens, 0.5 mg at bedtime), progesterone (100 mg at bedtime), and DHEA (50 mg in the morning). Dr. Braverman also gave Jackie a series of his own specially formulated PATH nutritional supplements which, in her case, included amino acids, zinc, magnesium, calcium, and antioxidants. She also took essential fatty acids in the form of borage and fish oils (400 mg, twice daily), niacin (500 mg, twice daily), and a complete vitamin B complex.

To help her sleep, Jackie took the amino acid tryptophan (500 mg) and melatonin (500 mcg) before going to bed. Despite her years of oversleeping, Jackie actually needed this assistance because, as she reduced her daytime sleeping hours and rebalanced her overall sleep/wake cycle, she at first had difficulty falling asleep at night. In addition, the serotonin-increasing effect of tryptophan would help alleviate Jackie's depression.

To reduce the symptoms of various allergies, Dr. Braverman gave Jackie an antihistamine formula containing the amino acid methionine, vitamin C, and the bioflavonoid (vitamin C helper) quercetin (130 mg). To help reduce her anxiety, Jackie used a cranial electrical stimulation (CES, SEE QUICK DEFINITION) device, applied to her wrist and forehead, for one hour every evening. The CES introduced a minute but therapeutic electrical current into her system as a way of improving her mood and state of mind.

"Mood and well-being are multifactorial and depend on healthy levels of hormones, nutrients, and electromagnetic fields," notes Dr. Braverman. His strategy for treating Jackie's depression was to balance the core hormones by recharging the brain nutritionally, hormonally, and electrically. "Jackie did everything possible to rebuild a healthy state of mind and body using natural means," he comments. Within the first two months, Jackie started feeling improvements and her depression began lifting; within another five months she was able to work again (and her hair grew in thicker, too), says Dr. Braverman.[13]

3) Serotonin Deficiencies

The average human body contains about 10 mg of the neurotransmitter serotonin—not a lot, seemingly, but if serotonin levels drop much below that, it can cause extreme mood changes. Low levels of serotonin have been associated with impulsive behavior, aggression, overeating (particularly carbohydrate cravings), depression, and suicide.[14] Drugs such as Prozac work to alleviate depression by rais-

For more about **Dr. Eric Braverman's program**, contact: PATH (Place for Achieving Total Health), 274 Madison Avenue, 4th Floor, Room 402, New York, NY 10016; tel: 212-213-6155; fax: 212-213-6188.

Cranial electrotherapy stimulation (CES) is a safe, nonaddictive use of microelectric impulses. CES stimulates the production of endorphins (pleasure-inducing molecules) in the brain by delivering, typically, 100 pulses per second of alternating current electricity from a packet-sized unit (weighing eight ounces) with ear-clip electrodes that apply the current across the patient's brain stem. CES is commonly used for treatment of insomnia, anxiety, depression, chronic pain, gastritis, substance abuse, and migraines, among other conditions.

As a supplement for depression, 5-HTP reportedly has many of the same beneficial effects as tryptophan, which is only available by prescription. Further, a study of 5-HTP found that it produced results similar to that of conventional antidepressants.

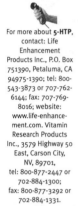

For more about **5-HTP**, contact: Life Enhancement Products Inc., P.O. Box 751390, Petaluma, CA 94975-1390; tel: 800-543-3873 or 707-762-6144; fax: 707-769-8016; website: www.life-enhance-ment.com. Vitamin Research Products Inc., 3579 Highway 50 East, Carson City, NV, 89701, tel: 800-877-2447 or 702-884-1300; fax: 800-877-3292 or 702-884-1331.

ing serotonin levels.

In the cases of Jackie and Margaret, you saw how natural antidepressants—amino acids—can more safely and effectively raise these levels. As mentioned previously, serotonin, or 5-HT (5-hydroxytryptamine), is made from the amino acid tryptophan. In the brain, tryptophan is converted into 5-hydroxytryptophan (5-HTP), and then to serotonin.

As a supplement for depression, 5-HTP, now available over the counter, reportedly has many of the same beneficial effects as tryptophan, which is only available by prescription.[15] Further, a study of 5-HTP found that it produced results similar to that of conventional antidepressants, according to Melvyn R. Werbach, M.D., of Tarzana, California. Researchers treated 25 depressed patients with either 5-HTP alone or in combination with a supplementary prescription drug that enhances the ability of the 5-HTP to reach the brain. Both groups experienced improvement in their depression within three to five days.[16]

Another study found that 5-HTP produced *better* results than did antidepressants. Study subjects with medically diagnosed depression received, three times a day, either 150 mg of a Prozac-equivalent or 100 mg of 5-HTP. After six weeks, the depression of participants in both groups had lessened, with the 5-HTP group showing slightly higher results in both the degree of improvement and the percentage of patients showing improvement.[17]

The mechanism by which 5-HTP raises serotonin may be superior to that of antidepressant drugs which simply pump serotonin into the system. "The employment of 5-HTP aims at providing the substate or metabolic precursor to serotonin while allowing the body itself to regulate the further steps in serotonin metabolism," states an article on the benefits of 5-HTP in *Let's Live* magazine.[18] In other words, supplementing with 5-HTP produces a closer approximation of what the body would do on its own.

Certain botanicals act as antidepressants as well. Blue-green algae boosts serotonin naturally because it is full of easily digestible amino acids, according to Dr. Christiane Northrup.[19] Dosages are variable, depending upon the individual. Dr. Steven Bratman reports that ginkgo (*Ginkgo biloba*), often used to aid mental alertness, can also relieve depression. He recommends a dosage of 40 mg to 80 mg, three times daily, of an extract standardized to contain 24% ginkgo flavonoid glycosides (the active ingredient). The antidepressant effect could take two to eight weeks, says Dr. Bratman.[20]

Perhaps the most well-known natural antidepressant is the herb St. John's wort (*Hypericum perforatum*) which, with its current popularity and the media attention it has received as a result, is fast approaching Prozac in public acceptance. In 1997, St. John's wort became the herb of choice for treating mild to moderate depression, known as dysthymia (see "A Depression by Any Other Name...," p. 206), following the release of the results of more than 25 clinical studies showing that St. John's wort reverses depression as well as or better than conventional antidepressant drugs. However, it is not recommended for severe suicidal depression, which needs a stronger intervention.

The active component of St. John's wort is hypericin which research has found works like chemical antidepressants to raise serotonin levels.[21] "Not only is the scientific data supporting [St. John's wort] reasonably good, my clinical experiences and those of numerous other practitioners using the herb in daily practice have convinced me that St. John's wort is a splendid option for mild to moderate depression," says Dr. Bratman.[22]

St. John's wort has the added advantage of producing no side effects other than possible light sensitivity (wear a hat and sunblock outdoors). Experts advise, however, that you should avoid combining it with prescription antidepressants. For mild to moderate depression, the standard dosage of St. John's wort recommended by many alternative medicine physicians is 300 mg three times a day. Most of the capsules now available over the counter are at or near that dosage. The herb is also available in health food stores in dried or extract form.

For more about **hypothyroidism**, see Chapter 1: Fibrocystic Breast Disease, p. 31, and Chapter 4: Chronic Fatigue Syndrome, pp. 180-183. For more about the **TRH and other thyroid tests**, see Chapter 4: Chronic Fatigue Syndrome, pp. 181-183.

4) Underactive Thyroid Gland

In addition to imbalances in hormones, amino acids, or brain chemicals, another frequent cause of depression is an underactive thyroid gland (hypothyroidism, SEE QUICK DEFINITION). The thyroid is possibly the most

St. John's wort is now the herb of choice for treating mild to moderate depression, based on the results of more than 25 clinical studies showing it reverses depression as well as or better than conventional antidepressant drugs.

QUICK DEFINITION

Hypothyroidism is a condition of low or underactive thyroid gland function that can produce numerous symptoms. Among the 47 clinically recognized symptoms: fatigue, depression, lethargy, weakness, weight gain, low body temperature, chills, cold extremities, general inappropriate sensation of cold, infertility, rheumatic pain, menstrual disorders (excessive flow, cramps), repeated infections, colds, upper respiratory infections, skin problems (itching, eczema, psoriasis, acne, dry, coarse, or scaly skin, skin pallor), memory disturbances, concentration difficulties, paranoia, migraines, oversleep, "laziness," muscle aches and weakness, hearing disturbances, burning/prickling sensations, anemia, slow reaction time and mental sluggishness, swelling of the eyelids, constipation, labored or difficult breathing, hoarseness, brittle nails, and poor vision. A resting body temperature (measured in the armpit) below 97.8° F may indicate hypothyroidism. Menstruating women should take the underarm temperature only on the second and third days of menstruation.

overlooked organ in the body. When it's not working properly, this gland in the neck can produce an astonishing number of health problems; thyroid problems are listed as a factor in all of the conditions covered in this book.

When the thyroid is underactive, everything in the body gradually becomes hypoactive as well, from circulation to libido. But as discussed in previous chapters, a large number of clinically severe thyroid conditions go undetected for long periods of time and some, regrettably, are never picked up. Along with this, people are often erroneously treated for chronic health conditions that are really based on the thyroid and that would respond well and quickly to a small dose of thyroid hormone.

For example, Stephen E. Langer, M.D., of Berkeley, California, a thyroid specialist, treated a patient who had been depressed for 60 years; yet when this man took thyroid hormone, his depression was gone within a month. Whatever his previous physicians prescribed focused on his depression only, but missed the underlying thyroid cause, so he was miserable for most of his life.

An underactive thyroid can affect almost every bodily function, producing symptoms as diverse as memory problems, chronic muscle pain, and slowed heart rate, but its main symptoms are depression and fatigue. The following case, featuring these symptoms, illustrates the common occurrence of hypothyroidism eluding testing and the dramatic recovery possible once the true problem is identified.

Success Story: Depression and Fatigue Reversed With Thyroid Treatment

Mona, 42, had suffered with depression and extreme fatigue for a year, waking in the morning, after eight to ten hours of sleep or more, feeling more tired than when she went to bed. During the day she often needed a nap. While she ate relatively little, Mona was steadily gaining weight (a classic symptom of hypothyroidism) and she also experienced bloating, constipation, and occasional abdominal pains; her skin was dry; her hair was thinning; and her menstrual cycles were irregular and preceded by PMS. Mona also reported that she had difficulty concentrating and was forgetful.

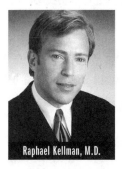

Raphael Kellman, M.D.

"Within two weeks Mona began to feel more energy and more alive," notes Dr. Kellman. "A few weeks later, her brain fog began to lift and her attention span was significantly better. In no time, she was back to her old self."

When Mona's conventional physician performed a routine thyroid hormone test (for T3 and T4 levels), the results came back normal. Although, on the basis of these results, she was advised to "rest and not worry," Mona thought otherwise, and sought a further thyroid test to measure TSH levels. But this test yielded normal results, too. Mona's doctor wrote her a Prozac prescription for her anxiety and depression.

To contact **Raphael Kellman, M.D.**: The Center for Progressive Medicine, 140 West 69th Street, New York, NY 10023; tel: 212-721-6633; fax: 212-721-6714.

When Mona consulted Raphael Kellman, M.D., founder and medical director of the Center for Progressive Medicine, in New York City, "her life seemed to be spiraling downwards," comments Dr. Kellman. "Her depression subsided a little on the Prozac, but her fatigue, weight, and other problems got worse." Dr. Kellman immediately ran the TRH thyroid test on Mona; her TSH level was 22, objectively indicating an underactive thyroid. He started Mona on Synthroid (a synthetic form of T4) and Thyrostim to convert T4 to T3.

"Within two weeks Mona began to feel more energy and more alive," notes Dr. Kellman. "A few weeks later, her brain fog began to lift and her attention span was significantly better. In no time, she was back to her old self and began noticing weight loss and thicker, fuller hair, and her skin was normal again. Soon her periods were more regular and her PMS became tolerable. Within six weeks of starting the program, Mona's depression was much better and her energy level was, in her words, 'The best I can ever remember.'"

In addition to causing depression on its own, hypothyroidism can

In treating an underactive thyroid, Dr. Feldman prefers not to use the synthetic form of thyroid hormone because, as the drug performs the gland's natural work, the thyroid shuts down. There is the risk of becoming dependent on the synthetic thyroid hormone for life, he explains.

worsen a problem that has its derivation in other causes, as exemplified by the following case in which the depression and fatigue accompanying the hormonal changes of childbirth were exacerbated by an underactive thyroid.

Success Story: Postpartum Depression Cured by Reviving Her Thyroid

Mara, 32, gave birth after an untroubled pregnancy, but three weeks after delivery, she began to notice a drop in her energy. Fatigue is typical for new mothers, but Mara had always been full of pep and was shocked by the dramatic change. By midafternoon every day, she needed a nap, and had to rest again in the early evening; in addition, she developed an intolerance to cold (a symptom of hypothyroidism). She was also depressed to the degree that she consulted a psychiatrist, who stopped short of diagnosing postpartum depression, but nonetheless suggested prescription antidepressants.

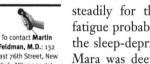

To contact **Martin Feldman, M.D.**: 132 East 76th Street, New York, NY 10021; tel: 212-744-4413; fax: 212-472-5139. For **#8THY**, contact: Nutri-West, P.O. Box 950, Douglas, WY 82633; tel: 800-443-3333 or 307-358-5066. For **Thyroid Plus** (also called N14), contact: Health Industries, 4745 State Route 94E, Murray, KY 42071; tel: 800-626-3386 or 502-753-2613; fax: 502-759-4536. For **Thytrophin PMG**, contact: Standard Process, 1200 W. Royal Lee Drive, Palmyra, WI 53156; tel: 800-848-5061 or 414-495-2122; fax: 414-495-2512.

Mara declined. However, her energy drain progressed steadily for the next three months. This continuing fatigue probably would still be considered normal, given the sleep-deprivation most new mothers experience, but Mara was deeply dissatisfied—she had a feeling something wasn't right. She sought the help of Martin Feldman, M.D., who practices in New York City.

Dr. Feldman had Mara do the basal body temperature test for thyroid function by placing a thermometer under her arm as soon as she woke up in the morning and before getting out of bed. Her temperature was lower (97.7° F) than the norm for this test, indicating some degree of thyroid sluggishness. However, a range of blood tests for Mara's thyroid function (T3, T4, TSH, and several others) came back normal. This is a common problem, observes Dr. Feldman. "The blood levels are fine, but the thyroid is not right."

Dr. Feldman also ran Mara through the Ragland

A Guide to Thyroid Hormones

The thyroid has four principal hormones: T1, T2, T3, and T4. Thyroid hormones are stored in the thyroid and released to the body as needed. T1 (mono-iodothyronine) and T2 (di-iodothyronine) are not considered especially active. T4 (thyroxine) contains iodine, is produced exclusively in the thyroid gland, and accounts for almost 93% of the thyroid's hormones active in all of the body's processes; its chief function is to increase the speed of cell metabolism, or energy conversion.

Iodine and the amino acid tyrosine are essential to forming normal amounts of T4. When the body requires more T3 (tri-iodothyronine), T4 can give up its iodine to form T3 which, while representing only about 7% of the thyroid hormone complement, has a greater biological activity by a factor of three to four times. About 80% of the body's T3 comes from converting T4, typically in the liver and kidneys.

The formation and secretion of T3 and T4 are regulated by thyroid-stimulating hormone, or TSH (thyrotropin), secreted by the pituitary gland in the brain. TSH, in turn, is directed by another hormone called thyrotropin-releasing hormone (TRH) which is secreted by the brain's hypothalamus gland. TSH blood levels are conventionally taken as the best index for thyroid dysfunction, both hypo and hyper (overactive). When thyroid function is low, TSH levels normally go up.

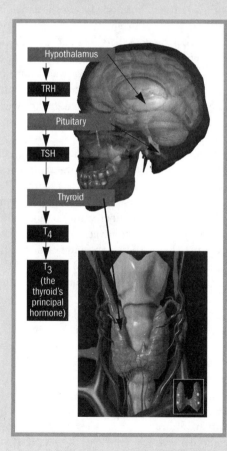

Hypothalamus

TRH

Pituitary

TSH

Thyroid

T$_4$

T$_3$
(the thyroid's principal hormone)

QUICK DEFINITION

A **glandular extract** is a purified nutritional and therapeutic product derived from one of several animal glands including the adrenal, thymus, thyroid, ovaries, testes, pancreas, pineal, and pituitary. It is prescribed by a physician for a person whose corresponding gland is underfunctioning and not producing enough of its own hormone. The various glands are part of the endocrine system which, along with the nervous system, coordinates the functioning of all of the body's systems.

For information on **testing your nutritional status**, see Chapter 4: Chronic Fatigue Syndrome, pp. 190-192.

Postural Blood Pressure test. For this, you rest horizontally for five minutes and your blood pressure is recorded, he explains. Then you stand up and your blood pressure is recorded again. In a healthy person, the values should remain constant or perhaps increase slightly. In Mara's case, her blood pressure dropped slightly indicating that her adrenal gland function was suboptimal, which would help explain her fatigue.

In treating an underactive thyroid, Dr. Feldman prefers not to use the synthetic form of thyroid hormone because, as the drug performs the gland's natural work, the thyroid shuts down. There is the risk of becoming dependent on the synthetic thyroid hormone for life, he explains.

For Mara's thyroid revival program, Dr. Feldman prescribed a liquid herbal blend called #8THY containing skullcap, parsley, uva ursi, and dulse. As a starting dose, Mara put five drops of the tincture in very warm but not boiling water, then let it sit for ten minutes to allow the alcohol in the tincture to dissipate. She drank this mixture three times a day, gradually raising the dosage to ten drops and finally 15 drops, three times daily.

Dr. Feldman also gave Mara the mineral selenium (200 mcg to start, building to 400 mcg, daily), the amino acid glutathione (variable dosage), and riboflavin (vitamin B2, 75 mg daily), all of which help in the conversion of T4 to T3. In addition, Mara took zinc picolinate (22 mg, then increasing) because zinc is part of the thyroid formation system; the amino acid L-tyrosine (500 mg, building to 1,000 mg, daily) to help produce thyroid hormone; the mineral rubidium (80 mcg daily in four divided doses) to support the L-tyrosine; and glutamic acid (variable dosage) to help the glutathione.

The third element of Dr. Feldman's thyroid revival program was a homeopathic sarcode called Thyroid Plus. A sarcode is a homeopathic preparation made from animal tissue or secretions, in this case, from an animal's thyroid. Thyroid Plus, which contains 11 different homeopathically prepared substances, comes in drop form and must be taken directly in the mouth, not mixed with water, says Dr. Feldman. Mara took this at the rate of five drops, three times daily, gradually building to ten drops and then 15 drops.

Finally, Mara took glandular extracts (SEE QUICK DEFINITION); specifically, Thytrophin PMG, which is thyroid hormone from cows processed to remove its thyroxine, making it a food, not a hormone, says Dr. Feldman. Mara took four tablets (45 mg each), then six, daily. Dr. Feldman emphasizes that the dosage and even the selection of a thyroid glandular is highly specific to the individual patient. Finally, to reset the adrenal glands, Dr. Feldman started Mara on an adrenal supplement.

After ten weeks on this multifaceted program, Mara's depression had disappeared and her energy was back to normal. Her basal body temperature registered normal as well, indicating that the hypothryoidism was no longer a problem. Had Mara gone on the antidepressants, she might have felt less depressed, but the real root cause, an underactive thyroid, would not have been addressed, comments Dr. Feldman.

5) Diet and Nutritional Deficiencies

Certain dietary practices and a diet lacking in sufficient amounts of the full range of nutrients required by the body can both cause depression. Dietary practices that contribute include frequent consumption of caffeine (found in coffee, tea, chocolate, and colas) or sucrose (found in baked goods, breakfast cereals, soda, and scores of other processed foods and beverages), says Dr. Melvyn Werbach. Food sensitivities and/or allergies can also be the culprits behind depression.[23]

Dr. Sherry Rogers suggests that depressed people stop consuming sugar, white flour products, alcohol, tea, coffee, soda, chocolate, processed foods, and chlorinated or fluoridated water, and also stop smoking. Any or all of these may be contributing to their depression.[24]

Leon Chaitow, N.D., D.O., of London, England, notes that another recently identified cause of depression is the excessive use of aspartame, the artificial sweetener widely used instead of sugar in diet colas and foods. "This is because aspartame is made up of amino acids and, when they are metabolized, they can cause an imbalance in brain chemistry because of their extreme concentration," Dr. Chaitow says.

Nutritional deficiencies can cause mood problems in a number of ways. If your body does not have the vitamins and minerals it needs to support the manufacture of brain chemicals such as serotonin, the level of brain chemicals drops and depression follows. If your thyroid gland doesn't have the nutrients it needs to work efficiently, hypothy-

Essential fatty acids (EFAs) are unsaturated fats required in the diet. Omega-3 and omega-6 oils are the two principal types. The primary omega-3 oil is alpha-linolenic acid (ALA) and is found in flaxseed (58%), canola, pumpkin, walnut, and soybeans. Fish oils, such as salmon, cod, and mackerel, contain the other important omega-3 oils, DHA (docosahexaenoic acid) and EPA (eicosapentaenoic acid). Linoleic acid or cislinoleic acid is the main omega-6 oil and is found in most plants and vegetable oils, including safflower (73%), corn, peanut, and sesame. The most therapeutic form of omega-6 oil is gamma-linolenic acid (GLA), found in evening primrose, black currant, and borage oils. Once in the body, omega-3 and omega-6 are converted to prostaglandins, hormone-like substances that regulate many metabolic functions, particularly inflammatory processes.

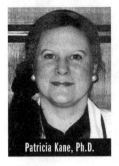

Patricia Kane, Ph.D.

When your diet no longer supplies the necessary raw materials—many of them derived from fats—for running the body efficiently, lots of things go wrong and the body—and brain—starts to shut down. Prozac is only a few more wrong meals away, says Dr. Kane.

QUICK DEFINITION

A **prostaglandin** is a hormone-like, complex fatty acid which affects smooth muscle function, inflammatory processes, and constriction and dilation of blood vessels, particularly in the lungs and intestines. In women, prostaglandins have a stimulating effect on the uterus. Essential fatty acids in the diet (omega-3 and omega-6, found in fish oils) provide the raw material for prostaglandin production; once ingested, these essential fatty acids can be converted to prostaglandins by nearly any cell in the body. Omega-6–derived prostaglandins (the most common type) can have either pro-inflammatory or anti-inflammatory properties, while most prostaglandins converted from omega-3 sources help reduce pain and inflammation. For proper body function, an appropriate balance of both types of prostaglandins must be maintained. Eating too many trans-fatty acids (found in processed foods such as margarine), for example, can interfere with fatty acid metabolism and thus reduce the body's production of prostaglandins.

roidism and its accompanying symptom of depression are the result. Similarly, if your ovaries and adrenal glands don't have the nutrients they need to produce hormones such as estrogen and DHEA, the consequent hormonal imbalances can create depression.

Deficiencies in certain nutrients have been specifically linked to depression, notably vitamin C, thiamine (B1), pyridoxine (B6), cobalamin (B12), niacin (B3), and folic acid.[25] Melvyn Werbach, M.D., of Tarzana, California, additionally cites biotin (in the B vitamin family) and riboflavin (B2), as well as deficiencies in the minerals calcium, copper, iron, and potassium. Both a deficiency and an excess of magnesium (found in nuts, legumes and whole grains) can cause depression, according to Dr. Werbach.

A lack of essential fatty acids (EFAs, see "A Fat Glossary," p. 230) is another factor in depression. **Patricia Kane, Ph.D.**, of Melville, New Jersey, explains the importance of these "good" fats and then relates a dramatic case history in which supplementation with EFAs and other nutrients reversed chronic depression in just four weeks:

Dietary Fats Can Cause—or Cure—Depression

If you study the diet of depressed patients, you often find they are making bad food choices, selecting foods that actually contribute, biochemically, to depressive states. In the interest of staying slim—this is especially true of women—butter and cream are rejected in favor of margarine and other hydrogenated (semi-solid) fats. Saturated hydrogenated fats (a category called trans-fatty acids) such as margarine create havoc in a person's neurochemistry, negatively affecting every system of the body. Using only, or mostly, hydrogenated fats leads to nutrient depletion because the body is not given the kind of fat it needs—essential fatty acids.

When your diet no longer supplies the necessary raw materials—many of them derived from fats—for running the body efficiently, lots of things go wrong and the body—and brain—starts to shut down. Prozac is only a few more wrong meals away. In the contrast between *trans*-fatty acids and *essential* fatty acids, you have the cause and cure of depression.

Trans or hydrogenated, manmade fats were synthesized originally to extend shelf life of commercial products. The production of trans-fatty acids for human consumption is the most devastating nutritional mistake ever made. In the effort to make foods last longer in the supermarket, all traces of essential fatty acids (such as omega-3s) are obliterated from processed foods, and trans-fats or partially hydrogenated oils take their place.

The absence of omega-3 essential fatty acids in Western diets has contributed to an alarming increase in a number of diseases that appeared only infrequently 100 years ago. A lack of the essential fatty acids and co-factors, such as minerals and vitamins, to handle fat combined with the consumption of trans-fats is more often the causal factor in obesity and cardiovascular disease than is eating cholesterol-rich foods. After all, the body *needs* some cholesterol.

> **The first order of the day is to study the depressed person's biochemistry. An imbalance in blood chemistry and fat metabolism owing to daily food choices can hold the answer to understanding the origin of depression.**

Rapidly accumulating evidence suggests that low or lowered cholesterol may be associated with increased non-illness related deaths, such as suicide, brought on by changes in the brain's biochemistry. Too little cholesterol and you are subject to depression. That's because cholesterol is needed to produce a cascade of crucial hormones (including pregnenolone, testosterone, progesterone, estradiol, estrone, and cortisol, among others) and hormones strongly influence mood. Cholesterol also assists in the absorption of essential fatty acids.

You also need fats (lipids) because, like proteins, they are building blocks of the body's essential structures. The brain is 60% lipids and the membrane of every cell is a thin envelope of fat. Fatty acids (the

For more about **testing nutritional status**, see Chapter 4: Chronic Fatigue Syndrome, pp. 190-192.

building blocks of lipids) contribute to the *fluidity* of this cell membrane, ensuring smooth traffic of nutrients and signals in and out of the cell.

Disturbances in fatty acid metabolism (its energy changes and chemical conversions) are reflected in every system of the body and can result in many physical and mental disorders, including depression. A trans-fatty acid sits like a heavy blob inside you, shutting down the fatty acid metabolism within the immune, endocrine, and central nervous systems, and replacing the good, necessary fats (omega-3s and omega-6s) with something harmful to health. You can't do anything with a trans-fatty acid except burn it for calories, and its activity poisons your system and generates an abnormal, undesirable biochemistry.

It is advisable then to *completely avoid* trans-fatty acids. As conventional medicine flounders in looking for the right brain chemical or link between the immune, endocrine, and central nervous systems to control depression, it has forgotten the *basis* of control of these systems—lipid metabolism. This metabolism, in turn, is controllable through targeted nutrition and correct dietary choices.

The first order of the day is to study the depressed person's biochemistry. An imbalance in blood chemistry and fat metabolism owing to daily food choices can hold the answer to understanding the origin of depression. As the following patient case shows, correcting the underlying biochemical imbalances and disturbed fatty acid metabolism can lift even a heavy depression.

Success Story: Reversing Three Years of Depression With EFAs

Sylvia, 29, had suffered from depression for three years. Initially, she had complained of chronic fatigue and mood swings as well; later, she reported digestive difficulties and food allergies. Although she had thus far avoided conventional drugs, she was on the verge of taking Prozac. After fruitlessly consulting several physicians, Sylvia found a doctor who had the insight to check her biochemistry. He ordered a detailed report on her blood chemistry and fatty acid status.

While I was not Sylvia's physician, I consulted on nutritional matters with her doctor. We relied on the CBC Blood Test Report which provides information on 44 different biochemical blood levels. We also used the Fatty Acid Red Cell Membrane, a test developed in 1997 to reveal the status of 67 essential fatty acids in the blood. It does so by examining their presence in the membrane of a single red blood cell. The goal of these tests is to give the physician a picture of the *whole* biochemistry, the checks and balances, suppressed and elevated values, specific to the patient.

Even a cursory look at Sylvia's blood chemistry in the CBC Blood Test Report revealed deeply imbalanced biochemistry. Most generally stated, Sylvia's blood status was an 80% match with the known "disease pattern" for depression, as correlated with the extensive database of previous reports maintained by the test's developers, Carbon Based Corporation, in Incline Village, Nevada. A second initial observation is that Sylvia's blood nutrient status deviated by 31% from the healthy norm.

We start to be concerned with deviations above 25%; these indicate inadequate nutrition. The higher the percentage of deviation, the more critically ill that person is; we have had many people with a 45% to 50% deviation who were literally only days from death. In Sylvia's case, her blood chemistry showed us that what Sylvia was eating was not supplying her nutritional needs. Trans-fatty acids and her low-fat diet were likely part of the problem.

The information provided by Sylvia's Fatty Acid Red Cell Membrane test completed the clinical picture of her depression by making the nature of her fats imbalance clear. Overall, the test showed that Sylvia had results out of balance by more than 25% for 29 categories; in 11 categories of specific fatty acid status, her results were graded "panic values," a situation which required medical attention. Her numbers indicated a suppressed ability to burn fat and impaired production of prostaglandins. The latter is often caused by a high intake of trans-fatty acids. The test also indicated significantly diminished immune capacity, again, probably due to the inadequacies of her diet.

The Dangers of Haphazard Prescribing

Haphazard supplementation—without the benefit of a detailed blood test—can be counterproductive, even dangerous. Sylvia's case highlights the importance of selecting treatment based on the facts gained from clinical testing. For example, her blood chemistry, and thus the underlying cause of her condition, would not have responded to St. John's wort, the increasingly popular herb given for depression. From another perspective we could say that if you supply the raw materials desperately needed by a depressed person's system, St. John's wort or a conventional antidepressant won't be necessary.

In prescribing for a complexly layered case of depression such as Sylvia's, you—both practitioners and lay or self-prescribers—need to exercise clinical intelligence, always bearing in mind the numerous checks and balances that exist among nutrients. Haphazard dietary

Nutrients to Lift Sylvia's Depression

The following list is not meant as a shopping list for all depressed patients; rather it indicates the nutrients specifically required to improve Sylvia's biochemistry.

- Free-form amino acids: five capsules with meals each morning and afternoon

- Buffered vitamin C: $\frac{1}{2}$ tsp taken one hour after each meal

- Similase: an enzyme; two capsules taken after each meal

- Multivitamin: one capsule, twice daily

- Bromelain: an anti-inflammatory; 500 mg, three times daily, taken before meals

- Evening primrose oil: six capsules daily, taken with high-protein meal

- Magnesium succinate: one capsule, four times daily

- Beta rutin: a bioflavonoid or vitamin C helper; 250 mg, twice daily

- AllerAid Formula II: selenium from kelp; 200 mcg, four times daily

- Magnesium citrate: 140 mg, twice daily

- Vitamin K: stimulates electron transfer and lipid metabolism; 200 mcg, four times daily

- Vitamin B complex: one capsule, twice daily

- Cetyl myristoleate: for arthritis symptoms; 260 mg, twice daily

- Folate/folinic acid: a member of the B vitamin family; 800 mcg daily

- Inositol: another member of the B vitamin family; 1,000 mg, four times daily

- Lipoic acid: 150 mg, twice daily

- Adenosyl-cobalamin: a form of vitamin B12; 1,000 mcg, twice daily

- Hypertonic Oral Electrolyte Concentrate: to restore electrolyte balance (SEE QUICK DEFINITION); one ounce mixed with any food except fruit or fruit juices, taken three times daily

QUICK DEFINITION

Electrolytes are substances in the blood, tissue fluids, intracellular fluids, or urine which conduct an electrical charge, either plus or minus. Examples include acids, bases, and salts, such as potassium, magnesium, phosphate, sulfate, bicarbonate, sodium, chloride, and calcium. Electrolytes provide inorganic chemicals for cellular reactions and control mechanisms, such as the conduction of electrochemical impulses to nerves and muscles. Electrolytes are also needed for key enzymatic reactions involved in metabolism, or the release of energy from food.

choices, even those made in the belief that they are *healthy* practices, can similarly produce biological chaos.

For example, believing it was good for her, Sylvia loaded herself with freshly squeezed orange juice every day, overlooking the fact that in so doing she was consuming a great deal of simple sugar. Once lipid metabolism is disturbed (as it was with her because she was eating no fats), merely eating a piece of fruit can upset it. Insulin, the hormone released by the pancreas to regulate blood sugar, begins to rise, and this upsets the production of enzymes which impact the activity of fats.

Similarly, Sylvia was eating a high-carbohydrate diet, also thinking it was good for her. Carbohydrates, too, can elevate insulin and lead to lipid problems by creating inflamed prostaglandins. I must emphasize that nearly every bodily function is involved in some way with fats, but through her ill-informed dietary choices, Sylvia was denying her system this vital controlling substance.

Correcting Sylvia's Diet to Relieve Her Depression

With precise information about Sylvia's biochemical status, developing a nutrient and dietary program was straightforward. Sylvia's problem was simple: we needed to supply her with good basic nutrients, especially nourishing fats, so her body could rebuild its proper biochemistry. Sylvia was given a specific schedule of supplements (see p. 228) and general dietary guidelines, the highlights of which follow:

■ Use liberal amounts of unprocessed sesame oil blended with Omega Nutrition coconut butter; similarly, use only avocado, sesame, almond, or grapeseed oils (cold-pressed).

■ Reduce carbohydrate intake, and avoid all refined sugars, processed foods, margarine, hydrogenated oils, and gluten-containing foods such as wheat, oats, and barley.

■ For better mineral density, increase the consumption of ground raw nuts and seeds (especially sesame), seaweeds, fish, tempeh (fermented soybeans), poultry, avocado, and legumes.

■ Consume more protein sources, such as chicken, turkey, duck, lentils, eggs, almonds, butter beans, shrimp, anchovies, mushrooms, and mussels. This enhances nitrogen retention; low nitrogen is one of the markers of depression. Protein intake should represent 30% of calories, specialized fatty acids 30%, and carbohydrates 40%.

■ When using grains, such as buckwheat, brown rice, or millet,

Patricia C. Kane, Ph.D., a nutritional biochemist, is author of *Food Makes the Difference* and director of nutritional biochemistry at the Kaplan Institute, in Orangevale, California. Dr. Kane can be contacted at: BodyBio Corp., S. Osprey Drive, Melville, NJ 08332; tel: 609-825-8338; fax: 609-825-2143. For more about the **CBC Blood Test Report** and **Hypertonic Oral Electrolyte Concentrate**, contact: Carbon Based Corporation, 920 Incline Way, 2C, Incline Village, NV 89451; tel: 800-722-8327 or 702-832-8485; fax: 702-832-8488; website: http://www.carbon.com; e-mail: cellmate@carbon.com. Carbon Based Corporation delivers the report to clients within 48 to 72 hours at a cost to practitioners of about $100. For more about the **Fatty Acid Red Cell Membrane test**, contact: Carbon Based Corporation East, Five Osprey, Millville, NJ 08332; tel: 609-825-2200 or 609-825-8333; fax: 609-825-2143. For **AllerAid Formula II** and **buffered Vitamin C**, contact: Allergy Research Group, 400 Preda Street, San Leandro, CA 94577; tel: 800-545-9960 or 510-639-4572; fax: 510-635-6730. For **bromelain, beta rutin,** and **lipoic acid**, contact: Ecologic Formulas, 1061-B Shary Circle, Concord, CA 94518; tel: 800-888-4585 or 510-827-2636; fax: 510-676-9231. For **Similase**, contact: Tyler Encapsulations, 2204-8 N.W. Birdsdale, Gresham, OR 97030; tel: 800-869-9705 or 503-661-5401; fax: 503-666-4913. For **Liquid Trace Minerals**, contact: Women's International Pharmacy, 13925 Meeker Blvd., Suite 13, Sun City West, AZ 85375; tel: 602-214-7700 or 800-699-8143; fax: 602-214-7708. For **Magnesium succinate**, contact: Champion Nutrition, 2615 Scanwell Drive, Concord, CA 94520; tel: 800-225-4831. For **Cetyl myristoleate** and **evening primrose oil**, contact: Hopewell Pharmacy, One West Broad Street, Hopewell, NJ 08525; tel: 800-792-6670; fax: 609-466-8222. For **folate** and **Adenosyl-cobalamin**, contact: Thorne Research, Inc., P.O. Box 3200, Sandpoint, ID 83864; tel: 800-228-1966 or 208-263-1337; fax: 208-265-2488. For **Inositol**, contact: Biotech, P.O. Box 1992, Fayetteville, AR 72702; tel: 800-345-1199.

A Fat Glossary

Lipid is a biochemical term for a fat or oil, which is one of the six basic food groups. Fats and oils are made of building blocks called fatty acids. Structurally, a fatty acid is a chain of carbon atoms with hydrogen atoms attached and an acid group of atoms at the end able to combine with phosphate (forming phospholipids). When three fatty acids attach to one molecule of glycerol, this makes a simple fat called *triglyceride*. The chain of carbon atoms can be short (2-6 atoms), medium (8-10), or long (12-30). Butyric acid, found in milk fat, butter, and cream, is a short-chain fatty acid. A fatty acid that has its full quota of hydrogen atoms is a *saturated fatty acid* (animal fats and hardened fats, solid at room temperature); a fatty acid with less than the full allotment of hydrogen atoms is an *unsaturated fatty acid* (many plant and fish oils, liquid at room temperature). When a fatty acid lacks only two hydrogen atoms, it is a *monounsaturated fatty acid* (such as oleic acid); and a fatty acid lacking four or more hydrogen atoms is a *polyunsaturated fatty acid* (linoleic acid). Unsaturated fats required in the diet are called *essential fatty acids* and include linoleic acid (an omega-6 oil), found in corn, beans, and some nuts and seeds (from souther climates).

A **trans-fatty acid** is a chemically and structurally altered hydrogenated vegetable oil (such as maragrine), in which the double bond linking hydrogen atoms is changed from a "cis" (atoms bonded on the same side of a chain) to a "trans" form (atoms bonded on opposite sides of a chain), considered more stable. Trans-fatty acid (TFA) composition of commercially prepared hydrogenated fats varies from 8% to 70% and comprise about 60% of the fat found in processed foods. It is estimated that Americans consume over 600 million pounds annually of TFAs in the form of processed frying fats. TFAs can increase the risk of heart disease by 27% when consumed as at least 12% of the total fat intake. TFAs also reduce production of prostaglandin (hormone-like substances which control all cell-to-cell interactions) and interfere with fatty acid metabolism.

Omega-3 and **omega-6 oils** are the two principal types of essential fatty acids, which are unsaturated fats required in the diet. The digits "3" and "6" refer to differences in the oil's chemical structure with respect to its chain of carbon atoms and where they are bonded. A balance of these oils in the diet is required for good health. The primary omega-3 oil is called alpha-linolenic acid (ALA) and is found in flaxseed (58%), canola, pumpkin, walnut, and soybeans. Fish oils, such as salmon, cod, and mackerel, contain the other important omega-3 oils, DHA (docosahexaenoic acid) and EPA (eicosapentaenoic acid). Omega-3 oils help reduce the risk of heart disease and impact the brain and immune system. Linoleic acid or cis-linoleic acid is the main omega-3 oil and is found in most plants and vegetable oils, including safflower (73%), sunflower, corn, and sesame. The most therapeutic form of omega-6 oil is gamma-linolenic acid (GLA), found in evening primrose oil. Once in the body, omega-3 and omega-6 are converted to prostaglandins, hormone-like substances that regulate many metabolic functions, particularly inflammatory processes.

soak them overnight in water then cook well and eat with protein foods (such as chicken) and Omega Nutrition oils.

■ Incorporate certain spices and herbs into the diet, such as fresh ground black pepper, thyme oil, and ginger; these foods contain substances that will help stabilize fats in the cell membranes.

■ Avoid all fats and oils containing very long chain fatty acids, such as mustard, peanut butter, peanut oil, and canola oil.

■ Avoid using pregnenolone, DHEA, or other supportive hormones until the fats status (such as low cholesterol) returns to normal.

■ Avoid eating foods which contain arachidonic acid (such as cream, meat, butter, egg yolk, and shellfish) if testing indicates that your levels are elevated.

Sylvia's improvement was swift and steady after the nutrient replenishment program was in place. Within two weeks of restoring the needed fatty acids, most of her symptoms had considerably abated, and after another two weeks, all signs of her depression, fatigue, digestive problems, and allergies had disappeared. Her case is a remarkable, but not unusual, demonstration of the link between nutrition and emotional and mental states. ■

6) Allergies and Sensitivities

Depression can also be strongly linked to allergies and food sensitivities, according to many alternative medicine practitioners, among them Priscilla Slagle, M.D., of Encino, California. Dr. Slagle cautions that allergies and toxicities from dietary habits (such as overconsumption of caffeine or sugar), exposure to chemicals (in water, air, food, and other sources), and drug reactions (including to antidepressants) can lead to depression in certain individuals. The case which follows shows how reversing these factors can alleviate depression, sometimes very rapidly.

Success Story: Allergy-Caused Depression Lifted

Lessa, 27, had given up on conventional mood-enhancing drugs by the time she visited Dr. Slagle for her depression. Suffering from frequent crying episodes and feelings of intense sadness, Lessa had already tried—and rejected—eight different antidepressant medications. "She tried all these mood-control medicines and had adverse reactions to even low doses of all of them," Dr. Slagle says. "She was hypersensitive." In addition to the depression, Lessa was suffering from a wide range of other ailments, including chronic fatigue, muscle weakness and pain, premenstrual cramps, insomnia, and gastroin-

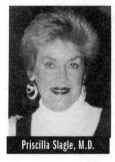

Priscilla Slagle, M.D.

Allergies and toxicities from dietary habits (such as overconsumption of caffeine or sugar), exposure to chemicals (in water, air, food, and other sources), and drug reactions (including to antidepressants) can lead to depression in certain individuals, says Dr. Slagle.

testinal disorders (bloating and irritable bowel syndrome).

Lessa's depression was a serious problem; her score on the Zung Depression Inventory Test, a questionnaire which measures the level of depression, ranked it as most severe. In order to address Lessa's depressed state, Dr. Slagle had to understand the total medical picture. "Lessa came to me for treatment of the mood problem. But when I treat the mood problem, I have to look at all the other things that are going on," explains Dr. Slagle.

She soon discovered that Lessa had been in and out of doctors' offices since childhood, suffering from recurrent ear infections for which she was treated with antibiotics, low blood sugar (hypoglycemia, see next section), anemia, and allergic sensitivities to chemical inhalants such as perfumes and hair sprays. Although Lessa had been skin-tested for several chemical sensitivities, she had never been tested for food allergies.

Dr. Slagle suspected that Lessa's "hypersensitivity" to her various antidepressant medications, not to mention her other medical conditions, might be caused by food allergies, some type of infection, or a combination of both. Laboratory tests confirmed these suspicions, revealing that Lessa was indeed allergic to a variety of foods: eggs, chicken, gluten, kidney beans, rye, soy, wheat, garlic, and all dairy products. She also had a severe case of candidiasis (an overgrowth of the yeast *Candida albicans*), which is often the result of repeated antibiotic use. To combat the allergies and help treat the candidiasis, Dr. Slagle put Lessa on a strict diet which cut out all food allergens and restricted her intake of sugar, alcohol, caffeine, and fruit. Drawing from conventional medicine, she prescribed Diflucan (a conventional antifungal) to further target the candidiasis.

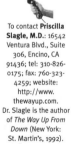

To contact **Priscilla Slagle, M.D.**: 16542 Ventura Blvd., Suite 306, Encino, CA 91436; tel: 310-826-0175; fax: 760-323-4259; website: http://www.thewayup.com. Dr. Slagle is the author of *The Way Up From Down* (New York: St. Martin's, 1992).

Based on the test results, Dr. Slagle then implemented a comprehensive nutritional supplement program. Lessa took L-tryptophan (1,500 mg daily) for her depression; for her premenstrual cramps, she took calcium and magnesium (250 mg of each, twice a day), vitamin B complex (25 mg daily), and a daily multivitamin designed for women. Dr. Slagle also suggested that Lessa improve her gastrointestinal function by supplementing with *L. acidophilus* (1 tsp of powder, twice daily), which is also helpful for candidiasis, and Similase, a plant-based digestive enzyme (one capsule, three times daily). Finally, for her chronic fatigue, Lessa took glutamine and L-tyrosine (3,000-4,000 mg daily of each), amino acids which improve physical energy and mental alertness.

Within two weeks, Lessa showed moderate improvement. A gradual lessening of her fatigue and muscle pain and weakness enabled Lessa to become more active, and the increased activity further contributed to her progress. After another two weeks, Lessa's gastrointestinal disorders had decreased dramatically, and she reported "significant improvement" in her overall mood.

At one point in the treatment, Lessa experienced a personal crisis and went off her diet. Many of her symptoms returned, but disappeared again soon after Lessa resumed her prescribed diet. Lessa soon found that as long as she continued to eat the correct foods, all of her symptoms disappeared completely. The experience helped Lessa see the degree to which food affected her emotional and physical state.

> **Lessa soon found that as long as she continued to eat the correct foods, all of her symptoms disappeared completely. The experience helped Lessa see the degree to which food affected her emotional and physical state, says Dr. Slagle.**

7) Low Blood Sugar (Hypoglycemia)

As with Lessa in the previous medical history, many patients who suffer from depression also have hypoglycemia (low blood sugar). In some cases, the hypoglycemia may even be the sole cause of the patient's depression, according to orthomolecular (SEE QUICK DEFINITION) psychiatrist Harvey Ross, M.D., of Los Angeles, California.

"Many times patients can feel depressed without being able to say why," says Dr. Ross. They may have accompanying symptoms of low energy, fatigue, irritability, and attacks of anxiety or fear, sometimes even to the point of developing phobias. Diabetes (hypoglycemia can be a precursor to adult-onset diabetes) may be part of their family history, but from a conventional medical standpoint there is nothing wrong with them, explains Dr. Ross.

While all of these symptoms are typical of hypoglycemia, this disorder, like hypothyroidism, is frequently overlooked. Sufferers often are referred to a psychotherapist or psychiatrist, but counseling does not alleviate their symptoms. Sadly, their depression and other disturbing symptoms could be eliminated fairly easily by a physician versed in the effects of nutrients on health, and hypoglycemia in particular, says Dr. Ross.

Hypoglycemia affects your mood through the wide fluctuations of blood sugar which characterize the disorder. Blood sugar, called glucose, enters the bloodstream after we eat a meal or snack. It is followed by a corresponding rise in insulin, which helps to transfer glucose into the body's cells. As this transfer proceeds, both glucose and insulin decline in the blood. When glucose reaches a certain low (approximately 60-65 mg of glucose per 100 ml of blood), we experience hunger and eat, thus beginning the cycle all over again. In a healthy individual, glucose and insulin rise and fall gradually in the blood. Charted over time, blood levels of the two substances appear as two smooth bell-shaped curves.

The changes in glucose and insulin levels in an individual suffering from hypoglycemia contrast markedly to that of the healthy individual. Dr. Stephen Langer describes the wild swings that characterize such disorders: "Your blood sugar leaps high, and you feel all's right with the world. Then comes the big insulin surge, your blood sugar drops, and you plunge from the mountaintops to the pits."[26] The rapid rise in insulin not only brings about a glucose "crash," but keeps blood sugar at a low level by preventing the delivery of "emergency glucose" from glycogen reserves stored in the liver.

QUICK DEFINITION

Orthomolecular medicine is an approach to medicine that uses naturally occurring substances normally present in the body, such as vitamins, minerals and amino acids, to create optimum nutritional content and balance in the body. The term was originated in 1968 by Nobel Prize–winner Linus Pauling, Ph.D. "Ortho" means correct or normal, and orthomolecular physicians recognize that in many cases of physiological and psychological disorders, health can be reestablished by properly correcting, or normalizing, the balance of vitamins, minerals, amino acids, and similar substances in the body.

In addition to managing glucose, insulin is used by the body to transport tryptophan which, as you know by now, is a building block of the brain neurotransmitter serotonin, the "happiness" chemical. When tryptophan and thus serotonin are in shorter supply, the brain demands immediate action—hence our desire for sugar, which delivers quick satisfaction by releasing insulin, which in turn delivers tryptophan and restores serotonin to the brain.[27] In effect, sugar works like an antidepressant, elevating serotonin, however temporarily.

Individuals who experience violent swings in their glucose levels are frequently victims to sudden and extreme changes in temperament. After eating, they feel bliss, a fleeting sensation that is often followed by a black mood. They become angry at others or themselves for no apparent reason. Although such emotional responses tend to be perceived as psychological in origin, for those suffering from a blood sugar imbalance, the problem is more biochemical than psychological.

As treatment for hypoglycemia and the depression associated with it, Dr. Ross typically recommends eliminating all sugar and processed foods and eating a high-protein, low-carbohydrate diet. He also advises "grazing" throughout the day; that is, instead of three large meals, eat three smaller meals and snacks every two hours between meals until bedtime. After the first four months on this program, patients are introduced to a maintenance diet that includes no more than three servings of fruit a day. Ideally, the patient will continue to refrain from processed foods and sugars, but may occasionally have a small amount of sugar. However, in times of increased stress, the patient is strongly advised to return to the stricter dietary program.

8) Stress and Weakened Immunity

All of the causes of depression we have discussed so far weaken the immune system which creates a cyclical effect of ill health, worsening the conditions underlying the depression. In addition, research has established a strong connection between mental states and immune function, so the depression caused by other factors is made worse by the weakened immunity. Depression itself compromises immune strength so the cycle is perpetual unless treatment intervenes at some point to break it.

Another factor which weakens the immune system is stress. Stress can be defined as a reaction to any stimulus or interference that upsets normal functioning and disturbs mental or physical health. It can be brought on by internal conditions, such as emotional conflict, illness, or psychological problems, or by external circumstances, such as work pressures, financial problems, loss of job or spouse, relocation, or traffic jams. Stress has become so much a part of modern life that many of us are not even aware we are experiencing it.

An estimated 70% to 80% of all visits to physicians' offices are for stress-related problems. Research confirms that high stress levels increase one's susceptibility to illness.[28] This is because stress overly activates the nervous system's "fight-or-flight" response. This was not meant to be a continual state and puts tremendous pressure on the immune system. It also depletes the body of valuable nutrients. Stress can also lead to hormonal imbalances which both directly and indirectly (by interfering with the immune system) contribute to depression.

For more about **serotonin**, see this chapter, pp. 215-217.

Hidden Sugars

If you have a tendency toward hypoglycemia, and you think it may be making you depressed, it's advisable to avoid eating sugar. However, many manufacturers have stopped using the word "sugar" in the list of ingredients on their sugar-containing products. To avoid the sugar stigma that could impact sales, they mislead consumers into thinking their product is sugar free by using a host of chemical synonyms, including:

- dextrose
- sucrose
- glucose
- fructose
- corn sweetener
- dextrin
- lactose
- maltodextrin
- maltose
- malt
- manitol
- sorghum
- sorbitol
- xylitol
- modified cornstarch
- high-fructose corn syrup
- fruit juice concentrates

Although all of these are sugars, fructose has the least severe insulin reaction and is therefore the preferable form, according to Anne Louise Gittleman, chair of the department of nutrition at the American Academy of Nutrition.[30]

For more about the **immune system**, see Chapter 4: Chronic Fatigue Syndrome, pp. 176-180.

As you can see, stress, weakened immunity, and depression are intimately linked. Alternative medicine physicians view this relationship as cyclical and research in the field of psychoneuroimmunology (PNI, SEE QUICK DEFINITION) over the last two decades confirms this view. The discovery of biochemical agents, called neuropeptides, firmly established the link between the mind (psycho), the nervous system (neuro), and the immune system (immuno).

Neuropeptides are known to affect mood; the most well-known of the neuropeptides are endorphins, which can have a pain-relieving and pleasure-inducing effect when released.[29] According to Dr. Leon Chaitow, neuropeptides are the key to changes in emotion because they increase or decrease the transmission of messages to and from the brain. Since neuropeptides are found throughout the body, not just in the brain, they also affect the functioning of the immune, nervous, and all other body systems.

If stress and lowered immunity are factors in your depression, the first step you need to take is to try to relieve some of the stress you are feeling. Without that, therapies to boost your immune system and address your depression will lose their effectiveness. High stress will just throw you back into the depression cycle again.

This doesn't necessarily mean eliminating the sources of stress in your life. Naturally, that would be ideal, but it's hardly possible, given the lives most of us lead. The secret is in how you deal with potentially stressful situations. People who have learned to handle stress efficently tend not to get depressed or lower their immunity. "This has been called the 'hardiness factor,'" says Dr. Chaitow. "It comprises a tendency to see problems as challenges not threats, having a commitment to involvement in society rather than having a sense of detachment from it, and having a feeling of control over life rather than a sense of being subject to the whims of fate."

According to Dr. Chaitow, these three elements can be learned via appropriate counseling and therefore the absence of one or all of them from a person's personality profile is not necessarily a permanent feature. "People can learn to cope with stress so that it does not negatively affect them," says Dr. Chaitow. This is also the basis of numerous healing modalities such as progressive relaxation, guided imagery, and biofeedback (SEE QUICK DEFINITION), which can be effectively used to treat both psychological and physiological disorders.

9) Toxic Exposure

Numerous studies have shown that exposure to heavy metals (such as mercury), solvents, paints, and other toxic substances and fumes can produce psychological symptoms including depression.[31] Toxic overload of the body weakens the immune system which, as established above, is directly tied to depression. Another mechanism of the link between toxic exposure and depression is the thyroid gland. Damage from toxins can slow thyroid function. As mentioned earlier, depression is a common symptom of an underactive thyroid gland.

Radiation is another poison that can damage the thyroid. Dr. John Gofman, M.D., Ph.D., director of the Committee for Nuclear Responsibility and professor emeritus in the Department of Molecular and Cell Biology at the University of California, states that radiation slows the thyroid. He studied the effects of the Chernobyl disaster (a nuclear reactor explosion in the mid-1980s in what is now the Ukraine) on human health and found that individuals exposed to the radiation from Chernobyl had symptoms virtually identical to that of hypothyroidism.[32]

Alarmingly, the toxin causing your depression may be in your mouth. If you have mercury dental fillings, you might consider being tested for mercury toxicity. Hair analysis or electrodermal screening are useful for this. These tests, along with urine analysis, can detect buildup of all kinds of toxins in

QUICK DEFINITION

Psychoneuroimmunology (PNI) is a medical concept that demonstrates on a biochemical level the assumption of a mind-body connection. Since the 1970s, PNI has documented the multiple interactions between the mind (psycho), nervous system (neuro), and cellular dimension (immunology) as they influence health; research in this field indicates that the body "listens" (and acts accordingly) to one's thoughts and emotions. On a biochemical level, the immune and nervous systems are linked by extensive networks of nerve endings in the spleen, bone marrow, lymph nodes, and thymus gland. These nerve connections serve to integrate the activities of the immune, hormonal, and nervous systems, enabling one's mind and emotional states to influence the body's resistance to a number of health conditions, from the common cold to cancer.

For more about **PNI and neuropeptides**, see *Alternative Medicine Guide to Cancer* (Future Medicine Publishing, 1997; ISBN 1-887299-01-7); to order, call 800-333-HEAL.

For more about **mercury toxicity and testing,** see Chapter 4: Chronic Fatigue Syndrome, pp. 183-184. For details on **detoxification,** see Chapter 1: Fibrocystic Breast Disease, pp. 35-39. For more on **Dr. Gofman's radiation research,** see Chapter 2: Breast Cancer, p. 65.

the body. If you think your depression may be in part caused by toxic exposure, the first step is getting one or more of these tests to identify the source(s) of the toxicity.

Once you have established the type of toxins involved, you can undertake the appropriate detoxification program. Detoxifying the body typically produces a worsening of symptoms as the toxins are flushed, so it is best conducted under the care of an alternative medicine practitioner. Detoxification methods include special diets, fasting, herbal and nutritional supplements, dry brushing of the skin, colonic irrrigation, and chelation therapy (for heavy metals, SEE QUICK DEFINITION).

10) Lack of Exercise

Exercise is an antidepressant, stimulating the release of endorphins, as in the runner's "high," a euphoric state that occurs during and after vigorous aerobic exercise. As mentioned in the section on stress, endorphins are one of the neuropeptides, chemicals in the body that influence our emotions. Endorphins make us feel relaxed, happy, and energetic. They also relieve stress, an important function in the prevention and relief of depression.

Another antidepressive action of exercise is the flushing of toxins from the body. Research has demonstrated that if we don't exercise aerobically and get oxygen to all parts of the body, our blood circulation and lymphatic drainage can become sluggish. Both are vital to the elimination of toxins, so when they are not functioning optimally, toxins build up in the body, a contributing factor in depression, as noted in the previous section.

The depressive effects of stress and toxic buildup can be ameliorated with aerobic exercise performed for at least 20 minutes four or five times a week, according to research. Weight training also can have antidepressive benefits. A study reported in the January 1997 issue of the *Journal of Gerontology* showed that in a group of 32 depressed people, 60 to 84 years old, those who exercised the most and the hardest showed the most improvement in mood.

One of the problems with depression is that it can seem impossible to summon the motivation or energy to engage in exercise. It is important to remember that exercise will make you feel better and it's vital that you get your body moving. It isn't necessary to engage in strenuous exercise in order to enjoy antidepressant benefits. Yoga and other forms of quiet stretching can also help reduce depression. Even a short walk is a start.

11) Light Deprivation

Lack of light can be as significant a cause of depression as any of the other deficiencies already covered. A decrease in the quality and quantity of light can affect one's mental state, according to pioneering photobiologist John Nash Ott, Sc.D. (Hon.).[33] Dr. Ott discovered that artificial lighting (incandescent or fluorescent) not only interferes with the body's optimal absorption of nutrients, but contributes to depression.[34] Research has demonstrated that by spending 90% of our lives indoors, in inadequate light conditions, we are causing, or worsening, a wide range of health problems, including depression and lowered immunity.[35]

Lack of light lowers serotonin levels. It also disturbs the melatonin (SEE QUICK DEFINITION) cycle of sleep and waking. When the morning light comes through your eyes, it sends a signal to the pineal gland via the optic nerve to stop producing melatonin, the lack of which causes you to wake up. Similarly, in the evening, the darkness will signal the pineal gland to begin melatonin production, which aids in sleep.

About midwinter when it seems the sun barely makes it into the sky, many people in the cold parts of North America begin to wish they were in the tropics or closer to the sun or that they could shake off the gloom that prolonged reduced sunlight seems to produce.

In recent decades, the winter blues have gained scientific credibility. Physicians now talk about SAD—seasonal affective disorder—the measurable negative effects that sunlight deprivation exacts on some people. In SAD, the lack of morning light throws the pineal gland off its schedule, affecting sleep and mood. The symptoms of SAD's winter doldrums (see "A Depression by Any Other Name…," p. 206) are no doubt familiar to many. In fact, it's estimated that over 10 million Americans experience SAD every year, according to the National Institute of Mental Health (NIMH), and another 25 million get some milder depressive symptoms on a seasonal basis. What does SAD feel like?

Typically, there is chronic depression and fatigue which may leave you bedridden; hypersomnia (increased sleep by as much as four hours or more per night) and reduced quality of the sleep, leaving you feel-

QUICK DEFINITION

Chelation therapy refers to a method of binding up ("chelating") toxins (e.g. heavy metals) and metabolic wastes and removing them from the body while at the same time increasing blood flow and removing arterial plaque. One type of chelation therapy involves the chelating agent disodium EDTA given as an intravenous infusion over a 3^1/$_2$ hour period. Usually 20 to 30 treatments are administered at the rate of one to three sessions per week. Chelation therapy is especially beneficial for all forms of atherosclerotic cardiovascular disease including angina pectoris and coronary artery disease.

CAUTION

Before beginning any exercise program, consult your physician to make sure it is advisable and that you don't have a serious physiological condition underlying your depression.

By spending 90% of our lives indoors, in inadequate light conditions, we are causing, or worsening, a wide range of health problems, including depression and lowered immunity.

ing less refreshed; and cravings for carbohydrates and candy, which can lead to sometimes significant weight gain. Women with SAD may report that their premenstrual symptoms are more aggravated. Similar seasonal behavioral changes, particularly increased sleep and variations in appetite, are seen in other mammals.

How does a shortage of sunlight cause these changes? According to naturopathic physician and educator Michael T. Murray, N.D., author of *Natural Alternatives to Prozac*, the cause may be in your hormones. "The key hormonal change may be a reduced secretion of melatonin from the pineal gland and an increased secretion of cortisol by the adrenal glands," explains Dr. Murray. These hormones also affect your mood; studies have found decreased melatonin and increased cortisol levels in depressed patients.

QUICK DEFINITION

Melatonin, a hormone produced by the pea-sized, light-sensitive pineal (pronounced pie-NEEL) gland in the center of the brain, regulates the body's internal clock, or circadian rhythm, which determines the 24-hour sleep-wake cycle. With aging, the peak in melatonin secretion is about one hour later than normal (normal peak secretion time is about 2 a.m.), and the maximum peak of melatonin is only one-half the level of young adults. Low melatonin levels have been associated with sleeping disturbances and light-related conditions such as seasonal affective disorder (SAD). Eating vitamin-and mineral-rich foods and increasing your exposure to bright light can improve the body's natural melatonin production.

Another theory about SAD holds that the body's internal clock—the circadian rhythm, or 24-hour cycle of sleeping and waking—is thrown off by the lessening of light during the winter. It's like a season-long case of jet lag. Melatonin is involved with this internal clock too, because it is released only during the night and directly influences your sleep cycles.

Obviously, one solution is to spend the winter in the tropics and leave your SADness in New York or Ottawa. But if that isn't an option, you can use any of several sunlight simulators to get more sunlight into you. Seventh Generation, Inc., a producer of environmentally safe household products in Burlington, Vermont, recently introduced a line of full spectrum light bulbs, which provide a "warmer," more natural light that closely resembles sunlight, according to the manufacturer. "Studies have shown that full spectrum lighting actually helps relieve eyestrain and improves a person's mood," says Jeffrey Hollender, president of Seventh Generation. "Everyone who has used them loves them and refuses to go back to harsh, ordinary bulbs."

Conventional light bulbs illuminate more intensely on the yellow part of the color spectrum. Our eyes are sensitive to this part of the spectrum, so these lights may cause some eye-strain and fatigue. Full spectrum light, on the other hand, is a balanced blend of all colors in the visible spectrum, closer to what we get from sunlight. "Full spectrum lighting, containing all wavelengths, sparks the delicate impulses which regulate brain and autonomic functions of the body, regulating these functions and maintaining health," states John Downing, O.D., Ph.D., director of the Light Therapy Department at the Preventive Medical Center of Marin, in Santa Rosa, California.

Not only can you change the lights bulbs in your indoor environment, you can cozy up to an artificial "sun" even while you work. The Happylite is a portable light box (made by Verilux, Inc., of Stamford, Connecticut) that provides 10,000 lux light (the same amount of light used in light therapy clinics) and provides a lens to block ultraviolet light and electromagnetic radiation. The unit weighs 11 pounds and measures 18" tall by 12" wide.

Verilux also sells full spectrum fluorescent tubes for office environments as well as light bulbs for the home. Office lighting can have an influence on productivity and stress level on the job, according to the manufacturer. The Verilux fluorescent lights use four rare earth phosphors (substances that emit light) to simulate a more balanced white light for the office.

Light therapy is designed to restore the natural 24-hour rhythm and normal hormone secretions through daily exposure to intense light. The lights used are usually fluorescent bulbs contained in a light box, with the light meant to recreate natural early morning sunlight.

Both the full spectrum light bulbs and the Happylite are practical low-cost applications which were based on research from the field of light therapy. This therapy is designed to restore the natural 24-hour rhythm and normal hormone secretions through daily exposure to intense light. The lights used are usually fluorescent bulbs contained in a light box, with the light meant to recreate natural early morning sunlight.

Most standard therapy protocols recommend two hours of exposure to 2,500 lux light daily. (Lux is a term used to measure the intensity of illumination; normal indoor light is 500 to 1,000 lux.) More recently, researchers have starting using 10,000 lux light for only 30 minutes daily, with 60% to 80% of patients showing improvement in

For more information on **light therapy**, contact: Society for Light Treatment and Biological Rhythms, Inc., 10200 West 44th Avenue, Suite 304, Wheat Ridge, CO 80033-2840; tel: 303-422-7905; fax: 303-422-8894. For sources of **full spectrum lighting**, contact: Seventh Generation, One Mill Street, Box A-26, Burlington, VT 95401-1530; tel: 800-456-1191 or 802-658-3773; fax: 802-658-1771. Verilux Inc., 9 Viaduct Road, Stamford, CT 06907; tel: 800-786-6850 or 203-921-2430; fax: 203-921-2427; website: www.ergolight.com. For a **light box**, contact: Enviro-Med, 1600 S.E. 141st Avenue, Vancouver, WA 98684; tel: 800-222-3296 or 360-256-6989.

their SAD symptoms.

The therapy is typically done first thing in the morning, with the patient sitting before the light box, with their eyes open but not staring directly into the light. Sometimes evening sessions are recommended instead of or in addition to the morning treatment. Patients can perform normal activities while undergoing therapy, so it can be done while at work. An initial therapy period of seven to 14 days is recommended to determine if the light therapy will be effective. Patients should never stare into the light during therapy and should be careful to choose light sources that screen out ultraviolet light. Researchers have observed that, within three days of full spectrum light therapy, people suffering from SAD are out of the depression and their hormonal levels and white blood cell counts have normalized. At the same time, discontinuation of the therapy produces a return of the symptoms in three to four days.

Dr. Christiane Northrup, M.D., prescribes light box therapy for many of her patients with SAD. She also urges everyone to get outside for at least 15 minutes a day. "Most of us (in the North at least) are at risk for at least a bit of SAD because we're often light-starved. Our society doesn't realize that natural light is a nutrient that naturally raises serotonin levels in our brains," says Dr. Northrup.[36] Replacing fluorescent lighting with full spectrum lighting can help counteract this problem.

Some physicians prescribe melatonin supplements along with the light boxes. The supplements help to normalize the body's own production of melatonin. Restoring proper sleep cycles can help alleviate the depression associated with light deprivation. Melatonin supplements are available at most health food stores. See your alternative medicine practitioner for information on dosages.

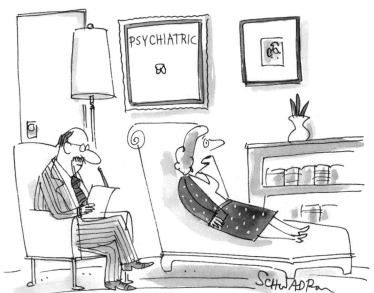

"OF COURSE I'M DEPRESSED. I LOST 67 POUNDS, AND THEN FOUND OUT I LOOKED BETTER FAT."

Endnotes

Chapter I
Fibrocystic Breast Disease

1 *The Merck Manual* (Rahway, NJ: Merck & Company), 1718-1719.

2 Carolyn DeMarco, M.D. "Women's Health." *Health Counselor* 7:4 (1995), 44.

3 From clinic handouts supplied by Katrina Kulhay, D.C., director of the Kulhay Wellness Centre, in Toronto, Ontario, Canada.

4 Susun S. Weed. *Breast Cancer? Breast Health! The Wise Woman Way* (Woodstock, NY: Ash Tree Publishing, 1996), 108.

5 Carolyn DeMarco, M.D. *Take Charge of Your Body* (Canada: Well Women Press, 1995), 155.

6 Christiane Northrup, M.D. *Women's Bodies, Women's Wisdom* (New York: Bantam Books, 1994), 295.

7 Ibid.

8 Susun S. Weed. *Breast Cancer? Breast Health! The Wise Woman Way* (Woodstock, NY: Ash Tree Publishing, 1996), 108.

9 *Physicians' Desk Reference* (Montvale, NJ: Medical Economics, 1995), 2205.

10 Mary Lou Ballweg. *The Endometriosis Sourcebook* (Chicago: Contemporary Books, 1995), 188.

11 J.E. Pizzorno and M.T. Murray, eds. *A Textbook of Natural Medicine* (Seattle, WA: John Bastyr College Publications, 1988-1989). Women's health expert John R. Lee, M.D., of Sebastopol, California, coined the term estrogen dominance.

12 John R. Lee, M.D. "Hormone Balance and Other Common Health Problems." *What Your Doctor May Not Tell You About Menopause* (New York: Warner Books, 1996), 40.

13 Paul Pitchford. *Healing With Whole Foods* (Berkeley, CA: North Atlantic Books, 1993), 133.

14 Carolyn DeMarco, M.D. *Take Charge of Your Body* (Canada: Well Women Press, 1995), 157.

15 Robert Garrison, Jr., M.A., R.Ph., and Elizabeth Somer, M.S., R.D. *The Nutrition Desk Reference* (New Canaan, CT: Keats Publishing, 1995), 194-195.

16 From clinic handouts supplied by Tori Hudson, N.D., of A Woman's Time: Menopause Options

and Natural Health, in Portland, Oregon.

17 Ibid.

18 Carolyn Dean. *Dr. Carolyn Dean's Complementary Natural Prescriptions for Common Ailments* (New Canaan, CT: Keats Publishing, 1994), 86.

19 M.A. Jansen and L.R. Muenz. "A Retrospective Study of Personality Variables Associated with Fibrocystic Disease and Breast Cancer." *Journal of Psychosomatic Research* 28:1 (1984), 35-42.

20 From clinic handouts supplied by Katrina Kulhay, D.C., director of the Kulhay Wellness Centre, in Toronto, Ontario, Canada.

21 John R. Lee, M.D. "Hormone Balance and Other Common Health Problems." *What Your Doctor May Not Tell You About Menopause* (New York: Warner Books, 1996), 251.

22 From clinic handouts supplied by Tori Hudson, N.D., of A Woman's Time: Menopause Options and Natural Health, in Portland, Oregon.

23 W.R. Ghent, et al. "Iodine Replacement in Fibrocystic Disease of the Breast." *Canadian Journal of Surgery* 36:5 (October 1993), 405.

24 Christiane Northrup, M.D. *Women's Bodies, Women's Wisdom* (New York: Bantam Books, 1994), 296.

25 Ibid.

26 Katherine Dedyna. "Iodine: Bosom Buddy." *Times Colonist* (September 9, 1997), D1.

27 From personal accounts by Jonathan Wright, M.D., of Kent, Washington, and chronicled in: John A. Myers, M.D. *Metabolic Aspects of Health* (Kentfield, CA: Discovery Press, 1979).

28 Christiane Northrup, M.D. *Women's Bodies, Women's Wisdom* (New York: Bantam Books, 1994), 296.

29 Tori Hudson, N.D. *Gynecology and Naturopathic Medicine* (Aloha, OR: TK Publications, 1992), Chap. 7, p. 1.

30 *Acupuncture Case Histories From China* (Seattle, WA: Eastland Press, 1996).

31 Chen Jirui, M.D., and Nissi Wang, M.Sc., eds. "Breast Masses." *Acupuncture Case Histories from China* (Seattle, WA: Eastland Press, 1996), 257-259.

32 Susun S. Weed. *Breast Cancer? Breast Health! The Wise Woman Way* (Woodstock, NY: Ash

Tree Publishing, 1996), 117.

33 Andrew Lockie, M.D., and Nicola Geddes. *The Woman's Guide to Homeopathy* (New York: St. Martin's Press, 1994), 219.

34 Judyth Reichenberg-Ullman, N.D. "Fibrocystic Breast Disease: A Case Example." *Resonance* (May/June 1993), 24-25.

Chapter 2
Breast Cancer

1 David Plotkin, M.D. "Good News and Bad News about Breast Cancer." *The Atlantic Monthly* (June 1996), 53.

2 The Breast Cancer Fund, 280 Second Street, Third Floor, San Francisco, CA 94105; tel: 415-543-2979; fax: 415-543-2975.

3 J.A. Petrek and A.I. Holleb. "The Foremost Cancer—Revisited." *CA: A Cancer Journal for Clinicians* 45:4 (1995), 197-243.

4 National Center for Health Statistics. *Vital Statistics of the United States, 1987, Vol. 2, Mortality, Part A.* DHHS Publication No. (PHS) 90-1101 (Washington, DC: U.S. Government Printing Office, 1990).

5 The Breast Cancer Fund, 280 Second Street, Third Floor, San Francisco, CA 94105; tel: 415-543-2979; fax: 415-543-2975.

6 U.S. Department of Health, Education, and Welfare. *Geomagnetism, Cancer, Weather, and Cosmic Radiation* (Salt Lake City, UT: U.S. Department of Health, Education, and Welfare, 1979).

7 John W. Gofman, M.D., Ph.D., and Egan O'Connor. *X Rays: Health Effects of Common Exams* (San Francisco: Sierra Club Books, 1985), 18. John W. Gofman, M.D., Ph.D. *Preventing Breast Cancer: The Story of a Major, Proven, Preventable Cause of the Disease* 2nd ed. (San Francisco: Committee for Nuclear Responsibility, 1996).

8 S. Wing et al. "Mortality Among Workers at Oak Ridge National Laboratory: Evidence of Radiation Effects in Follow-up Through 1984." *Journal of the American Medical Association* 265:11 (1991), 1397-1402.

9 "Breast Cancer Victims Unite." *San Francisco Examiner* (August 12, 1995), A14. "Energy Department Faces Vast Toxic-Waste Cleanup." *Marin Independent Journal* (September 18, 1995), A10. "Breast Health Update." *Energy Times* (July/August 1995), 67.

10 M.S. Wolff et al. "Blood Levels of Organochlorine Residues and Risk of Breast Cancer." *Journal of the National Cancer Institute* 85:8 (1993),
648-652.

11 The Burton Goldberg Group. *Alternative Medicine: The Definitive Guide* (Tiburon, CA: Future Medicine Publishing, 1995), 186.

12 M. Wasserman et al. "Organochlorine Compounds in Neoplastic and Adjacent Apparently Normal Breast Tissue." *Bulletin of Environmental Contaminants and Toxicology* 15 (1976), 478-484.

13 J. Westin and E. Richter. "Israeli Breast Cancer Anomaly." *Annals of the New York Academy of Sciences* 609 (1990), 269-279.

14 T.H. Maugh II. "Experts Downplay Cancer Risk of Chlorinated Water." *The Los Angeles Times* (July 2, 1992).

15 G.J. Judd. "Mass Fluoridation Causes Alarming Rise in Cancer Deaths." *Health Freedom News* (May 1995), 10.

16 C.B. Simone. "Carcinogens in Tobacco Smoke." In: *Breast Health* (Garden City Park, NY: Avery Publishing, 1995), 134.

17 C.B. Simone, M.D. *Cancer and Nutrition* (Garden City Park, NY: Avery Publishing, 1992), 15.

18 A.L. Weinstein et al. "Breast Cancer Risk and Oral Contrceptive Use: Results From a Large Case-Control Study." *Epidemiology* 2:5 (September 1991), 353-358.

19 Mary J. Minkin, M.D., and Carol V. Wright. *What Every Woman Needs to Know About Menopause* (New Haven, CT: Yale University Press, 1996), 111-112.

20 F.E. Leeuwen et al. "Risk of Endometrial Cancer After Tamoxifen Treatment of Breast Cancer." *The Lancet* 343:8895 (February 19, 1994), 448-452.

21 B. Rosenberg. "A Diner's Guide to Irradiation." *Science Digest* (September 1986), 30.

22 P. Croce. "Think Before You Sweeten." *Eating Clean: Overcoming Food Hazards* (Washington, DC: Center for the Study of Responsive Law, 1990), 52.

23 H. Dreher. *Your Defense Against Cancer* (New York: Harper & Row, 1988), 113.

24 M.F. Jacobson. "Undoing Delaney: FDA Allows Free Use of Dangerous Additives." *Eating Clean: Overcoming Food Hazards* (Washington, DC: Center for the Study of Responsive Law, 1990), 48-49.

25 S. Levine and P. Kidd. *Antioxidant Adaptation: Its Role in Free Radical Pathology* (San Leandro, CA: Allergy Research Group, 1986). Cited in: G.A. Strong. *Does Mercury From Dental Amalgam Contribute to Free Radical Pathology?* (Billings, MT: Strong Health

Publications, 1995), 30-33.

26 Committee on Diet, Nutrition and Cancer, Assembly of Life Sciences, National Research Council. *Diet, Nutrition and Cancer* (Washington, DC: National Academy Press, 1982).

27 P. Toniolo et al. "Consumption of Meat, Animal Products, Protein and Fat and Risk of Breast Cancer: A Prospective Cohort Study in New York." *Epidemiology* 5:4 (1994), 391.

28 B.L. Bloom, S.J. Asher, and S.W. White. "Marital Disruption as a Stressor: A Review and Analysis." *Psychological Bulletin* 85:4 (1978), 867-894. See also: L.L. LeShan. "An Emotional Life History Pattern Associated with Neoplastic Disease." *Annals of the New York Academy Sciences* 125:3 (1966), 780-793; B.L. Ernster et al. "Cancer Incidence by Marital Status: U.S. Third National Cancer Survey." *Journal of the National Cancer Institute* 63:3 (1979), 567-585.

29 S. Greer and T. Morris. "Psychological Attributes of Women Who Develop Breast Cancer: A Controlled Study." *Journal of Psychosomatic Research* 19:2 (1975), 147-153.

30 G.N. Rogentine, Jr., et al. "Psychological Factors in the Prognosis of Malignant Melanoma: A Prospective Study." *Psychosomatic Medicine* 41 (1979), 647-655. See also: S. Greer and T. Morris. "Psychological Attributes of Women Who Develop Breast Cancer: A Controlled Study." *Journal of Psychosomatic Research* 19:2 (1975), 147-153.

31 R. Grossarth-Maticek et al. "Interpersonal Repression as a Predictor of Cancer." *Social Science & Medicine* 16 (1982), 493-498. P. Dattore et al. "Premorbid Personality Differentiation of Cancer and Non-cancer Groups." *Journal of Counseling and Clinical Psychology* 48:3 (1980), 388-394. J.W. Shaffer et al. "Clustering of Personality Traits in Youth and the Subsequent Development of Cancer Among Physicians." *Journal of Behavioral Medicine* 10:5 (1987), 441-448.

32 Schimmel and Utiger. "Thyroid and Peripheral Production of Thyroid Hormones." *Annals of Internal Medicine* 87 (1970), 760-768.

33 Ann Louise Gittleman. *Guess What Came to Dinner* (Garden City Park, NY: Avery Publishing, 1993).

34 Hulda R. Clark. *The Cure for All Cancers* (San Diego, CA: ProMotion Publishing, 1993).

35 Dimitrios Trichopoulos, Frederick P. Li, and David J. Hunter. "What Causes Cancer?" *Scientific American* (September 1996), 82-83.

36 F.P. Perera. "Uncovering New Clues to Cancer Risk." *Scientific American* (May 1996), 54-62.

37 D. Trichopoulos et al. "Age at Any Birth and Breast Cancer Risk." *International Journal of Cancer* 31:6 (June 15, 1983), 701-704.

38 Virginia L. Ernster et al. "Incidence of and Treatment for Ductal Carcinoma *In Situ* of the Breast." *Journal of the American Medical Association* 275 (March 27, 1996), 913-918.

39 Norma Peterson. "Mammograms May Rupture *In Situ* Cysts, Causing Invasive Cancer." *Breast Cancer Action Newsletter* 38 (October/November 1996), 9.

40 *British Medical Journal* (February 1996).

41 C.J. Wright and C.B. Mueller. "Screening Mammography and Public Health Policy: The Need For Perspective." *The Lancet* 346 (July 1995); 29-32.

42 D. Plotkin. "Good News and Bad News About Breast Cancer." *The Atlantic Monthly* (June 1996), 82.

43 M.A. Helvie et al. "Mammographic Follow-up of Low-Suspicion Lesions: Compliance Rate and Diagnostic Yield." *Radiology* 178 (1991), 155-158.

44 National Women's Health Network Position Paper. *Mammography in Women Before Menopause* (Washington, DC: National Women's Health Network, 1993).

45 Ibid.

46 Nancy Breen and Martin L. Brown. "The Price of Mammography in the U.S.. Data from the National Survey of Mammography Facilitators." *The Milbank Quarterly* 72:3 (1994).

47 C.J. Wright and C.B. Mueller. "Screening Mammography and Public Health Policy: The Need For Perspective." *The Lancet* 346 (July 1995); 29-32.

48 S. Bogoch and E.S. Bogoch. "A Checklist for Suitability of Biomarkers as Surrogate Endpoints in Chemoprevention of Breast Cancer." *Journal of Cellular Biochemistry* Suppl. 19 (1994), 173-185.

49 P.E. Mohr. "Serum Progesterone and Prognosis in Operable Breast Cancer." *British Journal of Cancer* 73:12 (June 1996), 1552-1555.

50 Emile Bliznakov and Gerald Hunt. *The Miracle Nutrient Coenzyme Q10* (New York: Bantam, 1987).

51 *Energy Times* (January/February 1995), 12, 56. *Cancer Communication Newsletter* 1:1 (February 1995), 11. *Dr. Jonathan Wright's Nutrtition & Healing Newsletter* 1:1 (August 1994), 3-4. Information provided by Michael B. Schachter, M.D.

52 K. Lockwood et al. "Partial and Complete Regression of Breast Cancer in Relation to Dosage of Coenzyme Q10." *Biochemical and Biophysical Research Communications* 199 (1994), 1504-1508.

53 K. Lockwood et al. "Progress on Therapy of Breast Cancer With CoQ10 and the Regression of Metastases." *Biochemical and Biophysical Research Communications* 212:1 (1995), 172-177.

54 *Energy Times* (January/February 1995), 12, 56. *Cancer Communication Newsletter* 1:1 (February 1995), 11. *Dr. Jonathan Wright's Nutrtition & Healing Newsletter* 1:1 (August 1994), 3-4. Information provided by Michael B. Schachter, M.D.

55 "Adjuvant Use of the Béres Drops Plus in Oncological Diseases." Information provided by: BDP America, Inc., 4045 Sheridan Avenue #363, Miami Beach, FL 33140; tel: 305-861-3355; fax: 305-861-3366.

Chapter 3
Osteoporosis

1 John R. Lee, M.D. *Natural Progesterone: The Multiple Roles of a Remarkable Hormone* (Sebastopol, CA: BLL Publishing, 1993), 56.

2 Ann Louise Gittleman. *Super Nutrition for Menopause* (New York: Pocket Books, 1993), 68. L.G. Tolstoi and R.M. Levin. "Osteoporosis—the Treatment Controversy." *Nutrition Today* (July/August 1992), 6-12. Jodi G. Meisler, M.S., R.D. "Toward Optimal Health: The Experts Respond to Osteoporosis." *Journal of Women's Health* 7:1 (1998), 25.

3 Ruth S. Jacobowitz. "Making Noise About the Silent Disease: Osteoporosis." *éternelle* (Summer 1995), 18.

4 Ibid.

5 Susan E. Brown, Ph.D. *Better Bones, Better Body* (New Canaan, CT: Keats Publishing, 1996), 3.

6 Joel S. Finkelstein, M.D., "Osteoporosis," in *Cecil Textbook of Medicine*, 20th Ed., Vol. 2, edited by J. Claude Bennett, M.D., and Fred Plum, M.D. (Philadelphia: W.B. Saunders Company, 1996), 1379.

7 Susan E. Brown, Ph.D. *Better Bones, Better Body* (New Canaan, CT: Keats Publishing, 1996), 5, 32.

8 Joel S. Finkelstein, M.D., "Osteoporosis," in *Cecil Textbook of Medicine*, 20th Ed., Vol. 2, edited by J. Claude Bennett, M.D., and Fred Plum, M.D. (Philadelphia: W.B. Saunders Company,

1996), 1379.

9 Ann Louise Gittleman. *Super Nutrition for Menopause* (New York: Pocket Books, 1993), 88

10 Susan E. Brown, Ph.D. *Better Bones, Better Body* (New Canaan, CT: Keats Publishing, 1996), 48.

11 National Center for Health Statistics, Centers for Disease Control and Prevention, Hyattsville, Maryland. Eileen Hoffman, M.D. *Our Health, Our Lives* (New York: Pocket Books, 1995), 219. Vicki Hufnagel, M.D. *No More Hysterectomies* (New York: Plume/Penguin, 1989), 66.

12 The Burton Goldberg Group. *Alternative Medicine: The Definitive Guide* (Tiburon, CA: Future Medicine Publishing, 1995), 667. Vicki Hufnagel, M.D. *No More Hysterectomies* (New York: Plume/Penguin, 1989), 108.

13 Susan Love, M.D. *Dr. Susan Love's Hormone Book* (New York: Random House, 1997), 95.

14 Ibid., 244.

15 L.G. Tolstoi and R.M. Levin. "Osteoporosis—the Treatment Controversy." *Nutrition Today* (July/August 1992), 6-12.

16 Susan E. Brown, Ph.D. *Better Bones, Better Body* (New Canaan, CT: Keats Publishing, 1996), 4.

17 Susan E. Brown, Ph.D. *Better Bones, Better Body* (New Canaan, CT: Keats Publishing, 1996), 198-99. Susan Lark, M.D. *The Menopause Self-Help Book* (Berkeley, CA: Celestial Arts, 1992), 11. Linda Ojeda, Ph.D. *Menopause Without Medicine* (Alameda, CA: Hunter House, 1995) 95-100. Eileen Hoffman, M.D. *Our Health, Our Lives* (New York: Pocket Books, 1995), 152. *The PDR Family Guide to Women's Health and Prescription Drugs* (Montvale, NJ: Medical Economics, 1994), 371-375.

18 Susan E. Brown, Ph.D. *Better Bones, Better Body* (New Canaan, CT: Keats Publishing, 1996), 42-43.

19 B. Lees et al. "Differences in Proximal Femur Bone Density Over Two Centuries." *The Lancet* 341:8846 (March 1993), 673-675.

20 Susan E. Brown, Ph.D. *Better Bones, Better Body* (New Canaan, CT: Keats Publishing, 1996), 42.

21 John R. Lee, M.D. *What Your Doctor May Not Tell You About Menopause* (New York: Warner Books, 1996), 151.

22 "The Real 'Good News' for Osteoporosis Sufferers." *Bio/Tech News* Special Issue (Box 30568, Parkrose Center, Portland, OR 97294), 2-3.

23 Robert A. Ronzio, Ph.D. *The Encyclopedia of Nutrition & Good Health* (New York: Facts on File, 1997), 329.

24 D.P. Kiel et al. "Caffeine and the Risks of Hip Fracture: the Framingham Study." *American Journal of Epidemiology* 132:4 (October 1990), 675-684.

25 R.P. Heaney. "Calcium Bioavailability." *Boletin-Asociacion Medica del Puerto Rico* 79:1 (January 1987), 27-29. R.P. Heaney and R.R. Recker. "Effects of Nitrogen, Phosphorus and Caffeine on Calcium Balance in Women." *Journal of Laboratory and Clinical Medicine* 99:1 (January 1982), 46-55.

26 Susan Harris. "Caffeine and Bone Loss in Healthy Postmenopausal Women." *American Journal of Clinical Nutrition* 60 (1994), 573-578.

27 C. Coats, M.D. "Negative Effects of a High-Protein Diet." *Family Practice Recertification* 12:12 (December 1990), 80-94.

28 A.G. Marsh et al. "Vegetarian Lifestyle and Bone Mineral Density." *American Journal of Clinical Nutrition* 48 Suppl. 3 (September 1988), 837-841.

29 Melvyn Werbach, M.D. *Foundations of Nutritional Medicine: A Sourcebook of Clinical Research* (Tarzana, CA: Third Line Press,1997).

30 Susun Weed. *Menopausal Years: The Wise Woman Way* (Woodstock, NY: Ash Tree Publishing, 1992), 22.

31 J.A. Thom et al. "The Influence of Refined Carbohydrate on Urinary Calcium Excretion." *British Journal of Urology* 50:7 (December 1987), 459-464.

32 Robert Garrison, Jr., M.A., R.Ph., and Elizabeth Somer, M.A., R.D. *Nutrition Desk Reference* (New Canaan, CT: Keats Publishing, 1995), 242.

33 Susan E. Brown, Ph.D. *Better Bones, Better Body* (New Canaan, CT: Keats Publishing, 1996), 125.

34 "The Real 'Good News' for Osteoporosis Sufferers." *Bio/Tech News* Special Issue (Box 30568, Parkrose Center, Portland, OR 97294), 4.

35 Ibid., 7.

36 Robert Garrison, Jr., M.A., R.Ph., and Elizabeth Somer, M.A., R.D. *The Nutrition Desk Reference* (New Canaan, CT: Keats Publishing, 1997), 79-80.

37 M.S. Seelig. "Magnesium Deficiency with Phosphate and Vitamin D Excess: Role in Pediatric Cardiovascular Nutrition." *Cardio Med* 3 (1978), 637-650.

38 Susan E. Brown, Ph.D. *Better Bones, Better Body* (New Canaan, CT: Keats Publishing, 1996), 77-113.

39 Alan Gaby, M.D. *Preventing and Reversing Osteoporosis* (Rocklin, CA: Prima Publishing, 1994), 18.

40 Ibid.

41 Susan E. Brown, Ph.D. *Better Bones, Better Body* (New Canaan, CT: Keats Publishing, 1996), 65-67.

42 Ibid.

43 Christiane Northrup. *Women's Bodies, Women's Wisdom* (New York: Bantam Books, 1994), 451.

44 Brandon J. Orr-Walker et al. "Premature Hair Graying and Bone Mineral Density." *Journal of Clinical Endocrinology and Metabolism* 82:11 (1997), 3580-3583.

45 U.S. Congress, Office of Technology Assessment. *Effectiveness and Costs of Osteoporosis Screening and Hormone Replacement Therapy, Volume 1: Cost-Effectiveness Analysis* OTA-BP-H-160 (Washington: U.S. Government Printing Office, August 1995), 51.

46 Deanne Pearson and Lynne McTaggart. "Osteoporosis: A Load of Old Bones." *What Doctors Don't Tell You* 6:12 (March 1996), 1.

47 Susun Weed. *Menopausal Years: The Wise Woman Way* (Woodstock, NY: Ash Tree Publishing, 1992), 155.

48 John R. Lee, M.D. *What Your Doctor May Not Tell You About Menopause* (New York: Warner Books, 1996), 151

49 Deanne Pearson and Lynne McTaggart. "Osteoporosis: A Load of Old Bones." *What Doctors Don't Tell You* 6:12 (March 1996), 1.

50 R. Lindsay et al. "Bone Response to Termination of Oestrogen Treatment." *The Lancet* 1:8078 (June 1978), 1325-1327.

51 Jonathan V. Wright, M.D. "Natural Response." *Nutrition and Healing* (May 1995), 12.

52 "The Many Clinical Benefits of Natural Progesterone." *Life Enhancement* 30 (February 1997), 5.

53 Susan Love, M.D. *Dr. Susan Love's Hormone Book* (New York: Random House, 1977).

54 John R. Lee, M.D. *What Your Doctor May Not Tell You About Menopause* (New York: Warner Books, 1996), 151

55 John R. Lee, M.D. "Is Natural Progesterone the Missing Link in Osteoporosis Prevention and Treatment?"*Medical Hypotheses* (1991).

56 J.C. Prior et al. "Spinal Bone Loss and Ovulatory Distrubances." *International Journal of Gynecology and Obstetrics* 34 (1990), 253-256.

57 B. Uzzan et al. "Effects on Bone Mass of Long Term

Treatment with Thyroid Hormones: A Meta-Analysis." *Journal of Clinical Endocrinology and Metabolism* 81:12 (December 1996), 4278-4289.

58 Susan E. Brown, Ph.D. *Better Bones, Better Body* (New Canaan, CT: Keats Publishing, 1996), 162.

59 Johannes Bijilsma. "Prevention of Glucocorticoid Induced Osteoporosis." *Annals of the Rheumatic Diseases* 56 (September 1997), 507-509.

60 "The Real 'Good News' for Osteoporosis Sufferers." *Bio/Tech News* Special Issue (Box 30568, Parkrose Center, Portland, OR 97294), 6.

61 Ibid.

62 Ann Louise Gittleman. *Super Nutrition for Menopause* (New York: Pocket Books, 1993), 84

63 L.K. Bachrach et al. "Recovery from Osteopenia in Adolescent Girls with Anorexia Nervosa." *Journal of Clinical Endocrinology and Metabolism* 72:3 (March 1991), 602-606.

64 M.E. Nelson. "Hormone and Bone Mineral Status in Endurance-Trained and Sedentary Postmenopausal Women." *Journal of Clinical Endocrinology and Metabolism* 66:5 (May 1988), 927-933.

65 S.M. Wolfe, M.D., and the Public Citizen Health Research Group. *Women's Health Alert* (Reading, MA: Addison-Wesley Publishing, 1991), 124.

66 T. Lohman et al. "Effects of Resistance Training on Regional and Total Bone Mineral Density in Premenopausal Woman: A Randomized Prospective Study." *Journal of Bone and Mineral Research* 10:7 (July 1995) 1015-1024.

67 Peter Pietschmann. "Exercise and Physical Therapy in the Prevention and Treatment of Osteoporosis." *Osteoporosis* 18 (1996), 265-270.

68 J.E. Dook et al. "Exercise and bone mineral density in mature female athletes." *Medicine and Science in Sports and Exercise* 29 (1997), 291-296.

69 "Majority of Americans Spend Leisure Time Inactively." *Let's Live* (March 1996), 12. H.R. Yusuf. "Leisure-Time Physical Activity Among Older Adults." *Archives of Internal Medicine* 156:12 (June 24, 1996), 1321-1326.

70 National Institutes of Health Consensus Conference. "Osteoporosis." *Journal of the American Medical Association* 252:6 (August 1984), 799-802.

71 "The Real 'Good News' for Osteoporosis Sufferers." *Bio/Tech News* Special Issue (Box 30568, Parkrose Center, Portland, OR 97294), 5.

72 R.F. Klein. "Alcohol-Induced Bone Disease: Impact of Ethanol on Osteoblast Proliferation." *Alcoholism, Clinical and Experimental Research* 21:3 (May 1997), 392-399.

73 J.L. Gonzalez-Calvin et al. "Mineral Metabolism, Osteoblastic Function and Bone Mass in Chronic Alcoholism." *Alcohol and Alcoholism* 28:5 (September 1993), 571-579.

74 C. Cooper et al. "Water Fluoridation and Hip Fracture." *Journal of the American Medical Association* 19:32 (July 1991), 513-514. M.F. Sowers et al. "A Prospective Study of Bone Mineral Content and Fracture in Communities with Differential Fluoride Exposure." *American Journal of Epidemiology* 133:7 (April 1991), 649-660.

75 Gabriel Cousins, M.D. "Health Today." *New Frontier* (May 1994). Val Valerian. "On the Toxic Nature of Fluorides, Part 2: Fluorides and Cancer." *Perceptions* (September/October 1995), 30-37. George Glasser. "Dental Fluorosis: A Legal Time Bomb." *Health Freedom News* (July 1995), 40-46. John Yiamouyiannis. *Fluoride: The Aging Factor* (Delaware, OH: Health Action Press, 1993).

76 Susan E. Brown, Ph.D. *Better Bones, Better Body* (New Canaan, CT: Keats Publishing, 1996), 166.

77 Alan Cook. "Osteoporosis: Review and Commentary." *Journal of the Neuromusculoskeletal System* 2:1 (1994).

78 The Burton Goldberg Group. *Alternative Medicine: The Definitive Guide* (Tiburon, CA: Future Medicine Publishing, 1995), 776.

79 Lynne McTaggart. "Beating Osteoporosis Without Drugs." *What Doctors Don't Tell You* 6:12 (March 1996), 3.

80 Susan E., Brown, Ph.D. *Better Bones, Better Body* (New Canaan, CT: Keats Publishing, 1996), 238.

81 Ibid., 239.

82 Linda Ojeda, Ph.D. *Menopause Without Medicine* (Alameda, CA: Hunter House, 1995), 101.

83 Ibid.

84 M.T. Morter, Jr. "Osteoporosis!" *The Chiropractic Professional* (May/June 1987). M.T. Morter, Jr. "The Sodium Connection." *The Chiropractic Professional* (November/December 1987).

85 Ibid.

86 Jean Carper. "As Greens Go, Kale's Best of Bunch." *The Atlanta Journal/The Atlanta Constitution*

(August 44, 1994).

87 Raquel Martin, with Judi Gerstung, D.C. *The Estrogen Alternative* (Rochester, VT: Healing Arts Press, 1997), 102.

88 R.E. Rikli and B.G. McManis. "Effects of Exercise on Bone Mineral Content in Menopausal Women." *Research Quarterly for Exercise and Sport* 61:3 (September 1990), 243-249.

89 H.L. Wolfe. *Menopause: A Second Spring* (Boulder, CO: Blue Poppy Press, 1990), 151.

90 John R. Lee, M.D. "Significance of Molecular Configuration Specificity: The Case of Progesterone and Osteoporosis." *Townsend Letter for Doctors* 119 (June 1993), 558-562.

91 John R. Lee, M.D. "Osteoporosis Reversal: The Role of Progesterone." *International Clinical Nutrition Review* 10:3 (1990), 384-391. John R. Lee, M.D. "Is Natural Progesterone the Missing Link in Osteoporosis Prevention and Treatment?" *Medical Hypotheses* (1991). Personal communication with John R. Lee, M.D.

92 "The Many Clinical Benefits of Natural Progesterone." *Life Enhancement* 30 (February 1997), 11.

93 Alan Gaby, M.D. *Preventing and Reversing Osteoporosis* (Rocklin, CA: Prima Publishing, 1994), 272.

94 N. Appleton. *Healthy Bones: What You Should Do About Osteoporosis* (Garden City Park, NY: Avery Publishing Group, 1991), 61-62.

95 Ralph Golan, M.D. *Optimal Wellness* (New York: Ballantine Books, 1995), 398.

96 Ibid.

97 Susan E. Brown, Ph.D. *Better Bones, Better Body* (New Canaan, CT: Keats Publishing, 1996), 84-112.

98 U.S. Department of Health and Human Services, Public Health Service, National Institutes of Health. *Medicine for the Layman: Osteoporosis* (Washington: U.S. Government Printing Office).

99 Melvyn Werbach, M.D. *Foundations of Nutritional Medicine: A Sourcebook of Clinical Research* (Tarzana, CA: Third Line Press, 1997).

100 Suzanne G. Leveille et al. "Dietary Vitamin C and Bone Mineral Density in Postmenopausal Women in Washington State, USA." *Journal of Epidemiology and Community Health* 51 (1997), 479-485.

101 Ivor E. Dreosti. "Magnesium Status and Health." *Nutrition Reviews* 53:9 (September 1995), S23-S27.

102 Susan E. Brown, Ph.D. *Better Bones, Better Body* (New Canaan, CT: Keats Publishing, 1996), 239.

103 John R. Lee, M.D. *Natural Progesterone: The Multiple Roles of a Remarkable Hormone* (Sebastopol, CA: BLL Publishing, 1993), 40.

104 Alan Gaby, M.D. *Preventing and Reversing Osteoporosis* (Rocklin, CA: Prima Publishing, 1994), 273.

105 Susun Weed. *Menopausal Years: The Wise Woman Way* (Woodstock, NY: Ash Tree Publishing, 1992), 159, 190.

106 "The Real 'Good News' for Osteoporosis Sufferers." *Bio/Tech News* Special Issue (Box 30568, Parkrose Center, Portland, OR 97294).

107 Linda Ojeda, Ph.D. *Menopause Without Medicine* (Alameda, CA: Hunter House, 1995), 101.

Chapter 4
Chronic Fatigue Syndrome, Fibromyalgia, and Environmental Illness

1 U.S. Centers for Disease Control. "The Facts About Chronic Fatigue Syndrome" (August 1994). Internet website: http://www.cdc.gov/ncidod.diseases/cfs/facts.htm.

2 Ibid.

3 Jesse A. Stoff, M.D., and Charles R. Pellegrino, Ph.D. *Chronic Fatigue Syndrome: The Hidden Epidemic* (New York: HarperCollins, 1992).

4 Jacob Teitelbaum, M.D. *From Fatigued to Fantastic!* (Garden City Park, NY: Avery Publishing Group, 1996).

5 Don Goldenberg, M.D. Presentation to the 1994 American College of Rheumatology meeting. Dr. Goldenberg is Chief of Rheumatology at Newton-Wellesley Hospital, in Newton, MA, and Professor of Medicine at Tufts University School of Medicine, in Medford, MA.

6 M. Rosenbaum, M.D., and M. Susser, M.D. *Solving the Puzzle of Chronic Fatigue Syndrome* (Tacoma, WA: Life Sciences Press, 1992), 44

7 Neenyah Ostrum. "LEM: Exciting News for Good Health." *The New York Native* (July 31, 1989).

8 *HealthWatch* 4:3 (Summer/Fall 1994), 6. *HealthWatch* is available from: CFIDS Buyers Club, 1187 Coast VIllage Road #1-280, Santa Barbara, CA 93108; tel: 800-366-6056.

9 T. Prince et al. "Chronic Fatigue in a 43-year-old Woman." *Annals of Allergy* 74 (June 1995), 474-478.

Chapter 5
Depression

1 National Institutes of Mental Health, D/ART

(Depression/Awareness, Recognition and Treatment) website: http://www.nimh.nih.gov/newdart/index.htm. For additional information: D/ART, 5600 Fishers Lane, Rockville, MD 20857; tel: 800-421-4211.

2 Susan Swedo, M.D., and Henrietta Leonard, M.D. *It's Not All in Your Head* (San Francisco: HarperSanFrancisco, 1996), 176.

3 National Institutes of Mental Health, D/ART (Depression/Awareness, Recognition and Treatment) website: http://www.nimh.nih.gov/newdart/index.htm. For additional information: D/ART, 5600 Fishers Lane, Rockville, MD 20857; tel: 800-421-4211.

4 Steven Bratman, M.D. *Beat Depression With St. John's Wort* (Rocklin, CA: Prima Publishing, 1997), 27-31.

5 Barbara Strauch. "Firm Seeks to Promote Use of Prozac on Kids." *San Francisco Examiner* (August 10, 1997).

6 Harold M. Silverman, ed. *The Pill Book* (New York: Bantam, 1994), 394-395.

7 P.R. Breggin. *Toxic Psychiatry: Why Therapy, Empathy and Love Must Replace the Drugs, Electroshock, and Biochemical Therapies of the "New Psychiatry* (New York: St. Martin's Press, 1991).

8 Sherry Rogers, M.D. *Depression—Cured At Last!* (Sarasota, FL: SK Publishing, 1997).

9 Steven Bratman, M.D. *Beat Depression With St. John's Wort* (Rocklin, CA: Prima Publishing 1997), 48-50.

10 Ibid., 12-13.

11 Ibid., 9.

12 Priscilla Slagle, M.D. *The Way Up From Down* (New York: St. Martin's Press, 1992), 50.

13 From the patient records of Eric R. Braverman, M.D.

14 *Life Enhancement* 38 (October 1997), 5.

15 Ibid., 6.

16 K. Zmilacher et al. "L-5-hydroxytrptophan Alone and in Combination With a Peripheral Decarboxylase Inhibitor in the Treatment of Depression." *Neuropscholobiology* 20:1 (1988), 28-35.

17 Dallas Clouatre. "5-HTP and the Link Between Mood and Food." *Let's Live* (September 1997), 56.

18 Ibid.

19 Christiane Northrup, M.D. *Health Wisdom for Women* 2:5 (1995), 3-5.

20 Steven Bratman, M.D. *Beat Depression With St. John's Wort* (Rocklin, CA: Prima Publishing, 1997), 162-163.

21 Richard Huemer, M.D. "Allergies, Herbs and Blurred Vision," *Let's Live* (September 1997), 27.

22 Steven Bratman, M.D. *Beat Depression With St. John's Wort* (Rocklin, CA: Prima Publishing, 1997), v.

23 Melvyn Werbach, M.D. *Nutritional Influences on Mental Illness* (Tarzana, CA: Third Line Press, 1991), 123.

24 Sherry Rogers, M.D. *Depression—Cured At Last!* (Sarasota, FL: SK Publishing, 1997).

25 J.E. Pizzorno and M.T. Murray. *A Textbook of Natural Medicine, Vols. 1 & 2* (Seattle, WA: John Bastyr College Publications, 1989).

26 Barry Sears, Ph.D. *The Zone: A Dietary Roadmap* (New York: HarperCollins, 1995), 29.

27 Elliot D. Abravanel, M.D., and Elizabeth King. *Dr. Abravanel's Anti-Craving Weight Loss Diet* (New York: Bantam Books, 1990), 53-57.

28 *Harvard Mental Health Letter* 8:7 (January 1992). R.S. Lazarus and S. Folkman. *Stress, Appraisal, and Coping* (New York: Springer Publishing, 1984).

29 D. Healy et al. "The Thymus-Adrenal Connection: Thymosin Has Corticotropin-Releasing Activity in Primates." *Science* 222:4630 (1983), 1353-1355.

30 Ann Louise Gittleman, M.S. *Supernutrition for Women* (New York: Bantam Books, 1991), 68.

31 J.E. Pizzorno and M.T. Murray. *A Textbook of Natural Medicine, Vols. 1 & 2* (Seattle, WA: John Bastyr College Publications, 1989).

32 Lita Lee, Ph.D. "Hypothyroidism, A Modern Epidemic." *Earthletter* (Spring 1994), 1.

33 J. Ott. "Color and Light: Their Effects on Plants, Animals and People." *International Journal of Biosocial Research* 7-10 (1985-1988): 1-131.

34 J. Ott. *Health And Light* (Old Greenwich, CT: Devin-Adair, 1973).

35 P.A. Roos. "Light and Electromagnetic Waves: The Health Implications." *Journal of the Bio-Electro-Magnetics Institute* 3:2 (Summer 1991), 7-12.

36 Christiane Northrup, M.D. *Health Wisdom for Women* (November 1995).

Index

191
Irritable bowel syndrome, 18, 21

James, Mary, 142

Kane, Patricia, 224
Kava-kava, 193
Kellman, Raphael, 181, 219
Kells, John, 26, 181
Kelp, 23
Kidney, 121
Klinghardt, Dietrich, 74
Kotsanis, Constantine A., 163–68
Kulhay, Katrina, 19–22, 33, 50

Langer, Stephen E., 218, 234
Laya, Mary B., 87
Lead, 141, 151. *See also* Metals, heavy
Leaky gut syndrome, 186, 188, 197
Lee, John R., 40
    on bones, 113
    on calcium, 129, 132
    on enzyme deficiencies, 186
    on fluoride, 139–40
    on HRT, 134
    on osteoporosis, 128, 133–36, 143
    osteoporosis treatment, 119–21
    on progesterone, 137, 148–49
    on progesterone therapy, 41–42, 119
Lee, Lita, 25, 31, 172
L-glutathione, 37
Licorice, 21, 24
Lieberman, Shari, 161, 172–73
Lifestyle
    CFS and, 192–94
    osteoporosis and, 113, 115, 116, 146
Light, 240–41
    deprivation, 239–42
    sensitivity, 217
Light therapy, 166, 240–42
Lipid, 230
Lipomas, 15, 16, 49
Liver, 50, 205
    cleansing, 21, 38–39
    estrogen dominance and, 25
    function, 79–80
    role in FBD, 47
Loomis, Charles, 186
Love, Susan, 118, 135
Lugol's solution, 45, 46
Lumpectomy, 58
Lumps in breast, 14, 15, 16–17. *See also*

Fibrocystic breast disease
Lymph, 28
Lymph circulation, 19, 27
Lymphatic drainage, stimulating, 24, 36
Lymphatic system, 28, 29

Magnesium, 42, 124, 151
    iodine and, 45, 46
    osteoporosis and, 152
Magnet therapy, 195
Magnetism, harmful, 64
Malabsorption syndrome, 20, 21, 33
Malic acid, 189
Mammography, 17, 84, 86–88
    as breast cancer factor, 65, 86
Manic-depression (bipolar disorder), 206
Marcial-Vega, Victor, 103
Masculinization, 17–18
Mastectomy, 98
Medications. *See* Drugs
Melatonin, 180, 208, 211–12, 239, 240, 242
Menopause, 121, 206
    osteoporosis and, 114, 115
Menstruation
    bone health and, 117, 137
    breast pain during, 14
Mental factors in disease, 95–97. *See also* Emotion; Stress
Mercury toxicity, 19, 73–74, 164, 167, 183–84, 237
Meridians, 48, 74, 97, 122. *See also* Acupuncture
    herbs' effect on, 98
    teeth and, 75
Metabolism, 31
Metals, heavy, 141, 184, 212, 237
Methylxanthines, 21
Meyer's Cocktail, 197
Miasm, 82–83
Milk thistle, 21, 24, 50, 193
Minerals, 105, 108, 125, 133
    for bone mass, 124
Molecular residue, 83
Morter, Jr., M. T., 145
Moxibustion, 48, 50
Mucus, 28
Murray, Michael T., 150, 153, 240
Musculoskeletal system, 97
Myers, John, 45

NAET. *See* Nambudripad Allergy Elimination

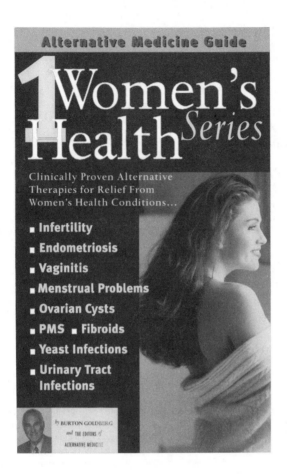

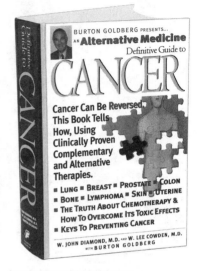

CURE YOUR HEADACHES...
USING NATURAL THERAPIES

If you suffer from headaches, this book could change your life. It is entirely possible that with this invaluable practical information, you may well put headaches behind you as something you once suffered from, but no more.

Robert Milne, M.D., and Blake More expertly guide you through the root causes and multiple treatment options for 11 major types of headaches, from sinus to migraine, cluster to tension.

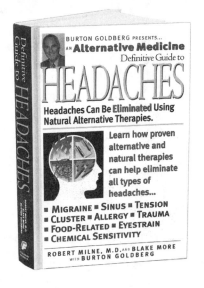

BURTON GOLDBERG PRESENTS...
AN **Alternative Medicine**
Definitive Guide to
HEADACHES

Headaches Can Be Eliminated Using Natural Alternative Therapies.

Learn how proven alternative and natural therapies can help eliminate all types of headaches...

- MIGRAINE ■ SINUS ■ TENSION
- CLUSTER ■ ALLERGY ■ TRAUMA
- FOOD-RELATED ■ EYESTRAIN
- CHEMICAL SENSITIVITY

ROBERT MILNE, M.D. AND BLAKE MORE
WITH BURTON GOLDBERG

We have made every effort possible to make this book practical and user-friendly for you. For a quick reference to headache types, symptoms, treatment options, use our Master Symptom Chart. If you suffer from tension headaches, turn directly to Chapter 6; if migraines are your millstone, see Chapter 7; and if you're not sure what type of headache you have, study the symptoms list in the Master Symptom Chart until you find the clinical term that best matches your condition.

No matter what kind of headache you used to have, after reading this book your head may never pain you again.

Hardcover ■ ISBN 1-887299-03-3
■ 6" x 9" ■ 525 pages

TO ORDER, CALL 800-333-HEAL

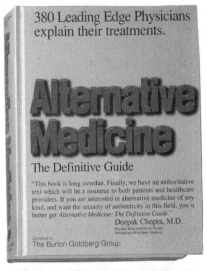

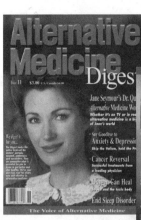
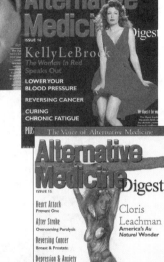
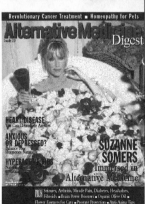
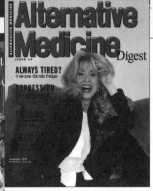

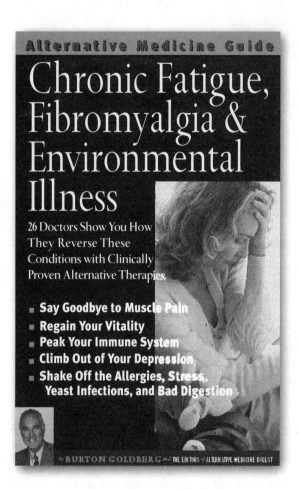

Alternative Medicine Guide

Chronic Fatigue, Fibromyalgia & Environmental Illness

26 Doctors Show You How They Reverse These Conditions with Clinically Proven Alternative Therapies.

- **Say Goodbye to Muscle Pain**
- **Regain Your Vitality**
- **Peak Your Immune System**
- **Climb Out of Your Depression**
- **Shake Off the Allergies, Stress, Yeast Infections, and Bad Digestion**

by BURTON GOLDBERG *and* THE EDITORS *of* ALTERNATIVE MEDICINE DIGEST

Chronic fatigue, fibromyalgia, and environmental illness can be permanently reversed using nontoxic alternative medicine treatments. In this book, 26 leading physicians explain the techniques and natural substances that brought complete recovery to their patients.

TO ORDER, CALL 800-333-HEAL

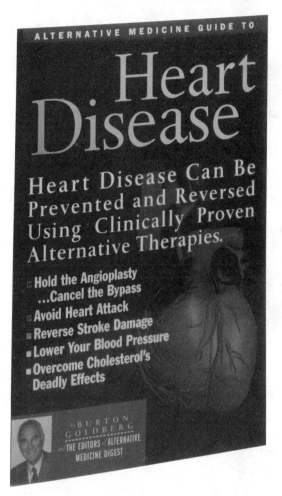

ALTERNATIVE MEDICINE GUIDE TO

Heart
Disease

Heart Disease Can Be
Prevented and Reversed
Using Clinically Proven
Alternative Therapies.

▫ Hold the Angioplasty
...Cancel the Bypass
▫ Avoid Heart Attack
▪ Reverse Stroke Damage
▪ Lower Your Blood Pressure
▪ Overcome Cholesterol's
Deadly Effects

by BURTON
GOLDBERG
and THE EDITORS of ALTERNATIVE
MEDICINE DIGEST

Save your heart from heart disease, attack, stroke, high blood
pressure, and the dangers of angioplasty, bypass, and other
invasive surgeries—12 top physicians explain their proven,
safe, nontoxic, and successful heart-saving treatments.

TO ORDER, CALL 800-333-HEAL

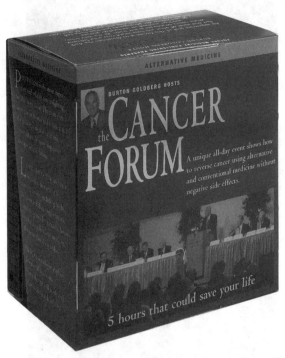

The Cancer Forum—five hours of lifesaving information from leading alternative medicine physicians who show you how to reverse cancer using alternative and conventional medicine without negative side effects.

Prevention is the most important and reliable cancer-fighting tool that exists today. The fact that cancer can be treated and reversed and that it can be detected early and prevented are the most significant messages of this forum.

Learn the latest proven, safe, nontoxic, and successful treatments for reversing cancer, including herbs, nutrition and diet, supplements, enzymes, glandular extracts, homeopathic remedies, and more, in this groundbreaking video.

TO ORDER, CALL 800-333-HEAL